W9-AXF-690 2022

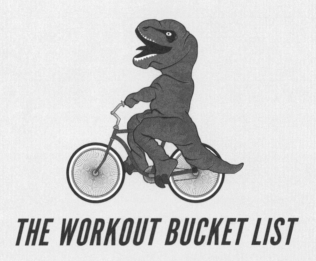

THE WORKOUT BUCKET LIST

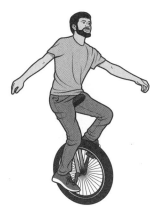

THE *WORKOUT BUCKET LIST*

Over 300 Life-Changing Races, Epic Challenges, and Incredible Hikes, Bikes, Lifts, and Runs around the World, in Your Gym, or Right in Your Living Room

GREG PRESTO

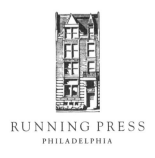

RUNNING PRESS

PHILADELPHIA

Neither these exercises nor any exercise program should be followed without first consulting a health care professional. If you have any special conditions requiring attention, you should consult with your health care professional regularly regarding possible modification of the activities contained in this book.

Copyright © 2022 by Gregory Presto
Interior and cover illustrations copyright © 2022 by Peter Sucheski
Cover copyright © 2022 by Hachette Book Group, Inc.

Hachette Book Group supports the right to free expression and the value of copyright. The purpose of copyright is to encourage writers and artists to produce the creative works that enrich our culture.

The scanning, uploading, and distribution of this book without permission is a theft of the author's intellectual property. If you would like permission to use material from the book (other than for review purposes), please contact permissions@hbgusa.com. Thank you for your support of the author's rights.

Running Press
Hachette Book Group
1290 Avenue of the Americas, New York, NY 10104
www.runningpress.com
@Running_Press

First Edition: April 2022

Published by Running Press, an imprint of Perseus Books, LLC, a subsidiary of Hachette Book Group, Inc. The Running Press name and logo is a trademark of the Hachette Book Group.

The Hachette Speakers Bureau provides a wide range of authors for speaking events. To find out more, go to www.hachettespeakersbureau.com or call (866) 376-6591.

The publisher is not responsible for websites (or their content) that are not owned by the publisher.

Print book cover and interior design by Josh McDonnell

Library of Congress Control Number: 2021938078

ISBNs: 978-0-7624-7206-2 (trade paperback), 978-0-7624-7208-6 (ebook)

Printed in China

1010

10 9 8 7 6 5 4 3 2 1

For Sara

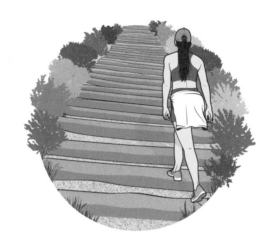

CONTENTS

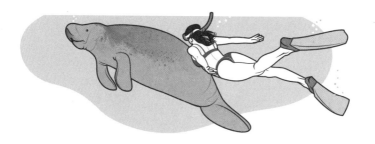

INTRODUCTION

If you've flipped open *The Workout Bucket List*, I feel as if I already know a little bit about you: You can relax on a beach, flop on the couch, or chill out in a hammock . . . but only for so long. Because you've got to *move*!

You've got to race to the top of a hill, bound from rock to rock like a kid, hike to a clearing to take in that incredible view, and leave no part of life untasted or untouched. You've got this one life to live, and you're going to squeeze every ounce of juice out of that sucker. And you're happy to get a little sweaty while you squeeze.

Sound like you? Or the version of you that you *want* to be? Then you've come to the right place.

The 300-plus workouts that follow will get you moving and motivate you. With this list, you'll explore the world, learn some history, and discover what your own body can achieve—the places it can take you, the feelings it can give you, the triumphs you can experience, and the ways it can connect you with friends, family, and the people you love. Whether you're a couch potato with big dreams or an Ironman triathlete, there are workouts here that you can try, succeed at, and have a blast doing.

How do I know? Because when I'm not writing about workouts, I'm trying them! I'm forever exploring adventurous physical experiences, and I've been sharing them with readers as a fitness journalist for publications like *Men's Health* and *Shape*, among others, for more than 15 years. So if you're looking for new, exciting ways to move your body, I've got ideas!

Maybe you're planning a summer road trip? Add in a stop to bike up (and probably fall down) America's steepest street, in my hometown of Pittsburgh. Or go for a run up Jerry Rice's training hill outside San Francisco. Or book a boat yoga class on the Chicago River.

Are you a sports fan? Try Steph Curry's pregame dribbling routine, or an NFL linebacker's workout favored by President Herbert Hoover. Are you a history buff? Sweat through a workout from the gymnasium onboard the *Titanic*. Are you a world traveler? Bike with zebras, use your body to power amusement park rides in Italy, or hike up a volcano and stare into a bubbling lake of lava. Can't leave town? Try a workout inspired by The Rock, the first woman to run the Boston Marathon, or a decorated Army veteran and *Dancing with the Stars* competitor.

Here's the rub: These workouts may or may not give you rippling abs. If that's what you're after, put this book down and find another one that promises you a washboard stomach. I can't promise *that*. But what I *can* promise is that whether you try 1, 20, or all 300-plus of the workouts that follow, you'll be happier, healthier, more confident, and amazed at what you can do and what the world around you has to offer. Your body is your passport to an endless universe of exploration. Think of *The Workout Bucket List* as your personal road map.

So let's get started—right now!

Pull up a chair and let's get fired up—not with a pep talk, but with some movement. Perch yourself on the front of the seat and sit tall with your feet apart and flat on the floor. Square your shoulders and suck in your gut. Let your arms hang loose at your sides. Now, thrust your head forward between your legs, as if you were trying to plant your forehead on the floor. Feel all the air push out of your lungs.

Once you're empty, come back up quickly. Throw your head up and back, eyes on the ceiling. Put a big smile on your face. Bring your shoulders down and back, like you're gripping a pencil between your shoulder blades. Feel the head rush and all that good stuff flying around your body. Repeat twice more, for a total of 3 reps.

That's a Magic Three, a pump-up method from fitness legend Jack LaLanne. In 1960, the TV host shared this exercise as his cure for what he called America's "pooped-out-itis."

Take Jack's advice: Throw your shoulders back, put on a big smile, and get your blood pumping. Feeling good? Great! Now get ready for some fitness adventure.

PART 1

WORKOUTS TO SEE THE WORLD

Exercise can take you places—literally, of course, if you're running or cycling. But moving your body can also mean moving all over this great big planet of ours. Whether it's for a race, a climb, or a sight to see, exercise can be the key that turns travel into adventure. These six chapters will help you turn that key and become a globe-trotting fitness explorer.

CHAPTER 1

DOIN' THE MOST ON THE EAST COAST

There are more than 300 million Americans, and we move in a million different ways in thousands of places. Chapters 1 through 5 are your guide to some of those movements that will help you explore our great nation, sweating and smiling from sea to shining sea. Start on the Eastern Seaboard with these Atlantic Coast adventures.

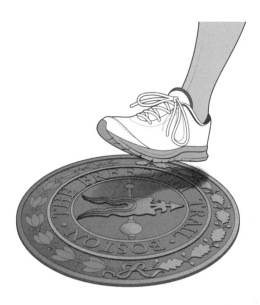

BEGIN AT AMERICA'S BEGINNING: EXPLORE THE REVOLUTION IN A 4K RUN

Cutting through the streets of Boston is a red line—a two-brick-wide strip that runs perpendicular to the rest of the city's brick-lined streets. It's more than a line, though: The two-brick path is a time machine that can take you on an instant tour of the American Revolution.

It's called the Freedom Trail, and it connects 16 sites across Boston that were integral in the founding of the US. Starting at Boston Common, the famed park that was converted into a militia training ground, the path winds through downtown Boston and across the Charlestown Bridge to Bunker Hill, site of the first major battle of the Revolution. Along the way, you'll pass America's first public school, where Benjamin Franklin was a student. It stops at Paul Revere's house, from which he started his historic midnight ride, and the Old North Church, where "one if by land, two if by sea" indicated the source of the oncoming British attack. There's also a Chipotle . . . which was once the Old Corner Bookstore, where works including *Walden* were first published and sold.

Each spot is marked with a Freedom Trail insignia on the ground, and walking to most—or all—of the sites is a popular tour. But for an even faster trip through 250 years of American history—and a chance to see which sites you'd like to revisit at a slower pace—run it! The Freedom Trail is only about 2.5 miles long. Grab a map and a brochure from www.thefreedomtrail.org (or their free Freedom Trail Walking Tour app), or pick up a print copy at Faneuil Hall, where the National Park Service operates a visitor center.

A LIGHTNING-FAST PHOTO TOUR OF DC ON TWO WHEELS

To give yourself more time to explore Washington and still get all the shots of your smiling family in front of the monuments and memorials of DC, tackle the National Mall on a bike instead of on foot, and leave the sweat-soaked, grumpy groups of walkers in your rearview reflector.

Capital Bikeshare offers simple, no-contract bike rentals at stations around DC. For $8, you can get a 24-hour pass to ride and park the bikes as many times as you'd like. Grab one by DC's Union Station, then follow this itinerary and ride the area's extra-wide sidewalks to do a complete monument photo tour—fast. The tour can be completed in less than an hour if you don't dawdle (and only slightly longer if you linger and take a few extra shots).

1. Pick up bikes at the Columbus Circle station—just around the corner from Union Station's northeast corner.
2. Walk your bikes out in front of the station to snap a photo in front of Union Station's dramatic neoclassical entrance, then turn around for a familiar view of the Capitol dome—in many movies, this is the shot used to show Congress.

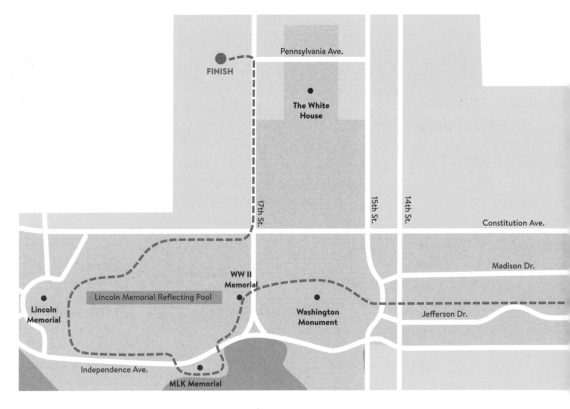

3. Ride down Louisiana Avenue, then turn left on Third Street NW until you're directly in front of the Capitol. Snap a photo here, then turn around for a breathtaking view of the Washington Monument—your next destination.
4. The Monument, at 554 feet, is the world's tallest obelisk. Look north from its hilltop for a view of the White House's South Lawn, and get a nice wide view of the Lincoln Memorial.
5. Head west from the Monument to the World War II Memorial.
6. Head south and make a right on the sidewalk in front of the statue of John Paul Jones on your way to the Martin Luther King Jr. Memorial. At MLK, you'll also get a postcard-perfect view of the Jefferson Memorial.
7. Take the sidewalks to the steps of the Lincoln Memorial—there are two Capital Bikeshare stations here, so you can park your bikes to head in and see Abe. (This may also be a good place to pause your tour. There's a refreshment stand by the memorial, and you can walk through the nearby Vietnam Veterans Memorial.)
8. If you want to continue snapping, head back along Constitution Avenue to 17th Street NW, then make a left—you're headed for the White House.
9. Park your bike at 18th Street and Pennsylvania Avenue, then walk back two blocks to pay a visit to the POTUS.

Congratulations! You've just done a daylong tour of DC in an hour!

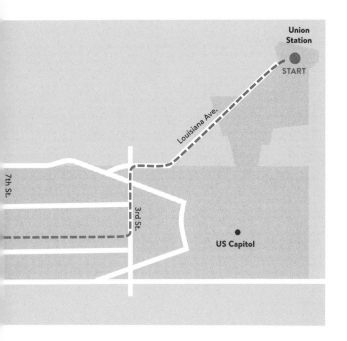

SEE THE BEST OF THE APPALACHIAN TRAIL WITH THESE DAY HIKES

There's no better way to take in the scenery of the eastern US than on the Appalachian Trail. Two million people hike sections of the trail each year, but only 1,000 people hike the whole thing at once—going from Georgia's Springer Mountain to Maine's Mount Katahdin (or vice versa) in a single, months-long camping trip.

For Gary Sizer, the through-hike was truly the adventure of a lifetime: He had dreamed about it for more than 20 years since his days as a 21-year-old Marine. Sizer saved for years before quitting his job, strapping on his backpack, and hitting the trail in Georgia. He finished the trek on his 45th birthday, after 153 days of Pop-Tarts and Clif Bars, gnarled toenails, and weeks of diarrhea. Don't have six months to hoof the whole thing? Sizer says these two hikes offer the best of the trail when all you've got is a day.

The Roan Highlands, North Carolina/Tennessee

Convenient parking can be found at the Carver's Gap trailhead, leading to 3 miles of exposed hiking that offers 360-degree views of the surrounding five peaks, or "balds"—tree-free outcroppings of ancient Appalachian rock. For a day hike, start at Carver's Gap, near Little Rock Creek, NC. Park by the trailhead, and head along the heavily trafficked gravel road for an easy hike to your first bald, Round Bald. Here, the trail becomes more rugged and the crowd thins out. Head for Jane Bald, then bear right at a fork in the trail to summit Grassy Ridge Bald. At just over 6,100 feet, this highest peak of the trio offers panoramic views of the highlands.

Pinkham Notch, New Hampshire, to Mount Washington

As through-hikers near the end of their epic journeys, they're faced with challenging hands-and-knees scrambling up more vertical rocks and crags. Mount Washington, the highest peak in the northeastern US, towers over them all. Its 6,288-foot peak stands near a place called Pinkham Notch, one of Sizer's favorite spots in the White Mountains.

The hikes around Pinkham Notch are scenic and numerous: You can follow the Appalachian Trail south from the Pinkham Notch Visitor Center (in Pinkham's Grant, NH) for about 1 mile to Glen Ellis Falls, or trek north along White Mountain Road to Thompson Falls—also about 1 mile away.

Or, climb the crown jewel of crown jewels: Take a full-day hike and summit the northeast's highest mountain, Mount Washington, with a trail that splits off the AT at Pinkham Notch. From the Pinkham Notch Visitor Center, head north along the Appalachian Trail to the Tuckerman Ravine trailhead. Follow the Tuckerman Ravine trail to the Lion Head trail, and turn right. Follow the rocky Lion Head's path to the top. Maps are available at the visitor center.

RUN THE CITY: THE BIG APPLE'S BEST ROUTES

The subway's fine for getting around, but if you really want to see New York—or any city, really—lace up your running shoes. You'll discover iconic views and glimpses of the town that are yours alone. Start your tour with these three routes.

Do NYC's most popular park loop

When Strava, the exercise tracking app, compiled America's most popular routes, New York's most-run loop wasn't in Central Park—it was in Brooklyn's Prospect Park. More than 180,000 Strava users have logged the flat 5K rings around the outside of the park, whipping past the lake and zoo. Start your run in front of the Central Library, where Flatbush Avenue intersects East Drive, which runs into the park. Where East Drive meets West Drive, take West—then just follow the loop back around.

Run across the Brooklyn Bridge

Foot traffic builds early, so you'll want to get going before rush hour (around 7 a.m.). To start from the Manhattan side, take the 4-5-6 subways to the Brooklyn Bridge station, then head for the intersection of Park Row and the Brooklyn Bridge promenade. If you beat traffic, you'll enjoy a wide (and wide-open) pedestrian path as you traverse the bridge a level above car traffic. The bridge drops you off at Brooklyn Bridge Park, where you can get a free early-morning workout on the fitness equipment at Pier 2.

Get an expert runner's view of the skyline

Claude Melm knows the streets around New York as well as any runner: He runs his commute home each weekday, logging almost a half-marathon between his midtown office and nearby Fort Lee, New Jersey. The run gives the 48-year-old time to train for three to five marathons a year without sacrificing family time. And one of his nightly routes gives him an incredible view of Manhattan's skyline.

Take the A train to the 175th Street Station, and head north toward 179th Street. Turn left to cross the George Washington Bridge into New Jersey. When you come off the bridge, turn left in scenic Fort Lee Historic Park, and take in views of the city on your left as you head south toward Edgewater, New Jersey.

In nearby Edgewater, turn around and run back north—past the bridge—into Englewood Cliffs for a break from the city's bustle (but not from its unique charms).

WORKOUT CONTINUES >>>

KEEP RUNNING!
TRAIN ON THE EAST COAST'S MOST POPULAR ROUTES

Despite what residents of the five boroughs might tell you, there *are* other cities on the East Coast—and they're just as much fun to run. Here are some of Strava's most popular routes in the East's biggest cities.

Boston: Run by Harvard's campus and get harbor views when you circle Pleasure Bay.
Run Boston like a top marathoner with this 5K that's frequented by some of the fastest distance runners in America. Begin in front of 640 Memorial Drive, along the Dr. Paul Dudley White Path. Head northeast, turning left to cross the river at Harvard Street. Once across, you'll make another left, putting you back on the Paul Dudley White Path, but on the river's opposite bank. Jog south until you're across the river from where you started.

Baltimore: Run north to Gunpowder Falls.
It's a little out of town, but the North Central Railroad Trail—one of many former railways–turned–running trails in the East—offers wooded views that have highlighted Maryland's oldest marathon, the NCR Marathon, since 1973. On this, the most popular Strava'd route in Baltimore, start from Paper Mill Road in Hunters Run. Head north on this ten-mile run into the Gunpowder Falls State Park.

Philadelphia: Work up a cheesesteak-worthy appetite along the river.

When you think of running in Philly, you probably think of Rocky. And we'll get to that soon (see "Do Road Work like Rocky," page 16). But the boathouses along the Schuylkill River—the same ones seen twinkling with lights in the intro to *It's Always Sunny in Philadelphia*—are just as iconic, and give this four-mile run a more serene, nature-infused feel than trotting through downtown.

To run this Strava favorite, start where the Falls Bridge meets West River Road. Head south toward the city, where you might see crew teams rowing along the river as you jog. Finish at—where else?—the Philadelphia Museum of Art, where you can bound up the steps like Rocky Balboa.

Washington, DC: Do a lap at Hains Point.

If you're visiting the capital, you've probably already got a plan to see the National Mall, and with the one-hour plan on page 4, you'll have plenty of time to check out other attractions around DC. Take a 5K loop around Hains Point, the knifelike peninsula at the confluence of the Potomac and Anacostia Rivers.

Start at the George Mason Memorial, a secluded, flower-studded garden on the Potomac River side. Then just stay on the well-paved path around the point—you'll get views of Reagan National Airport and its nearby waterfowl sanctuary. Run past duffers smacking golf balls on the island and finish at the foot of the Jefferson Memorial.

For more of Strava's most popular routes around the USA, turn to page 50 for Midwestern runs, and page 80 for routes in West Coast cities. Or, to find popular routes in your city, go to www.strava.com/heatmap.

BIKE (AND FALL DOWN) ON AMERICA'S STEEPEST STREET

Each Black Friday, masochistic cyclists in Pittsburgh bundle up and fall down 13 of the city's steepest hills in a race called the Dirty Dozen (yes, I know a dozen is 12). They finish on Canton Avenue, America's steepest street.

The street is absurd: Maybe 200 meters long, but pitched at an angle of 37 percent. It's so steep that it's closed for much of the winter because it's too dangerous to drive. In any weather, it's humbling to bike.

But it's worth it. You will sweat. You will fail. You will laugh. The neighbors will laugh (they say they don't mind). And whether you summit the hill or not, you will earn a big slice of pizza and a tall one to toast with any riding friends. If you make it to my hometown, give this hill a shot.

GET OUT OF THE LOOP: ICE-SKATE A 4.5-MILE TRAIL IN VERMONT

Skating an oval can be magical—at Rockefeller Center in New York, in the village below Half Dome in Yosemite, and at a thousand other rinks with unbelievable surroundings. But there's something especially enchanting about an ice-skating *trail*—slicing along a path as the scenery flies by.

America's longest skating trail is in Fairlee, Vermont, about a two-hour drive from Boston. There, the Morey Lake Resort's skating path stretches for 4.5 miles along the lake's perimeter, past quaint fishing villages with the wind whistling through the snow-covered trees, as youth hockey games get underway on plowed sections along the trail.

You don't have to stay at the resort to skate the path—skate rentals are $15, and the resort updates the ice's status each day on its Facebook page, www.facebook.com/lakemoreyresort. The path usually opens in late January.

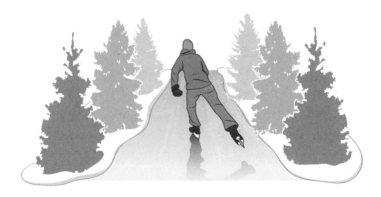

A t the summit of Popolopen Torne in the Hudson Valley, a pile of colorful rocks overlooks panoramic views of West Point and the Hudson River. It's a monument to deployed US service members, each rock a wish for their safe return by a climber who brought their stone from the bottom of the 942-foot mountain. Some are painted with the name of a soldier they're remembering, others with unit patches to honor a fallen veteran. Add to the pile and honor a veteran of your own: Grab some paint for your own stone, and make the 2-mile hike to this ever-growing tower.

Start your hike of the Popolopen Torne Loop by parking along Route 9W in either the lot at Fort Montgomery State Historic Site, or a hiker's lot at 701 Route 9W, Fort Montgomery, New York (each lot has a sign that it's there for hikers to park). From here, you'll walk across the 9W bridge's pedestrian lane to the Popolopen Gorge Trail. It's marked with red-and-white blazes.

Follow those red blazes for 1.6 miles until you meet a junction with a trail marked by blue blazes. You'll reach a footbridge, cross Mine Road, and have a half-mile to climb the 586 vertical feet to the summit—still following the blue blazes. Deposit your stone at the monument, honor your loved one and other veterans, and see the two memorial benches erected by Eagle Scouts by the cairn. Descend by continuing to follow the blue blazes to complete the loop.

Things to Know
- This trail isn't a breeze to navigate; download a map from a site like www.alltrails.com, and also use GPS to help you.
- The parking lot at Fort Montgomery State Historic Site closes at 5 p.m. If you start later, use the spillover hiker's lot at 701 Route 9W.

CLIMB THE CLIFFS OF MAINE ON 100-YEAR-OLD IRON RUNGS

Acadia National Park has breathtaking views—sheer granite cliffs, seas of pine, and tall ships pulling in and out of Bar Harbor—and a thousand ways to explore them. You could spend weeks hiking the Maine park's 150 miles of rocky trails, biking its 45 miles of carriage roads, rock climbing the vertical faces of Otter Cliffs, and stuffing your face with lobster to refuel for the next adventure.

For some of the most heart-pumping excitement in Acadia, grab some iron. Waldron Bates, memorialized on a plaque as the "Pathmaker" inside the park, came up with an ingenious, exhilarating way for explorers to reach many of Acadia's peaks: He and his fellow trailblazers of the early 1900s slammed iron rungs and ladders into exposed rock faces. Hoist yourself up the iron and you can get to the top of some of the most awe-inspiring views in the park—and get your heart rate pumping in the process.

These hikes aren't for the faint of heart or those afraid of heights, but for the sure-footed, they're must-dos. Grab a trail map, pack some water, and put these on your Acadia checklist.

The Beehive Trail
Perhaps the most-trafficked of the iron-rung routes, the route to the Beehive is a quick one. With many hikers venturing up from the nearby Sand Beach, small traffic jams can develop as unsuspecting hikers make their way up for incredible views of the sunbathers below. The rungs here are plentiful and the hike is short.

The Precipice Trail
The Precipice is everything you'll see at the Beehive turned up a notch—it's longer. It involves more rock scrambling up fields of square granite boulders. There's more exposure, steeper drop-offs, and the iron rungs—some of which are pretty far apart—seem to stretch endlessly into the sky. The Precipice is no joke! Get ready to sweat.

Beech Cliff Trail
The quietest of the bunch, the Beech Cliff Trail offers a unique experience—there aren't just rungs hammered into the stone, but whole metal ladders that help you traverse this clever route. At the top, you'll have incredible views of Echo Lake, where there's a beach waiting for you to have a post-climb dip in crystal-clear waters.

LET SCIENCE SAVE YOU FROM ROAD TRIP BACK PAIN

If you're going to become a bucket list–checking, active-life road warrior, you're going to spend a lot of time along America's scenic highways. But studies show that prolonged time in a car seat can lead to lower back pain, which could put an *ouch* in your otherwise active plans.

"If you don't change position or posture, it turns to pain," says Stuart McGill, one of the world's foremost experts on back pain. So if you're getting back pain from driving long distances, take breaks! McGill also suggests taking your wallet out of your back pocket, wearing looser pants while driving—since tighter pants can cause tight hips—and making your seat back more rigid. During your breaks, walk with a proud chest while swinging your arms at your shoulders—not your elbows—and try this simple stretch:

∞ Stand up in front of the car and push your hands toward the sky.
∞ Wait 10 to 20 seconds. The older you are, the longer you should hold.
∞ Then push your hands back a little bit. You'll notice a little more extension to your spine.
∞ Fully and deeply inhale. Fill the lungs and torso with air, "creating a pneumatic jack." You're jacking your rib cage off your pelvic floor, adding even more extension to the spine.
∞ Put your hands down and relax.

Performing this stretch on your rest breaks will measurably ease stress on the discs in your lower back. The stretch won't work for everyone, McGill says, as "there is no such thing as nonspecific back pain," and back pain associated with driving could actually be related to a tight psoas muscle. To find out the true causes of your specific back pain—and to build resilience to help reduce it—check out McGill's book, *Back Mechanic*.

CLIMB SEVEN PEAKS NAMED FOR SEVEN PRESIDENTS IN ONE DAY

The Presidential Traverse is a single hike that summits seven mountains named for former commanders-in-chief—Madison, Adams, Jefferson, Washington, Monroe, Eisenhower, and Pierce. It's a 20- to 24-mile hike through New Hampshire that includes climbing the five tallest mountains in the northeast US. You can do it in one day (but you'll probably want to do it in two).

That's not to say it's easy: The Traverse reaches 9,000 to 10,000 vertical feet along its route, and even in summer, can involve some unpredictable weather. The White Mountains of New Hampshire are the windiest range in the country, including Mount Washington, where hurricane-force gusts can be felt more than a hundred days a year.

Windy or not, Washington is one of the nation's most famous peaks, and along the other summits you'll find superb scenery to photograph on these 300-million-year-old mountains. On a clear day, views along the route extend into Vermont, and even Maine.

Things to Know

- Most hikers start on the northern end of the Traverse, at the base of Mount Madison, in order to climb the range's most difficult mountains—Madison, Jefferson, Adams, and Washington—while their legs are still fresh. Begin your hike at the Highland Center Lodge at Crawford Notch, where you can pick up maps and park.
- You *can* climb all seven peaks in one day, but two days is more manageable. There are three overnight huts along the route: Madison Spring, Mizpah Spring, and Lakes of the Clouds. The latter is closest to the middle—for $155, you can reserve a bed with dinner and breakfast in the bunkroom-style lodge and take a well-earned rest after conquering the first four peaks. Visit www.outdoors.org and click on "LODGING."

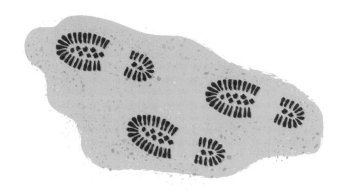

MAKE TRACKS ON AMERICA'S "BEST NATIONAL PARK HIKE"

It's not in the mist of Yosemite, in the volcanoes of Hawaii, or tramping through Yellowstone: America's "Best National Park Hike," according to readers of *USA Today*, is in West Virginia. The Endless Wall Trail, leading to panoramic views above the New River Gorge, took the honor—and it's easy to tread yourself and see why.

The 2.4-mile hike only takes about 90 minutes to complete, climbing through lush hemlock forests and rhododendron bushes so thick they create tunnels that hikers must sometimes crawl through—a delight in June when they're thick with pink and purple blooms. Continue as the trail zigzags along the cliff edge, rising a thousand feet above New River's dramatic gorge, where rock climbers scale the near-vertical sandstone above white-water rafters in the river below.

At the trail's summit, you'll reach Diamond Point, an overlook that makes the name of the trail obvious: The gorge's "Endless Wall" of sandstone stretches in both directions to the horizons, offering views more than a mile upstream and down before bending with the river. Your photos will be *epic*.

To get there: Point your GPS to the Endless Wall Trailhead in New River Gorge National Park. The trailhead is about 1.3 miles from the Canyon Rim Visitor Center, where you can pick up a map.

Things to Know

- Many hikers backtrack from Diamond Point, making the trail an out-and-back, but you can also finish the trail and walk about 0.4 miles along the road back to the parking lot.
- For a second day hike in the park, head for the Bridge Trail. It's less than a mile, but don't be fooled: This trail is steep, rocky, and strenuous. Your reward, though, is a breathtaking view of the New River Gorge bridge—the huge span depicted on West Virginia's state quarter.

DO ROAD WORK LIKE ROCKY THROUGH THE STREETS OF PHILLY

The training montages make *Rocky* movies iconic—that's partially from chasing chickens, but mostly a credit to the streets of Philadelphia. The city makes Balboa's runs memorable—and can make your own sightseeing through Philly inspiring, heart-pumping fun.

His runs range all over the city: In a 2014 article for *Philadelphia* magazine, Dan McQuade calculated the total distance of the *Rocky II* montage, the best run of the series. Put into a single run, the training session would go for 30-plus miles—too far for a boxer, and for most of us. I've run the whole route, and put together this "greatest hits" list for you. Removing a few locations that aren't that scenic or could be downright illegal, you're left with a run that's about 10K, and hits some of the most memorable spots along Rocky's route. Follow along with the map below and run through Philly like the Italian Stallion.

Stop 1: Rocky's House, 2313 South Lambert Street
This is the house where Rocky starts his run by jumping off the balcony onto the street. You should skip the jump—it's actually someone's house—but you can certainly check out the teeny-tiny, cute street where it's located. Because the street is so small, you're better off parking by Stephen Girard Park, about two blocks away.

Stop 2: Italian Market, Ninth Street
To get from Rocky's house to the Italian Market, you'll run northeast on Passyunk Avenue, then turn left on Ninth Street. At this corner, you'll run by Geno's and Pat's—the two most famous cheesesteak spots in Philadelphia. Make a note of this for your post-run feast. After turning left to head north on Ninth, you'll run through scenic neighborhoods of townhouses and through the Italian Market.

Stop 3: Independence Hall, 520 Chestnut Street
Make a right on Locust Street and cut through Washington Square Park to head for Independence Hall, at the corner of Chestnut and Fifth. Along the backside, you'll see the courtyard where Rocky hurdled a park bench while sprinting with a crowd of kids in tow. You can't run straight through Independence Hall, as Rocky does—that's been closed since 9/11—but you can see the famous spot where independence was declared.

Stop 4: Chestnut Street between Fifth and Broad Street
Rocky runs this section with kids in tow and American flags flying from buildings on either side. One difference you'll see: There are cars, so you can't run down the center of the street. Chestnut is also bustling with tourists, which could slow you down.

Stops 5 and 6: Philadelphia City Hall and "Love" Park

These aren't shown in Rocky's run, but they're Philadelphia landmarks—might as well get to them along the way. From Chestnut, make a left on Broad to head into the City Hall square. Run northwest from there to Love Park, where the much photographed "LOVE" sculpture sits. If you want a pic with the sculpture, you'll have to wait in line, so come back after your run.

Stop 7: Philadelphia Museum of Art Steps, 2600 Benjamin Franklin Parkway

From Love Park, you can't miss the Art Museum steps—it's about 1.5 miles away, a straight shot along Benjamin Franklin Parkway. Get there, and get up those steps!

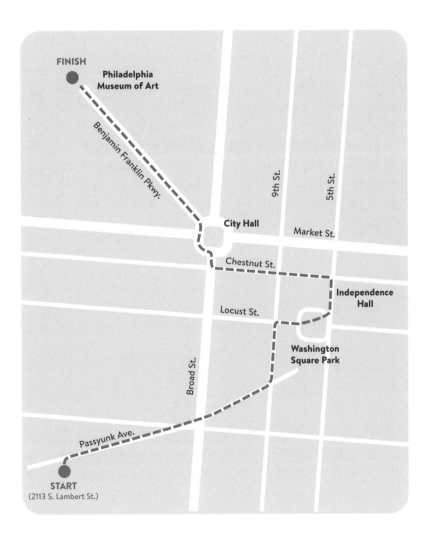

GO FOR A SPOOKY, SWEATY SPRINT UP *THE EXORCIST* STEPS IN DC

DC's spookiest tourist spot is far from the National Mall in a Georgetown parking lot. Rising at a seemingly impossible angle are the *Exorcist* steps, the 75-step staircase where (spoiler alert) Father Damien Harris falls to his death in the climactic ending of the 1973 classic horror flick.

The stairs are a blast to climb—impossibly steep, gloriously shaded from DC's intense summer sun, and quietly tucked away next to the 19th-century "Car Barn" building, where Georgetown's streetcars were once stored. Even walking up them can be tough, but the *Exorcist* steps have been used for intervals by local running clubs for years. Take their lead: Try to climb the steps at a run, then come down at a slightly slower pace. Try for at least 3 rounds and scare up an appetite for a post-workout feast.

The stairs are at 36th Street NW and M Street, in the lot west of the Car Barn.

BIKE VIRGINIA'S 300-YEAR-OLD GRAVEL ROADS

In a country where the landscape is constantly changing—that farm field from your youth is now a Walmart . . . that national monument is now an oil field—a road that's 300 years old is a rare treat. You can step into museums at historic locations, but riding these gravel pathways is a literal journey through time.

Loudon County, Virginia, about an hour from Washington, DC, has the largest and oldest intact network of gravel roadways in the US, used by millers and farmers, revolutionaries and presidents to get to town and to church, and to take products to market. The roadways of crushed rock still meander past horse farms, stone walls, Civil War battlefields, and sprawling farm fields.

You can find a map of these roads from America's Routes (www.americasroutes.com), a nonprofit dedicated to protecting them. Or you can join the annual Loudon 1725 Gravel Grinder, a series of organized 40-, 60-, and 80-mile rides along the historic gravel roadways. The rides are held each June, and start at $45 for registration. Visit www.ex2adventures.com.

Forget Times Square and the Statue of Liberty boat tour. Give yourself a fresh look at America's biggest city with this pair of "only in New York" workouts.

Hoop on hallowed ground at Rucker Park

If you try to step on the court during a pickup game at Rucker Park, you'll be laughed off the blacktop—the legendary streetball mecca has seen NBA players like Kareem, Dr. J, Metta World Peace, and more play pickup over the half-century since the Rucker Tournament was launched. If you don't have an Iverson-level crossover, you probably don't want to mix it up with the type of players lacing it up here.

That doesn't mean you can't shoot around at this hoops holy land, though: Just go early. Show up at Rucker in the morning, or in the early afternoon on a weekday, and you should be able to find space to shoot around, play a little Twenty-One, and soak in the atmosphere—can't do that at Madison Square Garden! And unlike MSG, if you stick around at Rucker, you're likely to see some good basketball: Take to the stands in the late afternoon or on a weekend to catch the real ballers in action.

If you're looking for a more mortal-friendly pickup game, head to Central Park: There are 12 courts at the North Meadow Recreation Center on 97th Street so you can find a game that's more your speed. Rucker Park is at West 155th Street and Frederick Douglass Boulevard. Take the B or D train to 155th Street, then walk south about a block.

Catch a big wave in the Big Apple

Not everyone can paddle the waters of Hawaii and California, so surfers across America will do anything to catch a wave—braving chunks of ice in the Upper Peninsula of Michigan, or chasing knee-high rolling waves in Cleveland. But the waves just outside New York City don't just tide surfers over—they're celebrated surf spots for beginners and veteran wave riders alike.

In the summer, avid surfers like my friend Shawn jump on the A train at 5 a.m. to get in 90 minutes on the water at the Rockaways before heading into work. Farther out on Long Island, in Montauk and on Long Beach, the waves get even bigger—there have even been pro surfing events held there.

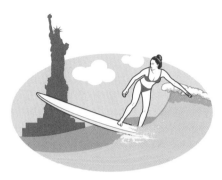

Things to Know

- If you want to surf in the city, Rockaway Beach is the closest option from Manhattan. To get there, take the A train toward Far Rockaway and get off at the Beach 60 Street or Beach 90 Street Holland stations, and walk south toward the beach. There are surf shops—and the Boarders New York Surf School—along the boardwalk. For Long Beach, you'll take the Long Island Railroad to Long Beach. Several of the surf shops are near the train station on East Park Avenue.

- Unfortunately, as one friend tells me, the best time to surf is "when it's the coldest." Hurricane season also brings big waves to the area. Check surf reports at www.surfline. com, and call local surf shops for more tips.

- You can buy boards at surf shops in Brooklyn, or rent a board and other stuff you'll need, like a wetsuit from Boarders Surf Shop in Rockaway Beach (www.boarderssurfshop.com) or from UnSound Surf Shop (www.unsoundsurf.com) or Long Beach Surf Shop (www.longbeachsurf.com) in Long Beach. Boards are $30–$50 per half-day at both locations. Boarders also offer lessons for $90 per person.

CHAPTER 2

SWEAT THROUGH THE SOUTH

Earn that barbecue, sweat off those grits, and make room for a slice of sticky-sweet pecan or Kentucky Derby pie: The South is scenic, historic, but most of all delicious. Work up an appetite as you see the sights with these 18 adventures.

START AT THE TOP: CLIMB THE TALLEST MOUNTAIN EAST OF THE MISSISSIPPI

You don't need carabiners or climbing experience to summit the tallest mountain in America's eastern half. Because it's just a third of the height of Denali, the US's tallest mountain, you can hike Mount Mitchell from bottom to top in under four hours wearing shorts and sneakers—and, if you're smarter than me, get a ride back without climbing down.

The flower-lined path of Mount Mitchell Trail stretches 6 miles from Black Mountain Campground to the summit, where you can look down at the surrounding Appalachian peaks that make the Blue Ridge Parkway one of America's most scenic drives. In fact, you could drive to the 6,684-foot peak—and you'll be joined at the top by many tourists who did—but the hike makes the view a crowning achievement that you can celebrate over a local pint at one of Asheville's many craft breweries.

Hiking the Mount Mitchell Trail from Black Mountain Campground is free. Park in the lot (just set your GPS to "Black Mountain Campground") and start from the campground office—the trail is across the road and well-marked by blue blazes. You'll hike for about two hours on an easy grade through tree roots and pine needles to another campground, which is your first landmark. It's about 90 more minutes to the top.

There's a parking lot up there and a concession area where you can grab snacks and water refills, and use a clean restroom. There are also shorter trails you can ramble around if you haven't had your hiking fill. Pro tip: If you have a friend who doesn't want to climb, save yourself the three-hour return trip—ask them to meet you at the top and drive you back down. Then buy them lunch.

AFTER YOU CLIMB, SQUARE DANCE IN THE STREETS

If you head to Asheville to summit Mount Mitchell or for some other outdoor adventure—kayaking, rafting, rock climbing—spend Friday night square dancing in the streets . . . in a circle.

In Waynesville, about 30 miles west of Asheville, summer Fridays are for Appalachian-style square dancing, where all dancers form a giant circle while pairs head to the center to perform moves like the "Wagon Wheel" and "Cage the Birdie." For the Mountain Street Dances, the town dusts the streets with cornmeal to give dancers a better grip for summer night hoofing. The coolest thing about the experience, though, may be the caller: Joe Sam Queen, a member of the North Carolina State House of Representatives, is the square dance caller—just as his grandfather was in the 1930s, when he called an Appalachian square for FDR. Visit www.downtownwaynesville.com for details and the summer schedule.

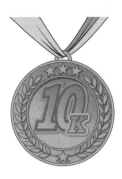

RUN IN THE WORLD'S LARGEST 10K

As many as 60,000 runners celebrate Independence Day with a 6-mile run through Atlanta at the Peachtree Road Race—the world's largest 10K. One reason: This 50-year-old event draws raucous crowds. Weaving through the streets of Buckhead into midtown Atlanta is easier when more than 100,000 people are there to root for you.

And you'll need the support: After 2.5 miles of downhill running, the course changes dramatically, pitting runners against Atlanta's most notorious climb—Cardiac Hill. It's "only" a 3.1 percent grade hill, but the Georgia heat and humidity, combined with the length of the climb—around three-quarters of a mile—leave many runners gasping at the top. You could get a boost from the crowd, though: As runners conquer this legendary will-maker, patients at the Shepherd Center, a spinal cord and brain injury hospital, will be cheering you on as you head for the finish in Piedmont Park. To sign up, go to www.ajc.com/peachtree.

CONQUER THE WORLD'S TALLEST CLIMBING WALL

An hour outside Atlanta, you'll find a different kind of high-rise: Towering over Historic Banning Mills, Georgia, is a 14-story rock climbing wall—the world's tallest. But newbies are welcome: The record-breaking climbing wall has nine different climbing lanes, with guided routes for climbing novices and experts alike. At the top: breathtaking views of the Snake Creek Gorge and Historic Banning Mills's zip-line system, which includes rides up to 3,400 feet long.

Climbs on the wall are $30 per person for an hour, or two hours for $40. Reservations are required. Go to www.historicbanningmills.com.

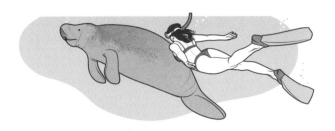

SNORKEL WITH MANATEES IN FLORIDA'S CRYSTAL RIVER

More than 120,000 people visit Crystal River National Wildlife Refuge each year to swim with the largest concentration of manatees in Florida. Snorkeling with these sea cows is especially incredible because the thousand-pound herbivores don't dart away. (Because they evolved in an area without predators, manatees don't have the type of predator-avoiding scurry you'll find with most other undersea animals.) You can't chase them down or touch them—that can actually incur a $100,000 fine—but if a manatee swims in your direction, you can relax near these giants as they hoover up as much as 10 percent of their body weight in seagrass.

The best time for manatee viewing is from late November through early March, and numerous companies offer guided snorkeling. Three- and 4-hour tours, with snorkeling gear, are available for $65–$75 per person. Visit https://fws.gov/refuge/Crystal_River/ for details on the sanctuary's seasonal hours and to find a tour operator.

GO SCOUTING FOR BIGFOOT IN A MAZE OF CYPRESS

Caddo Lake is an eerie wetland, a labyrinth of moss-covered cypress trees on the Texas–Louisiana border that's home to owls, alligators . . . and maybe Bigfoot.

Hundreds of Sasquatch sightings have been reported on Caddo, the second-largest lake in the South after Lake Okeechobee. Rent a canoe or kayak inside Caddo Lake State Park and explore more than 50 miles of paddling trails in the area, keeping your eyes peeled for owls, eagles, and, of course, any 8-foot stalkers hiding in the trees. Even if you don't spot a legendary creature, your surroundings will look legendary: You'll be weaving through gargantuan, half-submerged cypress trees, straight out of a fairy tale. For more info, visit www.tpwd.texas.gov/state-parks/caddo-lake. The park has hiking trails, fishing, and screened-in lodging—it's a bayou, so it can get buggy!

RUN IN THE FOOTSTEPS OF PIRATES TO THE FRENCH QUARTER AT DAWN

New Orleans's French Quarter is a legendary place to party, and—in the morning, at least—a memorable place to shake off the hangover and slip on your running shoes. The same streets that were teeming with tourists are blissfully quiet, letting you soak in the historic architecture in conditions that aren't yet face-meltingly humid. You can finish your run after a short rise up to the water, watching ships going in and out of port. It's a perfect way to center your mind and build your appetite for another evening of savoring crawfish tails and slurping hurricanes.

To mix a little history and fun with your run, take this route—the same path the notorious pirate Jean Lafitte and his followers took to reinforce Andrew Jackson's troops during the Battle of New Orleans in 1815. Begin at the Old Spanish Fort at Robert E. Lee Boulevard and Beauregard Avenue, and run west on Lee Boulevard. You'll run into the New Orleans City Park. Turn right on Marconi Drive—you'll run past the golf course and along the Orleans Canal south through the park for 1.5 miles. When you reach Orleans Avenue, turn left—head straight along Orleans until you reach Louis Armstrong State Park, a little more than 3 miles away. Cross through the park and exit on St. Peter, heading toward the water—you'll reach Jackson Square, where Lafitte and his men hooked up with the future president to join the fight against the British.

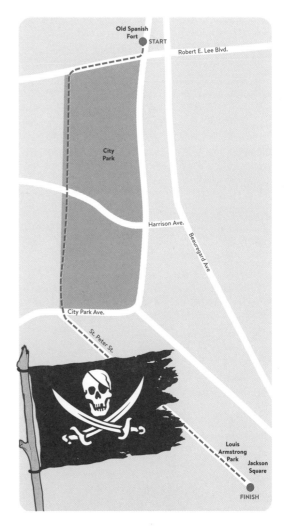

If you want more of a party with your run—you're in New Orleans, after all—a version of this same 9K route is run each March for the Jackson Day Race, a more than 100-year-old event. Reenactors dressed as pirates lead the way for one of the most affordable races in the US: Entry is only $25 if you get in early. Visit www.runnotc.org for details.

LIFT AT THE HOME OF THE "KING" OF BODYBUILDING

Fifteen years after he last won bodybuilding's top prize, Ronnie Coleman inspires the type of fanaticism that other swole beasts can only imagine. The seven-time Mr. Olympia winner is the subject of a documentary on Netflix, and is probably the only bodybuilder—except maybe Arnold—being quoted by NFL players in the weight room.

The quote? "Everybody wants to be a bodybuilder, but nobody wants to lift no heavy-ass weights."

Coleman's hard-core approach to training made him legendary—and videos of him will pump up even a novice lifter. If you're in the Dallas area, you can lift at Metroflex, the gym where Coleman built his prodigious bulk and continues to train in retirement. For $10, you can do a drop-in at this South Cooper Street establishment and train at this no-nonsense, extreme gym. Find a map to the gym at www.metroflexgym.com.

If you drop in, pay homage to Coleman with a workout in his signature style: high reps of heavy weights. Choose three to four exercises per body part and do 4 sets with a weight that's 75 percent of your one-rep maximum for each move. In each set, do 12 to 15 reps of the exercise.

Perform a warm-up set of each move, then perform 4 sets of 12 to 15 reps, each with a "heavy-ass" weight—one that's 75 percent of your one-rep maximum.

EXERCISE 1: Barbell Deadlift

1. Bend at your hips and knees to grab the barbell a little wider than shoulder width. Your feet should be flat on the floor.
2. Keeping your weight in your heels and maintaining the natural curve of your spine, pull the bar up as you thrust your hips forward and stand. The bar should remain close to your body as it comes off the floor.
3. Reverse the maneuver to return to start. Repeat.

EXERCISE 2: Barbell Bent-Over Row

1. Deadlift the weight off the ground (see above) so you stand holding the bar in front of you with an overhand grip, feet hip-width apart, knees slightly bent.
2. Push your hips back like you're opening a door behind you with your butt. This starts the hip hinge.
3. Keep pushing your hips back so that your back remains flat until it is nearly parallel to the floor with the weight hanging straight down from your shoulders.
4. Maintaining this flat back position, pull the weight toward your chest.
5. Lower the weight back to the starting position and repeat.

EXERCISE 3: Single-Arm Dumbbell Row

1. Stand with a firm bench on your left side. Place your left knee on the bench, then bend your torso forward and place your left hand on the bench to support your body. In this position, your upper body should be parallel to the floor.
2. Reach down and grab the dumbbell with your right hand, returning to this position where your body is parallel to the floor, with the weight hanging straight down from your right shoulder.
3. Maintaining that upper body position, pull your right arm straight up until your hand reaches the side of your chest.
4. Lower the weight back to the starting position and repeat. Do all your reps on this side, then switch sides and repeat.

EXERCISE 4: Standing Barbell Curl

1. Stand holding the barbell with an underhand grip slightly wider than shoulder-width.
2. Squeeze your butt and flex your abs during the movement to keep yourself from swinging your hips.
3. Bend your elbows to bring your hands up to your shoulders. Return to start and repeat.

EXERCISE 5: Seated Dumbbell Curls

1. Sit on a narrow bench with dumbbells at your sides, palms facing forward.
2. Curl the dumbbells up to your shoulders as you keep your torso upright.
3. Return to start and repeat.

EXERCISE 6: Preacher Bench Curl

1. Grab the bar with an underhand grip on the preacher bench.
2. Curl the bar up to your shoulders without swinging.
3. Return to start and repeat.

EXERCISE 7: Standing Cable Curl

1. Stand holding the straight bar cable from a low pulley with an underhand grip slightly wider than shoulder-width.
2. Squeeze your butt and flex your abs during the movement to keep yourself from swinging your hips.
3. Bend your elbows to bring your hands up to your shoulders. Return to start and repeat.

THE TENNESSEE BATTLEFIELD YOU CAN CLIMB

Most Civil War battlefields are just that: fields. Sure, history happened there, and a guide can show where a charge started and stopped, but they're mostly grass.

Lookout Mountain—as its name suggests—is different. It's a battlefield you can climb—and bike, rock climb, and horseback ride. The site of an 1863 Union victory nicknamed the Battle above the Clouds, Lookout towers over Chattanooga, just as it did when Major General Joseph Hooker's Northern army beat back the rebels. Today, though, there's something new: The Incline Railway, the world's steepest passenger train, ferries tourists up and down "America's Most Amazing Mile" for views of the city and the surrounding state forests.

You don't have to ride *up*, though: Here's one local's guide to hiking some of the mountain's 30 miles of trails, enjoying the train, and living la vida Lookout.

Park at Cravens House, a historic site of a local ironworker's home, where much of the fighting took place. Grab a map.

1. Hike the Cravens House Trail to the Mountain Beautiful Trail. Follow the signs to Point Park, a ten-acre memorial park that overlooks the battlefield and Chattanooga (admission is $7).
2. After walking around the paved paths of Point Park, walk south on East Brow Road to buy tickets and board the Incline Railway ($15). Take the scenic train trip downhill to the St. Elmo Historic District.
3. The historic district is dotted with microbreweries, restaurants, and ice cream shops. Refuel!
4. When you're done and have digested all those goodies, ride the train back to Point Park and hike back to your car.
5. Or, if you're up for a big hike, walk back: Head south on St. Elmo Avenue to the Guild Trail trailhead. Follow this paved trail to the intersection with TN-148 N. Make a sharp left, then look for "CRAVENS TERRACE." Follow it back to your car.

PADDLE THE MUDDY MISSISSIPPI LIKE HUCK FINN

Everything about the Mississippi River is big: its 2,300-mile length, its millions of gallons of water rushing into the Gulf of Mexico, and the innumerable legends and stories associated with America's largest waterway. To feel the enormity of it and live one of those stories on your own, go small. Float down Old Man River in a tiny craft, as Huck Finn did.

It won't be a raft like Twain's crew, but Quapaw Canoe Company in Clarksdale, Mississippi, will outfit you for a journey in the next best thing: A canoe. The 10-year-old company plans, outfits, and guides river adventures from one day to weeks long, complete with meals and shuttles from Clarksdale or Memphis. You'll wind down 20-mile-long bends in the mighty river on 29-foot-long, six-person canoes, past swirling eddies as large as a city block, through forests of willows to remote, wild islands. The experienced Quapaw guides help you and friends set up camp as they prepare meals like local fish and barbecue while spinning tales (tall and true) about the big, muddy river. It's an adventure straight out of one of the Great American Novels—and in our awesome modern world, you can book it online.

Prices vary based on how many paddlers you bring along. For a solo paddle, it's about $400 per day, including all meals and shuttles. That price falls between $50 and $100 per day for each person you add to your trip. Quapaw has all kinds of expeditions, but their most popular is a 101-mile trip, called Muddy Waters Wilderness. It's a five-day journey from Clarksdale that paddles past the childhood home of blues legend Muddy Waters. Visit www.island63.com for information and to book.

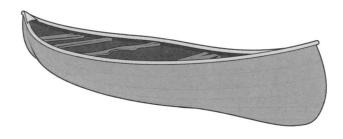

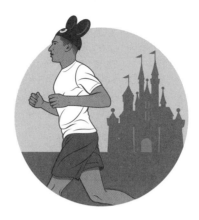

RUN THROUGH DISNEY WORLD . . . FOUR DAYS IN A ROW

Test your endurance and your sanity—all while giving your family a dream vacation. Disney World's Run Disney marathon is an event in itself, taking runners through all the Orlando parks in a single race. But for combination fitness-and-Figment fanatics, there's a bigger challenge: running four races through the parks on four consecutive days.

It's called the Dopey Challenge, and it's not clear if it's named for the dim-witted dwarf or the Mouse-loving masochists who take it on. The challenge: Run the Disney 5K, 10K, half-marathon, and marathon races all in a single year. These races are held over a single weekend, so Dopeys rack up 48.6 miles completing the challenge.

For the first three races, the parks are closed. You'll start as early as 5:30 a.m., cruising through the eerily empty streets of the Magic Kingdom and Epcot. But the marathon finishes when the parks have opened to the public, so the streets of Main Street USA and Tomorrowland are lined with cheering fans. There are also character stops where runners can pose with Mickey, Minnie, and, of course, Dopey. And you can even ride the rides during the race: Some runners duck into Space Mountain so they can grab a mid-ride picture while wearing their racing bib!

The Dopey Challenge is sanctioned by Run Disney and comes with a special finisher's medal. Depending on how early you register, the cost may be $590, $600, or $610.

Run Disney events are held every January, but fill up fast. Visit www.rundisney.com to sign up.

CLIMB INTO MISSISSIPPI'S "LITTLE GRAND CANYON"

About two hours from the Gulf of Mexico, the banks of the Pearl River have eroded, creating Red Bluff, a miniature Grand Canyon that grows with every rainfall. Striped with red clay and sand, the stunning, half-mile-wide canyon offers incredible views and photographs, and for those brave enough to descend 200 feet into the ravine, a strenuous, rewarding hike . . . maybe Mississippi's best.

Come prepared, though: Red Bluff is on private land and is unregulated. There are no rangers or safety precautions in place, and, more importantly, no bathrooms. There's also no sign, so praise Google for GPS: Point it to "Red Bluff Hike, Foxworth, MS" to find your way to the trailhead—about two hours from Gulfport, one hour from Hattiesburg, or just over two hours from New Orleans. Stop in nearby Columbia on the way for a bathroom break and grab a trash bag. Since the trail is public, some hikers have taken to leaving cans and other debris along the way. Leave this tiny treasure better than you found it—take out more trash than you bring in!

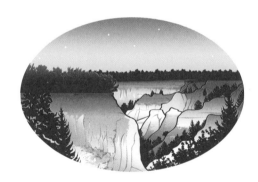

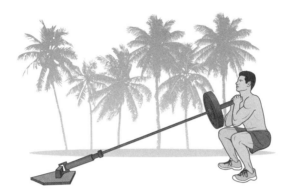

PERFECT YOUR BEACH BODY ON THE SANDS OF MIAMI BEACH

Outdoor gyms are the best: There's something exhilarating about sweating in the sun, trading in the cinder-block walls of a gym to stare out at a mountain vista while slinging barbells, doing pull-ups in the park, or gazing at the sea between sets. The greatest of these is probably Venice, California's Muscle Beach, where Arnold Schwarzenegger and other legends pumped it up. But the Calisthenic Park on South Beach in Miami Beach is a close second.

It's loaded with shiny, modern equipment: pull-up bars, parallel bars, rings, battling ropes, a heavy bag, a barbell land-mine press, and more. And it's right next to the volleyball courts—so you can show off while you get your sweat on.

If you head to Lummus Park—and you should—do this workout: It's designed using the equipment from the beach's gym.

First, warm up. Run around on the sand—you're at the beach! Get your heart pumping. Then:

Make Your Booty Pop: Do a Land-Mine Sumo Squat

Using the barbell land mine, where one end is affixed to the ground, stand with the end of the weight in front of you.

1. Spread your legs so your heels are slightly wider than hip-width apart, toes facing out.
2. Keeping an upright torso, push your hips back and bend your knees to drop your butt down toward the ground.
3. Grab the end of the barbell with both hands.
4. Press through your heels to drive back up to standing.
5. Squat back down and continue. Do 6 sets of 6 reps, resting 1 minute between sets.

Make Your Shoulders Look like Boulders: Do a Land-Mine Shoulder Press

Using the same apparatus, hold the weight in front of your chest with both hands, knees slightly bent, and your torso slightly angled toward the weight.

Use both arms to press the weight overhead without arching your back. Slowly return to start and repeat. Do 4 sets of 8 reps, resting 1 minute between sets.

Pop Your Pecs

Use the twisting push-up handles. But you don't need to twist them! By using push-up handles to create a neutral grip, where your palms face each other, you can perform more push-ups with less stress on your shoulders and wrists.

1. Put your hands on the handles, palms facing each other, and assume a traditional push-up position—your body should form a straight line from head to heels.
2. Maintaining this rigid body line, bend your elbows to drop your chest until it's even with your hands.
3. Press back to start. Do 3 sets to failure.

Put a Big Smile on Your Face

The smile is the most important part of any beach body—get it glowing by hopping on the Lummus Beach monkey bars. You'll work your arms, core, shoulders, and back, of course, but you'll come off the bars with a big smile, ready for a cool-off swim in the ocean before settling down for a beachside cocktail.

The Calisthenic Park is near Ninth Street and Ocean Drive, Miami Beach. Point your GPS to "Calisthenic Park South Beach."

RIDE CYCLING'S NEWEST MECCA: ARKANSAS

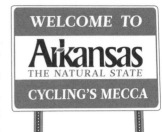

When you think of the world's great cycling destinations, you might imagine the canals of Amsterdam, the French Alps, or the boulders of Moab. Add Arkansas to that list: In the past decade, full-time trail crews in the Natural State's northwest have made the home of the Razorbacks a world-class haven for riders. The towns of northwest Arkansas now have hundreds of miles of trails branching off 36 miles of bike-friendly greenways, connecting the region.

The hub for this huge effort is Bentonville, the region's best-known city. The must-ride trail system in the area is the Slaughter Pen, which isn't as intimidating as it sounds—more than 20 miles of trails run through it, including beginner-friendly routes like the All-American Trail and the Seed Tick Shuffle. The trail system includes single-track mountain biking and sections of jumps, as well as tamer rides for beginners along rugged—but wider—stone pathways that wind through forest and sections of large-scale public art near the Crystal Bridges Museum of American Art. The museum's grounds are bike-friendly, making for unique photo opportunities with the art installations and architecture, including a classic Frank Lloyd Wright house on the campus.

Plan your own route within the Slaughter Pen with a map from OZ Trails, which builds and maintains many of Arkansas's amazing trails. Visit www.oztrailsnwa.com.

TRAIN WITH AMERICA'S BEST FITNESS CLASS INSTRUCTOR IN ATLANTA

In 2019, users of ClassPass—which lets users book classes at gyms around the world—booked more than 189 million hours of fitness classes. And the highest-rated teacher from all of those is in Atlanta. Claudia Fitzwater, the founder of Project: Body, has created a studio for women (sorry, fellow dudes) that combines cardio, strength, and flexibility in a space that rejects fat-shaming and is designed to welcome Black and brown bodies. And if the ridiculously high marks she's getting are any indication, it's working. Book a class with her while you're in Atlanta by visiting www.projectbodyatl.com.

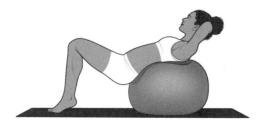

CLIMB 13 STORIES TO FLY DOWN AMERICA'S TALLEST WATERSLIDE

At the top of the Ko'okiri Body Plunge at Universal Orlando Resort, a trapdoor opens, dropping you 125 feet at a 70-degree angle into the pool below. How steep is that? Imagine you're standing on the face of a clock, and you're halfway between 11 and 12 . . . and sliding from there to the center of the clock at 60 mph.

If that doesn't get your heart racing, just getting to the top of this artificial volcano definitely will: There's no elevator, so you've got about 13 stories of climbing to psych yourself up—or try to calm yourself down—before reaching the upper platform, where the terrifying trapdoor is waiting to drop you for six seconds of screaming. Ride the slide eight times in a day, and you'll have climbed as high as the Empire State Building!

RIDE THE SOUTH'S MOST POPULAR BIKE TRAIL

The 9.4-mile White Rock Lake Park Loop Trail isn't just Dallas's most popular place to bike—the east side of the loop to the lake's southern tip is the most-logged bike route in the entire southern US on Strava, the popular GPS tracking app. More than 600,000 rides have been clocked on this stretch.

And no wonder: The path is wide and well-kept, and the views are incredible. The ride includes a stretch through the flora of the Dallas Arboretum, praised by no less than Martha Stewart. There are pelicans, beavers, and even wild parakeets flying around the endless trees, boats docked on the sun-dappled waters, and, around certain turns, dramatic views of the Dallas skyline. Stop for a water break at one of several picnic areas built by the Civilian Conservation Corps as part of President Franklin Roosevelt's New Deal during the Great Depression. As one avid rider says, "There is no bad mood that can survive this ride."

Begin your ride from the cyclists' parking lot on West Lawther Drive on the lake's western shore. To log your ride on the popular Strava segment, go for a clockwise route, heading left (west) from the parking lot before heading north.

HIKE 8 MILES TO GET TO YOUR HOTEL BED

The Smoky Mountain views are worth it!
Perched at 6,360 feet, near the peak of Mount LeConte in Tennessee, is LeConte Lodge—a rustic collection of guesthouses that are the highest lodging available in the eastern US. The catch: There's no road, so you'll have to climb the mountain to get there.

Visitors can choose from five different hiking trails, up to 8 miles long, to reach the lodge. The easiest route is the 6.7-mile Trillium Gap Trail, the same one used by packs of llamas to bring supplies to the lodge on Monday, Wednesday, and Friday. Stay for one of these days, and you can thank woolly camelids for providing the food and drink you'll enjoy at the top.

Those provisions are part of the reward for your dromedary-level climb. Guests at LeConte have both dinner and breakfast included with their room, with pancakes, grits, and rashers of bacon in the morning, and hearty fare like beef and gravy and chocolate chip cookies at night. And for an extra $12, enjoy all the wine you can drink during dinner hour.

Besides the grub, consider the views: Mount LeConte is the third-highest peak in the Smoky Mountains and sits high enough in the mist to offer brilliant, unencumbered sunrise and sunset views of the surrounding mountains.

The lodge books up about a year in advance at www.lecontelodge.com, at $158.50 per person, per night. But you can also visit on a day hike: The lodge offers lunch for $12 between noon and five, as well as baked goods to fuel your return hike.

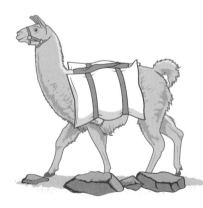

CHAPTER 3

MOVE IT
IN THE MIDWEST

When outdoor adventurers think of America, their minds go west: To the Rockies, the Badlands, or other elevated places. Don't fly over the Midwest. Its flat expanse is filled with surprises and fun, starting with an adventure hiding in one of its iconic farms.

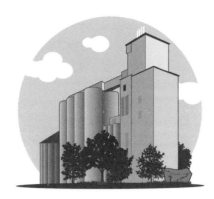

ROCK CLIMB *INSIDE* ABANDONED GREAT PLAINS GRAIN SILOS

Pancake-flat Indiana isn't where you'd expect to find a world-class rock climbing destination. But Upper Limits Gym in Bloomington is just that, thanks to its one-of-a-kind—actually, three-of-a-kind—climbing walls: a trio of grain silos.

Since 1995, routes have been being built inside these 65-foot tubes, letting climbers feel as if they're infiltrating a secret facility in *Mission: Impossible* or escaping the crazy Bane prison in *The Dark Knight Rises* while scaling more than 20 different top-rope routes. The facility also has an outdoor 110-foot wall, and gives even non-climbers the opportunity for an action movie experience: They can take an elevator to the top and rappel 120 feet down the facility's side.

An adult day pass is $16 and a complete rental package is $10. Visit www.upperlimits.com to check availability.

RACE THROUGH A 28-ACRE CORN MAZE

This may be the twistiest 5K on Earth! In Spring Grove, Illinois—near the Wisconsin border—you can wind through 28 acres at what Richardson Farm calls the world's largest corn maze (believe it or not, there's some debate over which maze is maziest). On race day, the path to the exit is clearly marked, with wrong turns marked off by tape. That doesn't make it easy: Racers have to navigate more than 250 turns to weave through 3 miles of stalks to get to the finish line. The winners still get through the maze quickly. In 2019, the race's top finishers ran 6:42 miles through the corn. The race is held each October. Visit www.richardsonadventurefarm.com for details.

Not in the Midwest but still want to run a corn maze? Bob's Corn & Pumpkin Farm near Seattle holds a similar event each year. Visit www.bobscorn.com to learn more.

RUN A LAP OF THE INDY 500

You may not ever get behind the wheel like an Andretti, but at Indianapolis's Mini-Marathon, you can run a lap of the world's most famous race track: the Brickyard.

On the first Saturday of May, more than 35,000 runners race across Indianapolis with an IndyCar leading each group from the starting line. But it's around the halfway mark that makes this mini an iconic American race: You'll run inside Indianapolis Motor Speedway for a 2.5-mile lap on the same track where the "Greatest Spectacle in Racing" takes place. Many runners sacrifice a few seconds from their half-marathon time to follow an Indy 500 tradition: bending down to smooch the bricks at the starting line.

After that, it's a fast, flat course through the streets of downtown Indianapolis, finishing with—what else?—checkered flags.

Registration is $65. Visit www.indymini.com for details. A double-dip bonus for sports fans: The Mini-Marathon's Expo is on the field of Lucas Oil Stadium, home of the Indianapolis Colts.

RUN ON FOOTBALL'S MOST SACRED GROUND

The "frozen tundra" of Lambeau Field is an NFL landmark and legend. It's the longest continuously used stadium in football and has been home to some of the most epic and frigid games the sport has ever seen. And if you run the Green Bay Marathon, you can run on this hallowed ground.

Here's the good news: The ground won't be frozen at all. The race is held in May of each year, so it's shorts weather for the small race, with about 1,700 runners doing the full marathon in 2018. After a short run through the city and some small crowds, the race thins out more than most big-city marathons, so it's a peaceful run along the water and through town until you get near the finish. Before you're done, you'll run into the stadium and do a lap around the legendary field. But you don't have to run 26 miles for your Lambeau Lap: Whether you run the full marathon, the half-marathon, or even just the 5K, the stadium run is included.

Registration fees range from $85 in early January up to $140 during the weekend of the race. Details at www.cellcomgreenbaymarathon.com.

PLAY BALL AT THE FIELD OF DREAMS

If you build it, they will come, right? Well, they built it, and you can go to the baseball field constructed for *Field of Dreams*. The outfield "wall" is still just cornstalks and Kevin Costner's farmhouse is a museum that's open almost every day. The best part: You can play ball on the field, and it's free.

Visitors bring bats, balls, and gloves to the field almost every day for games of pickup baseball, and anyone can join in. If you're willing to "go the distance" and make the drive to Dyersville—about three hours from Des Moines, two hours from Madison, Wisconsin, or almost four hours from Chicago—you can take the field, too, for a few innings at third base, a few swings at the plate, and a daylong celebration of the game.

The field is located at 28995 Lansing Road, Dyersville, IA, 52040. It's open 359 days per year, and it's free to park your car and play. There are, however, some days with special events, so check the website to make sure your day is available: www.fieldofdreamsmoviesite.com. While you're there, you can see if the farmhouse is available for a tour during your visit: You need to give 24 hours' notice.

WALK ACROSS THE MISSISSIPPI RIVER WITHOUT GETTING WET

At its mightiest points, the Mississippi is more than 10 miles wide, 200 feet deep, and pumps 600,000 cubic feet of water per second down its more than 2,300 miles. But at Minnesota's Lake Itasca, where that rushing river gets started, you can walk across America's longest river without getting your socks damp.

The hike to the source of the Mississippi, about 100 miles east of Fargo at Lake Itasca State Park, is only about a half-mile trip. The trail is wide and usually crowded—more than 500,000 people visit each year. Plunking down the park's $7 entry fee and braving the crowds is worth it, though, to take in the beginning of this mighty river—and to rock hop across its 30-foot width, so you can say you've crossed the Mississippi on foot!

Of course, half a mile isn't much of a workout. So once you've gotten the obligatory selfie at the sign indicating the river's source, head out for a longer hike. Take the Aiton Heights Fire Tower Trail for an easy mile-long hike that ends at the titular tower. Wait in line to climb it and get 360-degree views of five or more of Minnesota's 10,000 lakes.

CANOE THE NIOBRARA RIVER TO STARGAZE IN THE WIDE-OPEN PLAINS

Most coastal Americans take in the open expanses of the Great Plains quickly—either looking down at patchwork quilts of farms from above, or zooming past amber waves of grain on an interstate. Get a slower perspective (and a workout . . . and some of the best dark-sky stargazing you'll ever see) on board a canoe in Nebraska's Niobrara River.

Two hundred miles west of Sioux City, Iowa, the Niobrara flows through the prairie toward the Missouri River. It's a peaceful paddle past more waterfalls than you'd expect in such a flat expanse—there are 230 falls along the river's 500-odd miles. And if you camp along the way, you're in for what one globe-trotting friend said was the most epic, star-studded sky he'd ever seen.

Things to Know

- Canoes and kayaks can be rented in nearby Valentine, Nebraska, for as little as $40 per day. Visit the National Park Service's page on Niobrara (www.nps.gov/niob) for a list of local outfitters.
- Bonus excursion: If you're up for a drive the next day, head 150 miles west to Alliance, Nebraska, to visit Carhenge—an exact replica of Stonehenge . . . but made of old cars.

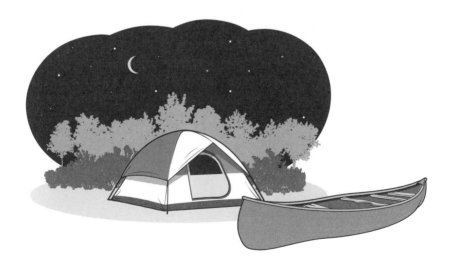

JOIN THE WORLD'S BIGGEST BIKE PARTY

What do people do in Iowa when it's *not* a presidential campaign year? They farm, sure. But they also RAGBRAI.

The [*Des Moines*] *Register*'s Annual Great Bicycle Race Across Iowa (that's the "RAGB-RAI") is the world's largest bike-touring event. Tens of thousands enter a lottery months in advance, looking for one of 8,500 spots for seven days of cycling west to east across the state. Along the way, RAGBRAI-ers will stop overnight to camp in tiny towns with names like Storm Lake, Maquoketa, and Fort Dodge.

But it's not all super-competitive drudgery—it's just the opposite, and that's the reason to get in that lottery. RAGBRAI is a thousands-strong, two-wheeled party. Teams with names like Antiques Road Show (made up of senior citizens, of course) cycle in matching shirts and even costumes as they're chased by colorful buses. Riders stop to do silly things, like adorn roadkill with Mardi Gras beads on their way to the next town. When the crowds arrive after a daily ride of 60 to 80 miles, locals welcome them with free slices of pie and pork for sale in just about every permutation imaginable—sliders, pulled pork, bacon on a stick, and so many others that some riders have said they actually *gained* weight during the 500-mile ride.

RAGBRAI is held each July, finishing on the last Saturday of the month. Spots in the race are chosen by lottery: Registration is open from November through March at www.ragbrai.com. Winners of a spot in the ride are announced starting on May 1, and must pay $175 for a seven-day pass.

Things to Know

- RAGBRAI is mostly a camping event, as the stopover towns are small. You can register to have a support vehicle of friends come along for an additional $40. You have to be in a group of at least three people to have a vehicle, though.
- You can bring a bag: A baggage service, included with registration, will tote a 50-pound bag from town to town so you don't have to carry everything you'll need on your back.

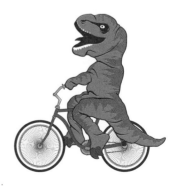

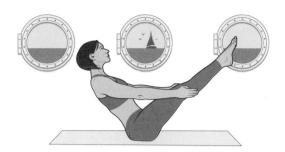

DO BOAT POSE ON A BOAT

Gaze over the fingers of your warrior pose at the neo-Gothic spires of Tribune Tower, look up from your crescent lunge at the Hancock Building's antennas, and flow through downward dog as you float down the Chicago River. Each spring and summer, the Windy City's classic architectural tours give passengers a twist—literally—with boat yoga.

Similar to other novelty classes, like goat yoga, a morning of asanas on the water may not be the best or toughest yoga class you've ever taken, but it's definitely the best combination boat ride, architecture tour, and stretch session you'll ever experience. So get on board!

Boat yoga classes are held on weekend mornings starting in May, continuing throughout the summer. They're $35 and you'll need your own mat. Visit www.cruisechicago.com for a schedule and to book.

WALK ON FROZEN LAKE SUPERIOR TO MAGICAL CAVES OF ICICLES

At Apostle Islands National Lakeshore on the northern tip of Wisconsin, extra-cold winters form fairy tale–worthy ice caves that would impress Elsa. Waterfalls freeze in place and pinprick-thin icicles dangle precariously from caves along the waters of Lake Superior—which is frozen so solid that visitors can hike up to 3 miles each way to visit the glimmering wonders of these fleeting caverns.

The conditions have to be right, though—and "right" means downright *frigid*. The winter has to be cold enough for the ice caves to form and the lake to freeze. And that doesn't happen every year: From 2016 to 2020, the caves weren't even accessible. So when they are, it's a potentially once-in-a-lifetime trip across the frozen surface of Superior. Book a stay in nearby Bayfield, bundle up, and bring shoes with serious traction. The National Park Service suggests wearing shoes with spikes if you can.

You can usually find out if the caves will be accessible by late January. Call the "Ice Line" at 715-779-3398 (extension 3) for details, or check out the park's Facebook page at https://www.facebook.com/apostleislandsnationallakeshore/.

RACE WITH THE WORLD'S BEST AT AMERICA'S PREMIER CROSS-COUNTRY SKI EVENT

The American Birkebeiner is the kind of race people plan their lives around for months: The almost 50-year-old 50K event draws more than 7,000 cross-country skiers to northeast Wisconsin after they've spent the better part of a year running, stair-climbing, cycling, and skiing to build up the endurance needed for this massive celebration of snow. Beginners and pro racers alike compete on the same course, in the same race, with a $20,000 purse on the line.

That's a bit of hyperbole: The "Birkie" is divided into ten waves at the start, and those in the back waves don't have much chance of posting a winning time—the challenging hill climbs can become traffic jams as faster skiers in the back catch up with slower racers in earlier waves. And first-time racers are automatically slotted into that final, slowest wave.

A tip from Birkie veterans to enjoy your first time out: Don't race the full-length event on your first try. Instead, do the shorter Kortelopet, a smaller, 26K event on the same course. Your time in the Korte will let you enter faster waves in the full Birkie the following year.

The Birkie (and Kortelopet) are held each February in Hayward, Wisconsin, about 150 miles from Minneapolis. The registration fee starts at $150. Find details and register at www.birkie.com.

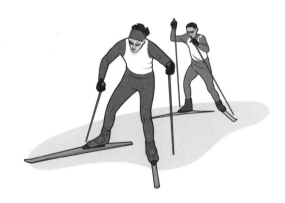

LEARN TO ICE CLIMB IN THE CHICAGO SUBURBS

Ice climbing looks epic: Slamming ice axes and spiked crampons into a literal frozen waterfall is the stuff of Coors Light commercials. But it also looks impossible to try: Where the hell are you going to find a frozen waterfall? Who will lend you a pair of ice axes or spikes for your shoes? And who's going to teach you to use that stuff so you don't die?

The answer: A guy an hour south of Chicago will teach you in his backyard—on a human-made wall of ice. In Monee, Illinois, the "Nice Ice Ice Climbing" wall towers more than 30 feet over the suburbs, so you don't have to be a master adventurer or a beer commercial actor to scale a frozen cascade. Made by pumping water over a climbing wall of wood, the tower puts the bone-chilling winter winds of Illinois to good use and creates a safe atmosphere for Midwestern weekend warriors to get high. Lessons—with gear included—are $75 and available by appointment only. Visit www.chicagoicetower.com to check conditions and book.

CLIMB THE BACK OF THE PRESIDENTS' HEADS AT MOUNT RUSHMORE

The monument might be out front, but the adventure is at the back of Mount Rushmore— there are more than 800 rock climbing routes in the Rushmore National Memorial, including a number of famous fun climbs right up the back of Teddy's head.

Even with punny names like the Emancipation Rockphormation and Garfield Goes to Washington, these climbs are not to be taken lightly: Most are rated 5.8 or higher, meaning they're not for total novices. But there are climbing routes—and climbing experiences—for every level in the park. What a "What I Did This Summer" story to share! Load up the station wagon and head for the (Black) Hills to tackle this adventure.

Things to Know

- Summer weather is great, but fall's even better. Overall, May through October is ideal for climbing.
- Beware holidays and bikers: Some of the climbing routes are closed for Memorial Day and Independence Day weekends. And in the first half of August, South Dakota is much more populated than normal: The annual Sturgis Motorcycle Rally can make lodging harder to find, and the deafening sounds of hundreds of Harleys will be cutting through the hills as you climb.
- Get a guide: The Sylvan Rocks Climbing School offers guided climbs in Rushmore Memorial. An eight-hour day for a single person is $360 with equipment, with the per-person prices going down for bigger groups. Visit www.sylvanrocks.com.

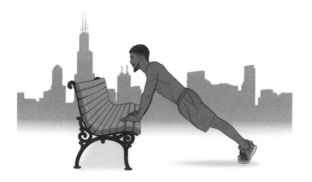

GET A TOTAL-BODY WORKOUT ON CHICAGO'S LAKE SHORE

Lake Shore Drive is already one of the ultimate locations for a run or bike ride—travel south along the lakeside path and you'll get picture-perfect views of the Windy City's skyline, enjoy breezes off the lake, and see dogs frolicking on the beach.

Take a detour from the lakefront path at Diversey Parkway and head a block away from the lake to turn your run or ride into a full-body sweat session. There's an outdoor calisthenics gym at the corner of Lake Shore and Diversey, just south of the driving range, with pull-up bars, monkey bars, ladders, and ropes, just waiting to get you ripped—and build up an appetite for a thick slice of deep dish. Play around and create your own workout, or try this five-move circuit routine before heading back out on your run.

Perform one set of each exercise, then do one chin-up, and move to the next exercise in the sequence. Do 3 to 5 total rounds, resting as little as possible between sets.

EXERCISE 1: Incline Push-Up (8 reps per round)
Assume the classic push-up position, but with your hands on one of the bars: Your hands should be directly beneath your shoulders, your body forming a straight line from head to heels.

1. Maintain this rigid body line as you bend your elbows to lower your chest toward the bar.
2. Press back to start, maintaining the straight body line. After each set, jump up to a bar and do one or two chin-ups. Then move to the next exercise.

EXERCISE 2: Inverted Row (5 to 8 reps per round)

1. Lie beneath one of the bars that's around hip height. Reach your arms up and grab the bar with an overhand grip that's slightly beyond shoulder width. Create a straight body line from head to heels, with your heels resting on the ground and your torso suspended in the air.
2. Keeping this rigid body line, pull your chest to the bar by squeezing your shoulder blades together and then bending your elbows. Try to pull your nipple line toward the bar, rather than bringing your fists to your armpits.
3. Control your body as you lower back to the starting position. After each set, jump up to a bar and do one or two chin-ups. Then move to the next exercise.

EXERCISE 3: Lateral Duck-Under (5 reps on each side in each round)

1. Stand to the right of one of the bars that's around waist height.
2. Squat down and take a big lateral step under the bar with your left leg. Place your left foot on the other side of the bar and bring your body under the bar.
3. Bring your right foot under to meet your left leg. Reverse the movement to return to start. Again, do one to two chin-ups after each set.

EXERCISE 4: Supported Single-Leg Squat (3 to 5 reps per round)

1. Stand to the left of a vertical pole. Lightly place your left hand on the pole. Bend your right knee slightly and lift your left leg off the ground in front of you at a 30- to 45-degree angle.
2. Keeping your back flat and your core braced, push your hips back to lower into a single-leg squat, lowering until your right thigh is parallel to the ground. Use the pole only for balance and only as needed.
3. Press through your right heel to stand back up. Do all your reps, then switch sides. After your set, do one to two chin-ups.

EXERCISE 5: Slant-Board Sit-Up (8 to 10 reps per round)

Using one of the slant boards in the calisthenic area, do sit-ups. Cross your arms over your chest so you don't pull your neck and keep your back flat throughout the movement. Do one to two chin-ups after each set.

THE RACE WHERE EATING DONUTS MAKES YOU FASTER

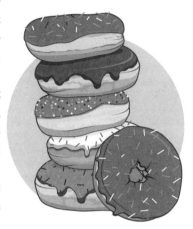

Forget packs of goo. If you want to bike faster, down some donuts—at least, that's the idea behind the Tour de Donut. At the annual August race in Troy, Ohio, riders along the 40-mile course visit two donut stops. For every delicious ring they can stomach, their race time is reduced by five minutes.

It sounds like a gimmick that serious riders would skip, but the race's winners really fill their stomachs: At the 2017 edition, the winner of the men's 19 to 50 age group, Yasir Salem, ate 44 donuts, taking nearly 4 hours off his official time. He finished with a time of *negative* 50 minutes.

If you've got an iron stomach and thighs of steel, chasing Salem may be the event for you. Visit www.thetourdedonut.com to be one of the 2,000 eater-riders next August.

HIKE IN TWO COUNTRIES—AND SEE 100,000 FLOWERS—IN ONE DAY

The International Peace Garden in Dunseith, North Dakota . . . is also in Manitoba, Canada. Founded in 1932 and home to more than 100,000 flowers in peak bloom, the garden straddles the border. While you're there, you can cross at will—creating the unique opportunity to hike in two countries on the same day.

The garden, which was created to promote "international friendship," has more than 10 miles of hiking and biking trails on both sides of the border, as well as a 13-foot working clock that's made of more than 2,000 living flowers. Two countries, one day—just bring your passport. You'll need it to get back through customs as you leave the garden. (Yes, really.)

The garden is in fullest bloom in the summer: Vets of the experience say August is the best time to visit. Entrance is $20 per car.

If hiking isn't fast enough for you, there's now a triathlon in the garden each July—so you can race across the border. Visit www.peacegardentriathlon.com for details.

HIKE WITH BISON IN TEDDY ROOSEVELT'S BADLANDS

Let's give North Dakota the respect it deserves: The oft-forgotten state is home to some of the most breathtaking scenery in the nation. The striped, weathered rocks and rivulet-scarred erosion of the Badlands so enchanted Theodore Roosevelt that he made it his refuge after the tragic death of his first wife, busying himself ranching, hunting, and taking in the gobsmacking beauty surrounding him to get over his grief.

That time appreciating the great expanses of the Dakotas inspired Roosevelt to create the National Park system—and, eventually, inspired that system to turn his former ranches themselves into a National Park. Appropriately named Theodore Roosevelt National Park, it's comprised of two sections near his two ranches in the Badlands. Between the two sections runs the Maah Daah Hey Trail, the longest continuous single-track mountain bike trail in the US. The 144-mile stretch of Dakota ranchland has become a bucket list ride for two-wheel fanatics.

If 144 miles sounds a little long, head to the less-visited North Unit of TR's park: The Caprock Coulee Trail will let you experience the magical Badlands that enchanted the 26th president. Sagebrush, prickly pear cactus, and the dramatic striping and piping of the coulee walls all feature prominently on this four-mile hike, where bison, coyotes, feral horses, and pronghorn antelope roam.

To learn more about this remote, unspoiled landscape, go to www.nps.gov/thro.

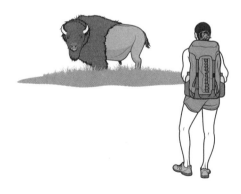

THE MIDWEST'S MOST POPULAR LAKE RUNS

If you don't share your run on social media . . . did you really run? For thousands of Strava fans who use the app to log their training, that's a no. But even if you aren't touting your latest mile time online, you can benefit from those who do: The most popular Strava routes are a shortcut to exploring the best runs in the cities of the Midwest. And—no surprise—they're all around some of the region's amazing lakes.

Chicago: See the Beach, Zoo, and Skyline in One Run

The most popular segment in the Windy City, of course, is a run up the perfectly paved lakefront path along Lake Michigan. This Strava segment travels north, from Diversey up to Bryn Mawr, but running south is even better—you'll stride directly toward the city skyline, with the Hancock building and the rest of Chicago's iconic architecture growing larger as you go. You'll run past several beaches of dogs and sunbathers (well, in the summer), as well as boats at Belmont Harbor. A quick side trip onto Fullerton Avenue can take you through the Lincoln Park Zoo, or stay on the path to see if you run into a Chicago Cub—I've seen several pitchers out for off-day runs on this stretch over the years.

Minneapolis: Loop Lake Calhoun

In the land of 10,000 lakes, this one's the most popular to run around. More than 8,400 runs have been logged around this tree-lined lake, with its views of the Minneapolis skyline. And there are some fast runners on that list—the loop's fastest recorded time is 16:01 for a 5K.

St. Louis: Run around Creve Coeur Lake

For reasons lost to history, the lake's name means "broken heart," but its 4-mile paved path won't leave your ticker—or your ankles—breaking. To log this run as a segment, start at the parking area just off Marine Avenue, and head left (southeast) around the lake for a 3.8-mile run past a waterfall, through woods, and along the shores of this onetime resort lake.

Detroit: A 10K at Stony Creek Lake

It's not exactly downtown—at 26 Mile Road, it's a marathon's distance north of the city center—but the six-mile loop at Stony Creek Lake is worth the trip for a break from city traffic and to get a taste of Michigan's wilder side. Stony Creek Ravine Nature Park has open meadows full of butterflies and statuesque oaks, and, like any Michigan lake, it's teeming with waterfowl.

For more of Strava's most popular routes around the USA, turn to page 8 for East Coast runs and page 80 for routes in West Coast cities. Or, to find popular routes in your city, go to Strava.com/heatmap.

CHAPTER 4

MAKE TRACKS IN MOUNTAIN TIME AND THE AMERICAN SOUTHWEST

The Rockies and the Southwest sport views that will take your breath away. Let them leave you out of breath, too: Don't just see these places. Move through them on these adventures.

JUMP OFF A WATERFALL IN THE GRAND CANYON

Sounds pretty amazing, right? It is—you'll fly from a 60-foot waterfall before splashing into turquoise waters set against the burnt-sienna sandstone of the western Grand Canyon—but you'll have to work pretty hard to get to Beaver Falls.

For starters, you'll need a permit, and you'll need to register for it early. Three-day, two-night permits for camping in Havasupai Indian Reservation become available in early February, costing $650. If you want a bit more luxury, there's a lodge: Reservations for the following year open in June of each year and run about $400 per night.

You'll also need to hike: From the Hilltop Area, where most hikers leave their cars along the canyon walls, it's about a seven-mile hike to the campground's check-in. To avoid the heat of the day, many campers arrive at the parking area the night before and sleep in their cars, leaving for the morning hike around 3 a.m.

After the check-in point, you'll hike another 2 miles to the campground. Nearby are 3 sets of waterfalls—Mooney Falls, Beaver Falls, and Havasu Falls, each cascading into pale blue pools, many of which you can swim in. Trekking around Mooney Falls includes a crawl through a dark cave and some slippery ladders and ropes that can get a bit scary, even for experienced hikers. But it's worth it: Mooney Falls's beauty draws rave reviews, even eclipsing those of Havasu Falls.

Havasu Falls is too high, at 125 feet, for jumping. But both Beaver and Mooney Falls have jumping points where you can splash down into an oasis of blue. Visit www.havasupaireservations.com to book.

Things to Know

- To get a good campsite spot, start early! The spots are first-come, first-served.
- Bring tear-proof bags for your food: Squirrels have been known to chow down on campers' stores.
- Don't forget your headlamp!

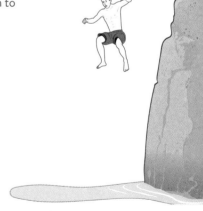

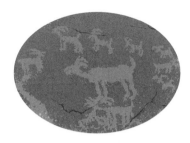

SEE 1,500-YEAR-OLD STONE ETCHINGS ON AN ARIZONA HIKE

It sounds like something out of a fantasy quest: "Hike the hieroglyphic trail at Superstition Mountains." But it's real! This cactus- and wildflower-lined, three-mile trek east of Phoenix winds up the Superstitions past intricate petroglyphs etched into the basalt rocks by the Hohokam Indians around 500 CE.

The trail to the glyphs is pleasant and relatively easy—navigable, but rocky as it gradually builds. After taking the fork north—follow the signs—you'll hike along an inclined ridgetop for a half-mile before dropping down into the looser rocks of the Hieroglyphic Canyon. This section provides something of a challenge—there can be a bit of rock climbing as you enter the canyon at the finish, but there's a reward: a crystal-clear waterfall, and a look at those ancient pictographs.

Things to Know

- To get there, point your GPS to "Hieroglyphic Trailhead, Gold Canyon, Arizona." The trailhead is at the end of East Cloudview Avenue, a few turns from US-60, the "Superstition Freeway."
- The parking lot at the trailhead on Cloudview Avenue fills up early. Start first thing in the morning if you can, and, if the lot is full, wait for a spot: Cars are towed for parking on the street.

THE BEST RIDES IN AMERICA,
ACCORDING TO THE WORLD'S BEST LONG-DISTANCE CYCLIST

If you want to know the most fun, most beautiful places to bike, there's no one better to ask than Lael Wilcox. She rides more than 20,000 miles per year—almost the circumference of the Earth!

Wilcox is the world's best ultra-endurance cyclist, meaning she rides races that would make Forrest Gump blush—2,750 miles down the length of the Continental Divide in 17 days, or 4,400 miles from Oregon to Virginia in 18 days. She crushes the other racers—men and women—in these unassisted events, sleeping just a few hours each night and carrying everything she'll need on board her bike.

When she's not racing, Wilcox is still in the saddle, guiding tours in Arizona or taking on ambitious riding projects. Basically, she's seen—and ridden—it all. These are two of Lael's must-ride trails in the US:

Denali Park Road, Denali National Park, Alaska

In 2017, Wilcox rode every mile of every road in Alaska—a love letter to her home state. Her favorite ride in America's biggest state was the peaceful 92-mile gravel road into Denali National Park. No cars are allowed: Tourists must come on foot, on a bike, or in a tourist bus.

During Alaska's long summer days—around the summer solstice, the sun shines 24 hours a day—the ride can be done in a single day. Bikes are available for rental at several shops outside the park gate, including Denali Outdoor Center (www.denalioutdoorcenter.com), where a 24-hour rental is $40.

If you don't think you have the legs for a 92-mile ride, you can shorten the journey by starting at Savage River, where the paved road ends and the gravel begins. The park's Savage River Shuttle offers this 15-mile trip for free, or you can drive your car to this spot and park. You can also camp along the road for a Lael-style multi-day trip: There are campgrounds at mile 35 and mile 85. See Denali's official website (www.nps.gov/dena/planyourvisit/cycling.htm) for more details.

Montezuma Pass, San Rafael Valley, Arizona

Just 2 miles from the US-Mexico border, this wide-open grassland trail runs along a well-maintained road that's almost traffic-free—it's used mainly by border patrol agents, ranchers, and cyclists, many guided by Wilcox herself. Lael guides in this area with a company called the Cyclist's Menu, and says climbing Montezuma Pass is her favorite spot to guide.

To access the pass, you'll start at the Coronado National Memorial's Visitor Center (4101 East Montezuma Canyon Road, Hereford, AZ; www.nps.gov/coro). Ride 3 miles along a paved road before coming to the Montezuma Pass trailhead sign. From here, a dirt road climbs the pass for 2 miles to an overlook point where you can take in stunning views of the San Pedro and San Rafael River valleys.

HOW WILCOX STAYS STRONG ENOUGH TO RIDE 4,000 MILES

How does Wilcox ride for thousands of miles in these races? To keep herself on the saddle for weeks-long races, Wilcox does strength, cardio, yoga, and core maintenance work when she's not on her bike. If you want to ride longer and stronger, try her daily workout:

1. **PUSH-UPS:** 4 sets of 25 reps. In each set, do 10 narrow-grip push-ups, with elbows pinned to your sides, and 15 wider-grip push-ups.
2. **JUMP ROPE:** 2 sets of 10 minutes of jumping. Stretch your calves for a minute between sets.
3. **FOUNDATION TRAINING VIDEO:** A 12-minute workout video. Check it out on YouTube by searching "Foundation Training original 12 minutes."
4. **FOREARM PLANK:** 4 planks of 2 minutes each, with 1 minute rest between planks.
5. **FOUR-MILE RUN.**

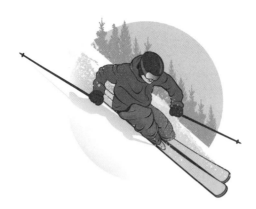

GET A TASTE OF WILD SKIING . . . WITHOUT THE AVALANCHE RISK

I f you've always dreamed of skiing untouched powder in the wilderness but don't know where to start—or the risk of an avalanche gives you pause—go "sidecountry" instead: Hike the ridge at Bridger Bowl, the oldest ski area in the Bozeman, Montana area.

For "sidecountry" skiing, ski areas create terrain areas and runs that are avalanche controlled, but out of the reach of ski lifts—so you're in for a hike. At Bridger Bowl, you'll need an avalanche transceiver and the legs and lungs for a 15-minute hike at 8,800 feet. The result, according to one local friend: "You shred the powder that those who stay on the groomers will never know about. It's easily the closest thing to out-of-bounds snowboarding I've ever done, since I have no avalanche training."

Talk to locals and the ski area guides to find out where to go and which safety precautions to take. This type of ski terrain is less risky than truly wild backcountry skiing, but it's still dangerous. Visit www.bridgerbowl.com for more details.

CLIMB 2,000 FEET IN LESS THAN A MILE

Just outside Colorado Springs is Manitou, a quaint town of antiques shops and gold rush–era buildings. Rising above the town like a spire is the Manitou Incline, a funicular railway turned mega-steep staircase. Climbers gain 2,000 feet of elevation in less than a mile along 2,744 steps that appear, at times, to go straight up. The Incline inspires crazy feats, with locals trying to scale it hundreds of times in a single year.

Go up once and you'll see why: The Incline tests you, then rewards you with the kind of crystal-clear vistas that make any trip to the Rockies breathtaking. It will probably take you longer than the record 17 minutes, 45 seconds to reach the top (my time: 40 minutes), but once you do, soak it in, catch your breath, take a few selfies, then follow the advice of one of my fellow trailgoers: "Let's get some beers."

The Incline is free to climb and $5 if you park at the Incline base. There's free parking elsewhere, but it's worth it to be right at the trailhead.

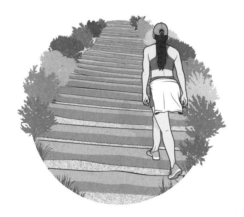

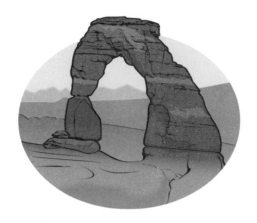

HIKE, BIKE, AND RAPPEL THROUGH AN AMAZING MOAB WEEKEND

For a combination of adventure and awe-inspiring natural beauty, Moab may be America's premier destination. Situated between two of our most scenic National Parks—Arches and Canyonlands—this red-rock Utah town has become a magnet for mountain bikers and a haven for hikers, climbers, trail runners, canyoneers, and more. And, due to its popularity, its rough edges are rimmed with little luxuries—high-end steakhouses, craft cocktail bars, gourmet coffee—that can help you recover from adventure and rope everyone into the fun. Here's a sample starter itinerary to make the most of a Moab weekend.

Day 1: Hike to the Fiery Furnace or to Utah's Most Famous Arch

These are two of Arches' most iconic hikes: The Delicate Arch is depicted on Utah's license plate, making it the state's most recognizable landmark—and it doesn't disappoint. The three-mile hike climbs about 480 feet over totally exposed, bright-red stone, with rocks for kids and kids-at-heart to climb on along the way. It's likely to be crowded at the arch, where you'll have to wait to get your photo taken underneath—but the surrounding scenery makes it an easy, enjoyable wait.

The Fiery Furnace hike is another iconic trek, with narrow sandstone canyons, arches, and towers that burn bright red at sunset—thus the area's name. This hike presents two challenges: You'll need to book a permit in advance, and, as a result of the multitude of canyons and arches, it's easy to get a little lost. Solve both with one move by booking a ranger-led hike up to six months in advance so you'll have your permit *and* a guide to the area. Visit www.recreation.gov/ticket/facility/234668 to book.

Day 2: Explore Epic Canyons

With just a little hiking—and a lot of gear and help from a guide—you can rappel into narrow slots throughout Moab, rubbing your hands across centuries of rock, slipping into keyhole gorges and under suspended boulders, and even swimming in waters trapped in canyons. Two must-try canyons are Ephedra's Grotto, a giant rain gutter with sheer faces of layered rock, and Chamisa Canyon, with water-filled pools for swimming and wading. Cliffs and Canyons Moab is a top guiding service in the area. Visit www.cliffsandcanyons.com to book.

Day 3: Ride One of the World's Most Celebrated Mountain Biking Trails

Moab boasts more than 2,000 miles of mountain bike trails, part of the reason it's considered one of the globe's premier places to ride. And one of its most celebrated trails, the Whole Enchilada, is crowded for a reason—it's on every rider's bucket list.

The Whole Enchilada really does have it all. Starting from an alpine pass above the tree line, the 27-mile path covers every type of riding and scenery available in Moab in one magical 8,000-foot descent—you'll pass through sandstone canyons, over red rock and black soil, ride on wide, paved paths and trickier singletrack across bare rock and through thick evergreen forest. The trail allows for riders of multiple skill levels to feel the thrills—the jumps are not mandatory to make it down, and wider dirt roads and paved paths can take riders away from the tight switchbacks of singletrack when needed.

The popularity of the trail provides one big bonus: shuttles. Companies like Porcupine Shuttle and Moab Cyclery can get you to the top, saving you 30 miles of climbing—so all you have to do is ride down, finishing back in town.

While this would be an all-time blockbuster weekend, it barely scratches the surface of this red rock playground. Visit www.discovermoab.com to gawk at the scenery and dream up even more.

SQUEEZE THROUGH GAPS AND DEFY DEATH IN ONE OF AMERICA'S LARGEST CAVES

Caving will leave your heart pounding, your core sore, and your grip aching. You'll be squeezing your body through gaps so small you'll *swear* they're impassable, sliding along edges above drops into total blackness and crawling under rocks that feel like they'll crush your rib cage if you turn the wrong way. Even for a claustrophobe like me, it's a chance to see an Indiana Jones–worthy world while seeing how far your body can go.

There are caving opportunities all over the Lower 48, but one of the most stunning and strenuous is within Wind Cave, near Rapid City, South Dakota. The third-longest cave system in the US, Wind Cave is also our nation's most unique—the maze of passages doesn't feature stalagmites and stalactites, but is the world's most extensive "boxwork" cave. This lacy rock formation creates spiderweb-like cave walls seen almost nowhere else on Earth.

For a death-defying, explorer feel, book the Wild Cave Tour. The four-hour experience will have you climbing up and down cave walls, cramming yourself through cracks, and pushing yourself to the limit—all with the help of a National Park guide who can run you through the necessary moves, step by step.

Cave tours in Wind Cave are only available in the summer months. The Wild Cave Tour is $30. Visit www.nps.gov/wica for details.

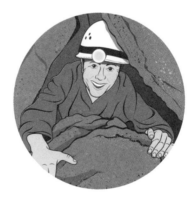

BUCKET LIST HIKES AT ZION NATIONAL PARK

Zion's soaring red-and-pink sandstone and too-blue-to-be-true skies have inspired poetry, lofty prose, and 2.8 gazillion Instagram photos. Utah's jewel is on many an American traveler's bucket list. If you're among them, these two hikes are musts for your Zion experience.

Angel's Landing

You'll be hanging from a chain that's bolted into a mountain, taking in some of the most dramatic scenery in the US—it's no wonder that Angel's Landing is one of the park's most talked-about hikes.

Beginning from the Grotto trailhead in Zion Canyon, you'll "only" hike 5 miles round trip, but those miles climb more than a quarter-mile into the azure Utah sky. You'll hike 21 tight, steep switchbacks, named Walter's Wiggles (for Walter Reusch, who supervised the creation of the trail). From the Wiggles, you'll arrive at Scout Lookout, where there are dramatic views and a restroom—which you might need as you look up at the trail's final half-mile. It's *steep*, and you'll be grateful for the chains. As one climber told me, "You'll meet your maker" and be humbled—but it's well worth the climb.

Important: Bring water! This hike is steep and it's hot, and no water is available once you leave the trailhead.

The Narrows

Zion's most popular hike offers the opposite challenge—there's *tons* of water. Traveling through a slot canyon lined with waterfalls and cascading wildflowers, the Narrows "trail" is actually the Virgin River, a shallow waterway that runs through the park. Hiking up to 16 miles of the river involves splashing and wading in cool water up to your ankles, shins, or even waist. But don't worry: This hike is accessible for just about everyone who can walk, and is a great option for families with children.

Most hikers tackle the Narrows from the "bottom up," starting at the Temple of Sinawava. To get there, you'll need to ride a shuttle into Zion Canyon, about a 45-minute ride. From here, you'll walk on the Riverside Walk for a mile—basically a sidewalk stroll—before entering the river. Then, river-hike as far north as you'd like. Many try to make it to Orderville Canyon, about a two-hour hike upstream, where the canyon is at its narrowest.

Visit https://www.nps.gov/zion/index.htm for maps and more information.

JOIN AMERICA'S LARGEST MASS-START BIKE RIDE

Get to Tucson in November to join America's biggest biker gang: Nine thousand riders take to the streets for rides of 25, 50, or 100 miles in Arizona's second-largest city. And it's easy to see why: *Bicycling* magazine ranked Tucson the second-best city in the country for a reason. The weather is gorgeous.

But that's not the only reason El Tour de Tucson, held the week before Thanksgiving, draws such a crowd. The ride offers stunning mountain views on a route through saguaro cactus–dotted desert, creek crossings, and a climb into the foothills of the Santa Catalina Mountains. For first-time long-distance riders, the course is relatively flat, with some climbs for the 100-mile distance. There's plenty of water and snack stations, spaced between 7 and 12 miles apart. And if you've got friends or family who are less ambitious about their mileage, the event's "Fun Rides" offer 1-, 4-, and 10-mile options.

The catch: The race costs $200 to enter. Pricey, sure, but you get to join America's biggest bike party. Registration starts in March each year. Visit www.perimeter bicycling.com for details.

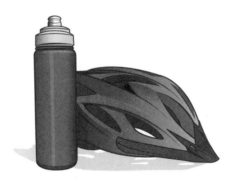

Colorado's 53 mountaintops of 14,000 feet or more—known as "14ers"—inspire adventurers from around the globe to summit their Rocky peaks. Too many adventurers, if you ask locals and experienced mountaineers. Even the most remote, difficult-to-climb 14ers are teeming with people.

Enter the state's 500-plus 13ers: same thin air, same challenges, fewer people. And Grizzly Peak, the tallest 13er, has a secret: It used to be a member of the 14,000-foot club, before being demoted. At 13,988 feet, this peak between Aspen and Leadville is Colorado's 54th-highest peak. And you can summit it in a day.

The path to the peak of Grizzly is Class 2, which means there could be some loose rocks, and you may need to put your hands down on the ground occasionally for balance—but the climb doesn't require specialized equipment. Two exceptions: a map and compass. Class 2 climbs may involve some route-finding, meaning the trail may not be perfectly marked.

That's not to say it's easy. The 800 feet of climb from 12,500 feet to 13,300 is a loose, rocky "battle" that one climber called "ball-bustingly tough." Other than that stretch, though, the 8-mile round-trip climb is mostly hiking, and offers stunning views of the Sawatch Range and the nearby Collegiates. It may not have the cachet of climbing a 14er, but this peak will give you a taste of the truly wild West, with fewer crowds.

Things to Know

- McNasser Gulch Trailhead can be reached in the summer by two-wheel-drive vehicles at the junction of South Fork Lake Creek Road and FS-394. Park here, and follow the East Ridge route.
- The air is thin, so you'll need to take this climb slowly. Get started early so you can reach the peak before noon.
- The weather can change quickly, so pack warm clothes and rainproof gear, even if the forecast is sunny.
- If route-finding gives you even a twinge of doubt, play it safe: Hire a guide. Companies like Aspen Alpine Guides (www.aspenalpine.com) can help you get up and down the peak safely.

RUN A MARATHON THROUGH TATOOINE

It may not have two suns, but the Death Valley Trail Marathon really does run across Luke Skywalker's home planet. Just a 2.5-hour drive from Las Vegas, the race tracks through the same valley where R2D2 and C3PO are first seen in *A New Hope*.

Of the marathons he's run in 42 different states, Scott Moran says the Death Valley Trail is his all-time favorite—and not just because he's a *Star Wars* superfan. Moran, who chronicles his state-by-state runs on www.scottrunsamerica.com, says the scenery is one of a kind: "It's bizarre . . . like being on the moon."

The fact that the event is small and secluded adds to the otherworldly feeling: The race has a cap at just 250 participants. Runners are driven out to the starting line in buses and set to run the trail course through the desert. There are a few water and aid stations along the course, but otherwise it's just you and the other few runners on the course, Moran says.

The fact that it's run in December is key to making the race so enjoyable. You're in Death Valley, after all. Unlike the infamous Badwater Ultramarathon, which is run in scorching summer heat, the Death Valley Trail Marathon is held in the winter, when mere mortals (and droids) can hoof in the steps of the Skywalkers.

Registration begins for the next year's race almost immediately after the previous one finishes. The price starts at $160 and increases in price as more runners register. Visit www.raceroster.com.

Things to Know
- Buses shuttle participants to the start from a place called Furnace Creek Inn & Ranch, a hotel in Death Valley. There are other hotels nearby, including the event's headquarters, The Oasis at Death Valley.

CHAPTER 5

PLAY OUTSIDE ON THE PACIFIC COAST

The American West was built on big dreams of adventure, dappled in sunshine—and, depending how far north you go, rain. Manifest your own destiny: Go west, my friend, and get active in some of our nation's most iconic spots.

PICK UP SOME GOOD VIBRATIONS SKATING LA'S BEACH WALKS

From the glittering mansions of Laguna Beach to the sideshow acts on Venice Beach to the exquisite homes of Malibu, the beach towns of Southern California are among the most beautiful in the world. And there's no more California way to see them than gliding on a pair of skates down the winding beach paths that line the Pacific.

Start on the north side of the Santa Monica Pier and grab some skates—Sea Mist Rentals (1619 Ocean Front Walk) and other companies nearby rent them for around $20 per day. Then head south along Ocean Front Walk. You'll pass gorgeous towns like Hermosa, Manhattan Beach, and Venice, where you can stop to watch the kick-flips and flying acts at Venice Skatepark or watch lifters at Muscle Beach—or you can join them!

Aside from a quick inland roll around the marina at Marina del Rey, you can just hug the coastline, weaving past Will Rogers State Beach before finishing your skate, 18 miles later, in beautiful Redondo Beach. Bite into a juicy burger at the Slip Bar or enjoy some seafood overlooking the ocean, then grab an Uber back to Santa Monica for around $27 (you can also take two buses for $3–$4, but that'll take close to two hours for the return trip).

Things to Know
- Most novice skaters travel at 8 to 10 mph, so you'll probably need two to three hours for each of these skates.
- Bring a bag for your shoes—that way, you can change out of the skates for lunch and the ride back.

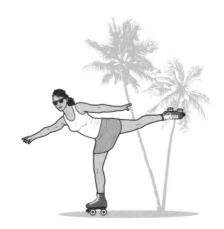

CATCH A GIANTS GAME IN A KAYAK

This one's a must for any baseball fan: kayaking to McCovey Cove, the area in San Francisco Bay just outside the wall of Oracle Park, home of the Giants. Since 2000, this area has hosted a different way to watch a ball game—from a kayak. It's a floating party, with boaters drinking, paddling, and hoping for a Giants slugger to smash one out of the stadium and into the water.

Many game-day kayakers launch from Pier 40, a ten-minute paddle from the Cove. This is one of the easiest launch points to find parking, and rental shops, such as City Kayak (www.citykayak.com), are located nearby, renting one-person boats for $60–$80.

The atmosphere is more than worth the trip. Ted Berg, a former baseball writer for *USA Today Sports*, paddled out during the 2014 World Series and said the experience was one of the highlights of his career.

The atmosphere may not be the flotilla that Berg encountered for a regular-season game in August, but the party's still going. And you can join the radio-toting party without getting your phone wet. Many kayak rental shops offer a waterproof radio you can bring along to join the chorus.

But don't go there counting on catching a home run ball. As of the end of the 2018 season, only 125 homers have splashed down in the cove, an average of one every 11 home games.

Don't worry about the ball. Enjoy the day. Berg suggests cruising around the bay for an hour or so before the game to soak up the sun and the sights before settling into the cove for a nine-inning party.

What You Need
- Clothes that can get wet: Many kayakers wear board shorts.
- Sunscreen, sunglasses, a hat, and a jacket: It's San Francisco! It always gets a little cold.
- Some snacks and drinks: There are no hot dog vendors in the water.

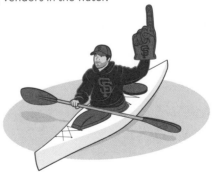

POUND SOME OREGON PAVEMENT LIKE STEVE PREFONTAINE

For the uninitiated, Steve Prefontaine was one of the greatest American middle-distance runners ever. He owned every American record from 2,000 meters to 10,000 meters. He ran a four-minute mile nine different times and finished second at a 1972 5K in Rome . . . just four days after he finished fourth in the same event at the Munich Olympics.

But it was his tragic death from a car accident at age 24—and the intensity with which he ran beforehand—that made him America's running rock star. Prefontaine was said to have never lost a race in team practice. His cocksure competitiveness helped launch Nike's success for fellow Oregon Duck Phil Knight; he was profiled in two feature films; and he inspired the creation of the annual Prefontaine Classic, one of the premier track meets in the world.

Another smaller event, the Prefontaine 10K, is held each September in his hometown of Coos Bay, Oregon. The event follows a favorite training run of Prefontaine's, running past his childhood home, a monument erected in his honor, and his high school track. Register for the race at www.prefontainerun.com for $35, or, if you go on a running pilgrimage at a different time of year, run this similar course yourself:

1. Begin at South Fourth Street and Anderson Avenue in Coos Bay. Head west on Anderson.
2. Turn right on 7th Street, then bear left on Central Avenue.
3. At Harmony United Methodist Church, Central Avenue bears right and becomes Ocean Boulevard SE. Stick with it for 3 miles.
4. Turn around at Ocean Boulevard SE and Norman Avenue. Head back toward the start.
5. Where Central Avenue meets 7th Street, continue south on 7th to Elrod Avenue. Turn right on Elrod.
6. Prefontaine's childhood home is on Elrod between 7th and 11th. Once you pass it, turn left on 11th Street to head south.
7. Turn left on Ingersoll Avenue to finish at Marshfield High at the Prefontaine track.

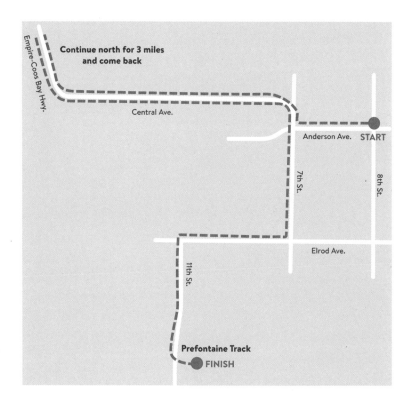

Can't make it to Coos Bay? You can try one of Prefontaine's preferred training workouts at your local track. It's called the "30-40" and was among the Oregon legend's favorites.

Start by warming up. Then run 12 laps—that's 3 miles—around the track, running the first half of each lap 25 percent faster than the second half of the lap. For Prefontaine, that meant the first half of the lap was done in 30 seconds, while the second half was done in 40 seconds—thus, the "30-40" workout. For a more manageable speed, try doubling that to start: Run the first half of every lap in one minute, and the second half in 1:20. Continue for 12 total laps.

SURF WAIKIKI AT DUSK

Waikiki Beach is the most popular surf break in the world for good reason: It's a wide-open, safe space to learn the ropes and catch your first wave. It doesn't hurt that its white sand beaches tumble into some of the clearest waters you'll find anywhere, with the high-rises of Honolulu towering over the surf.

But that beautiful setting means the beach is slammed—and the waves often so crowded you can smash into other surfers trying to catch one. One local's solution for an unforgettable Waikiki experience: Surf at dusk.

The break will be completely cleared out by then, as other surfers will need to return their rental boards. Rent one that you can keep overnight, and head out for a less crowded experience that's also got a look few others experience. You'll see the beach and the hotels all lit up, and the mountains in the backdrop.

On a beach that boasts unforgettable views that have been photographed a million different ways, you'll enjoy your own—and get a workout at the same time.

GET A PUMP WHERE THE LEGENDS OF *PUMPING IRON* LIFTED

Muscle Beach in Venice, California, helped build the most celebrated bodies in the history of lifting: Arnold Schwarzenegger and his training partner, Marco Columbu, would have impromptu bench press competitions here, and trained alongside legends like the original *Hulk*, Lou Ferrigno. In 2008, ESPN named it one of the 100 most important venues in sports.

Unlike the other 99, you can participate, and you don't have to be in line to star in a *Pumping Iron* sequel to do so. The outdoor gym, just steps from the Venice Beach boardwalk and loaded with plates, bars, dip stations, and more, is open to the public. A day pass to lift at this legendary bodybuilding destination is just $10. The gym opens at 8 a.m. each day—come early if you're bashful about lifting with a crowd, then stay after your session to see if you can catch a glimpse of a modern legend chasing a pump.

Visit the Venice Beach Parks and Recreation Office at 1800 Ocean Front Walk, Venice, California, to get a pass and more info.

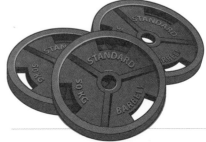

ROCK A VEGAS VACATION WITHOUT EVER PLACING A BET

The real thrills in Las Vegas are off the Strip. Just a few miles from the casino floors are breathtaking canyons, world-class rock climbing, dusty rock paths leading into thick pine forests, and mountaintops with wraparound vistas—including views of downtown Las Vegas and the Strip. Here's a trio of outdoor recommendations from Vegas locals for an incredible long weekend—no betting required.

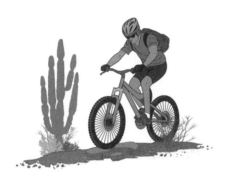

Mountain Bike at Red Rock Canyon

Just 20 minutes from the Strip, Red Rock Canyon National Conservation Area is like a miniature Grand Canyon, offering natural beauty that outstrips (get it?) almost anything you've seen before: There's desert landscape featuring the canyon's signature crimson rock formations, a pine forest with hidden waterfalls, and a 13.5-mile road ringing the sprawling expanse.

The canyon offers world-class mountain biking around this road and in the canyon, and local shops will not only outfit you with gear and guide your ride—they'll pick you up from your Vegas hotel and drop you off when you're finished. Try McGhie's for the complete experience. Visit www.mcghies.com or go to www.redrockcanyonlv.org for more biking ideas.

WORKOUT CONTINUES >>>

While You're There, Scale Some World-Class Climbing Routes

Red Rock is also one of the country's premier climbing destinations—beginners and wannabe Alex Honnolds alike can scramble all day up multiple pitches on innumerable faces, boulder on sandstone, and more. Besides Red Rock, there are limestone caves that can be climbed an hour north at Mount Charleston.

You don't have to bring your own gear to get started. Red Rock Climbing Center (www.redrockclimbingcenter.com) and the Mountain Guides (www.themountainguides.com/location/redrock) both offer gear rentals and guided climbing days and weekends. Guiding and gear from both are available for $300 per person for a full day of climbing.

Earn Unparalleled Views of Vegas on a Steep Climb

For a perfect photo of the grand scale of Sin City—whether it's bathed in neon at night or sprawled out in front of you under the scorching sun—head for Frenchman Mountain. Just 25 minutes from the Strip, this is one of the toughest hikes in the Vegas area, tracing an extremely steep gravel road up the 4,000-foot mountain. But the views at the top are worth every step. By day, you can see the casinos to the southwest, and Nellis Air Base to the northwest, complete with planes taking off and landing. At night, the entire valley is bathed in light and neon.

The hike is 4.4 miles and features wildflowers and that signature Vegas heat—so if you're climbing in the warmer months, bring plenty of water and start early. Point your GPS to the Frenchman Mountain Trailhead, park, and follow the gravel road.

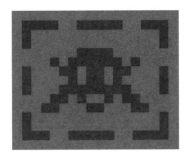

HUNT SPACE INVADERS ON THE STREETS OF SAN DIEGO

Look up at the right building in San Diego and you'll see a visitor from another world—a tiny, tiled Space Invader. As part of a 2010 exhibition coordinated by the Museum of Contemporary Art, the street artist Invader plastered 21 of these 8-bit aliens—some small, some huge—across the city. If visitors walked a specific path to find them, they'd draw a giant GPS invader with their footsteps.

Many of the aliens have been removed in the decade since, but spotting Space Invaders is still a delightful treasure hunt and makes for a memorable tour of the city. Use this checklist on foot or on a bike to zigzag around downtown, zapping (and snapping) eight invaders as you cover around 5 miles.

1. Museum of Contemporary Art, Kettner Boulevard and West B Streets: Start where the exhibit started! Look up for a white alien on a blue field.
2. Park Boulevard and G Street: There's a big black invader on the Art School building.
3. F Street and Seventh Avenue: Look for a red invader on a computer monitor.
4. C Street and Sixth Avenue: There's a little red invader on a field of white with a blue border. He's posted on some gray bricks on the corner of a 7-Eleven.
5. F Street and First Avenue: Across from Horton Plaza, look for a red invader with a blue outline.
6. Horton Plaza Walkway: A white invader on a blue background is on a stairway bridge.
7. New Children's Museum, Island and Front: There's a red invader on a blue background here.
8. Second Avenue at Interstate 5: Just behind the Sheraton Four Points Hotel, look for a white invader on red on a bridge pillar.

You can spot Space Invaders in other cities, too! Invader has placed his tiles in more than 75 cities around the world, including New York and Miami. Check out a map at www.space-invaders.com.

HIKE TO THE HOLLYWOOD SIGN

The Hollywood sign is an LA icon—and behind those big white letters, there's a hell of a view. Standing behind the 45-foot aluminum capitals, the towers and lights of Los Angeles spread out below and the blue waters of the Pacific glint in the background.

You can hike there. You *should* hike there. At the end of Canyon Drive inside Griffith Park, there's a small parking lot with a gated trailhead. (Search Google Maps for "Griffith Park Hollywood Sign Trail.") Park here and hike north.

Around 1.8 miles into the hike, make a left at a three-way junction with Mulholland Highway. In another half-mile, you'll come to another junction. Keep to the right to stay on Mulholland Highway. Soon, you'll come to a junction with a paved road—Mount Lee Drive. The top of Mount Lee's your goal.

Take a right onto Mount Lee Drive and get ready to sweat: The last mile is really steep. At the top, you'll see it—the back of the Hollywood letters. You'll have to look through a fence, since it's illegal to go right up to the letters, but it still offers a killer view. Go a little higher to get an unfenced view for a photo, then head back down.

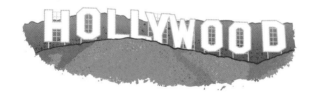

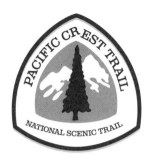

GO *WILD* ON THE BEST OF THE PCT

The Pacific Crest Trail may not be as famous as its eastern cousin, the Appalachian Trail, but the West Coast mega-trail attracts more thru-hikers each year: In 2019, 7,800 people obtained permits to see the entire stretch of mountains, valleys, deserts, and grasslands between Canada and Mexico, while only about 3,000 hiked the entirety of the AT.

No doubt many long-distance trekkers were inspired by the gorgeous views in *Wild*, the 2014 film starring Reese Witherspoon based on Cheryl Strayed's memoir. You might not have 94 days to hike, as Strayed did—or even more to tackle the entire PCT—but you can still enjoy its splendor. These hikes offer some of the best of the 2,650-mile expanse when you've only got a day to hit the trail.

Carson Pass, California

It's a wildflower paradise: In midsummer, flowers with apt names like "paintbrush" bloom everywhere in the volcanic soil of this pass east of Sacramento. The PCT stretches through this area between Yosemite and Lake Tahoe, offering day hike opportunities—a favorite is an 8-mile out-and-back to the peak of Round Top.

Start at the Carson Pass parking lot (after paying a $5 fee at the information station) and head south along the PCT. After a half-mile, you'll rise out of the trees into fields of wildflowers. Follow the trail to the top of 10,300-foot Round Top, taking in the views of blue-green Winnemucca Lake and the surrounding mountains as you relish your triumphant climb on the knife's edge of the peak.

WORKOUT CONTINUES > > >

Columbia River Gorge, Oregon

Enjoy views of Oregon's second-tallest peak, Mount Jefferson, as you explore the country's largest national scenic outdoor area—and marvel at a 74-foot waterfall along the popular and well-marked Dry Creek Falls Trail. The falls are spectacular, crashing into a natural amphitheater of sheer basalt.

Park at the Bridge of the Gods trailhead. From there, you'll pick up the PCT going north—you'll walk about 100 yards on a road and under the freeway and continue on the Crest Trail, which is also the Gorge Trail at this point.

Climb gradually from here through maples and firs as you trek the 2.2 miles to Dry Creek Falls. Along the way, you'll pass over another road (under some power lines), enjoying forest wildflowers like columbines in spring, and be challenged by a fairly steep climb near the end. Your reward: the secluded, picturesque falls, cascading in the otherwise quiet amphitheater.

Crown Point, Washington

This 7.5-mile loop, halfway between Yakima and Seattle, showcases views of Mount Ranier and leads hikers through valleys of blooming wildflowers. There's even a chance to glimpse an elk or a mountain goat along the way.

To get there, park at Parking Lot C of the Crystal Mountain Ski Area and pick up the trailhead for the Bullion Basin Trail (#1156). After about 2.5 miles of forest hiking on a gradual climb, you'll reach the PCT. Head south on the trail to straddle the hill's ridge and take in views from all sides as you make your way to Crown Point. After 2.7 miles, hook up with the Silver Creek Trail. Take this trail back to return to your car.

CLIMB AMERICA'S TALLEST STAIRCASE

Murphy Ranch, outside Santa Monica, California, was home to a pro-Hitler group of Americans, the Silver Shirts, who hoped to hunker down on their 55 acres until the Germans won World War II. Before the war even ended, the FBI swooped in and arrested them. The land was sold to an artists' colony and later to the city of Los Angeles.

Today, it's one of the funkiest hikes on the West Coast, a tour through abandoned structures that have been taken over by weeds and layers of graffiti. To get down to the ravine containing these run-down bunkers, you'll need to take stairs—lots of them. The Murphy Ranch East Stairway has 512 steps—the longest unbroken staircase in the US, according to www.publicstairs.com, a wonderful website that really exists.

How to get there: Find a place to park east of Capri Drive on Casale Road and hike west. This road turns into the Sullivan Fire Road at a sharp corner. Around the half-mile mark, you'll pass through a yellow gate. Hike another 0.6 miles until you reach a gap in the chain-link fence. The stairs descend from here. (If you're unsure of where to go, enter "Murphy Ranch East Stairs" in your GPS.)

Head down the steps and descend 200 feet in about 0.1 mile. Then take a look around—snap some photos of graffiti-strewn buildings and wander around the compound. Some hikers avoid the stairs on the way back up, making a loop. But if your knees are up for it, come on: Climb the nation's tallest staircase. You're 512 steps from the top!

THEN GO EVEN BIGGER: CLIMB 2,830 STAIRS IN VANCOUVER

Every summer, Vancouver's Grouse Mountain turns from a ski resort into Mother Nature's StairMaster—the Grouse Grind, a 1.8-mile hike that gains 2,800 feet and climbs 2,830 stairs through the Canadian forest to the mountain's summit, challenging more than 150,000 hikers per year.

The unofficial record for the climb is just under 24 minutes, but most hikers take 90 minutes to two hours. But when they get to the top, they're treated to the best thing to ever happen at the top of any mountain climb: They don't have to walk back down. For $15 on weekdays or $20 on weekends, hikers can save their knees and book a ticket on the Skyride, a ski gondola that ferries passengers back to the base.

The grind opens at different times each summer. Visit www.metrovancouver.org to confirm that it's open, and go to www.grousemountain.com to pre-book your Skyride ticket.

GO TO THE BEST SPIN STUDIO IN AMERICA

Forget SoulCycle: Of the 30,000 boutique studios around the country, users of ClassPass, the behemoth of fitness class booking, say that GritCycle's six studios in Los Angeles are the best in America. Visit www.gritcycle.com to sign up, or book a class via ClassPass while visiting LA.

THE NUMBER ONE BIKE RIDE IN AMERICA'S NUMBER ONE BIKE CITY

Portland, Oregon, is the most bike-friendly city on the continent, and second only in the world to Amsterdam—and that's not by accident. The city has worked for 15 years to make itself palatable to pedals, resulting in 300 percent growth in two-wheeling since the early '90s—and Portland-weird events, like the World Naked Bike Ride, popping up throughout the city. To further encourage riding, the local government even provides free guides to cycling the city.

If you take one of Portland's premier short rides, the 11-mile Sellwood Bridge Loop, you'll finish with a sprint along the West Coast's most popular segment on Strava, the GPS tracking app. More than 250,000 rides have been logged on the 1.6-mile segment Bridge to Bottom in the middle of this loop. The complete route is mostly on bike paths, with little street riding. You'll enjoy green spaces along the Willamette River and finish at Oaks Bottom Wildlife Refuge, where you can hop off to stroll through 163 acres and check out scores of great herons.

1. Begin at the south end of Sellwood Park, where you'll find bathrooms for a pre-trip break. Cross the Sellwood Bridge going west.
2. Turn right after the bridge and head north on the Westside Greenway Trail. Pass through Willamette Park, the aerial tram, and the Salmon Springs Fountain in Waterfront Park—a street-level fountain that's popular for cooling off in the summer.
3. Continue north to the Steel Bridge. Turn right to cross it.
4. Turn right down the Eastside Esplanade.
5. When you reach the Ross Island Bridge, get ready to sprint: From here to the Oaks Bottom Wildlife Refuge is the Bridge to Bottom segment.
6. Finish at Oaks Bottom Wildlife Refuge.

Find more Portland rides—with free maps of *tons* of loops—at www.portlandoregon.gov/transportation/39402.

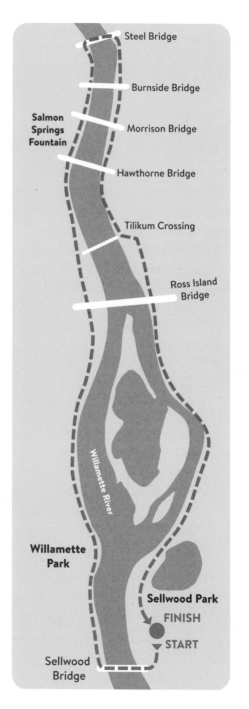

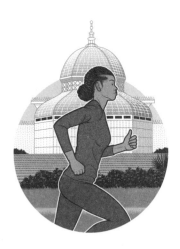

BEST IN THE WEST: STRAVA'S MOST POPULAR RUNNING ROUTES

From hiking to kayaking to biking to lifting, there are so many incredible ways to experience the Pacific Coast. But, for me, it's tough to beat exploring a city on foot. And I'm not alone—just as in the rest of the country, thousands of runners log runs up and down the left coast using apps like Strava. So run—and explore—like the locals do: These are some of the most popular routes in some of the region's biggest cities.

San Francisco: Ramble through Golden Gate Park

The Bay Area might be the best place to run anywhere—plenty of challenging hills, gorgeous views of mountains, parks, and the Golden Gate Bridge, and just-right weather that won't have you overly bundled or caked in sweat. No surprise, San Fran's most popular run is through Golden Gate Park—more than 36,000 people have logged this one. Start where Stanyan Street meets JFK Drive and follow Kennedy west—you'll run past SF's Botanical Garden, loaded with trees from the Pacific Coast, South Africa, Madagascar, and more. You'll cruise by boats on Stow and Spreckels Lakes, Frisbee-flingers on the disc golf course, and finish on the beach. If you've still got energy, head north, and follow the coast to the Golden Gate Bridge via nearby Presidio Park.

Oakland: The Lake Merritt 5K

Lake Merritt is America's oldest wildlife refuge, a heart-shaped lagoon near the city's Financial District that's been protecting different species of ducks, geese, and cormorants since the 1800s. It's also almost exactly a 5K loop, with a wide, well-kept path for locals training for their next big race. Soak up some city views as you take the loop yourself, then stop in the park's Bonsai Garden, where you can see tiny trees that have been growing for as long as 1,600 years.

Seattle: Loop Green Lake, Then Grab Some Grub

Green Lake, north of Seattle's downtown and abutting the Woodland Park Zoo, offers a bit of outdoor adventure without leaving the city—or its amenities. It's almost a perfect 5K to loop the lake. Start in front of Starbucks on East Green Lake Drive, and head north to loop the lake for the city's most popular run. The best part? When you're done, there are tacos, burgers, and other four-star fare waiting to be your post-run refuel.

Los Angeles: Run a 5K around the Rose Bowl

More Strava users have gone for a run down Santa Monica's beaches, but you might have more fun doing that on roller skates (see page 66). Instead, tackle LA's second-most-popular route—a nearly perfect 5K around one of America's most fabled stadiums. To log the segment, start south of the Rose Bowl, where Seco Street meets Rose Bowl Drive. Head east, then make a left on Rosemont Avenue. Continue north up and around the Brookside Golf Club. Hang another left at West Washington Boulevard, and a final left on West Drive before returning to the start.

For more of Strava's most popular routes around the USA, turn to page 8 for East Coast runs and page 50 for routes in Midwest cities. Or, to find popular routes in your city, go to Strava.com/heatmap.

CHAPTER 6

GRAB YOUR PASSPORT

It's a big world beyond our borders—volcanoes to climb! Canyons to explore! Homemade human-powered amusement parks to play in! There are 195 countries on Earth, and this chapter is your guide to start pinning the globe with your own active explorations.

THE WORLD'S NUMBER ONE BUCKET LIST REQUEST: RUN WITH THE BULLS

If this one's on your bucket list, you already know the deal: They release the bulls on the streets of Pamplona, and you run away. The bulls' hooves pound. Your heart pounds. You hopefully survive. You celebrate, post on social media, and, one day, tell your grandchildren.

It's the logistics that you may not know. And according to Nate Scott, a former colleague who ran with the bulls in 2016, "It's not obvious at all what to do." Here are some quick FAQs:

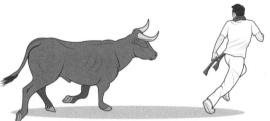

Do you have to plan a whole year in advance?
If you want to get a hotel room in Pamplona, where the festival is held, yes. But if you want to save some scratch or be more spontaneous, as Nate was, you can drive into town from elsewhere before the bulls are released between 7 and 8 a.m. The run doesn't cost anything, and you don't need to preregister. You don't even need the ubiquitous red handkerchiefs you've seen in videos of these runs. Just show up early in the morning on one of the seven days of the July San Fermin Festival and you can run.

So I just stand by the start?
No. Police and other festival officials corral everyone near the starting line before the bulls are released, but once they've done so, you can start anywhere along the half-mile course to the stadium entrance, where the running ends. Nate suggests not standing too close to where the bulls are actually released.

Nate and Mrs. Nate started two-thirds of the way along the course. If you're too close to the entrance to the stadium, people on balconies may heckle you. But they're 19-year-olds, drunk on red wine at 8 a.m., and you will not be dead. So take the heckling with a grain of salt.

Okay, so how do I not die?
Besides starting a little farther down the course, Nate suggests remembering two things that no one warned him about: First, be aware that the ground is very slick. Its cobblestones are covered in wine and vomit from Pamplona's version of Mardi Gras. So be aware of your footing.

Second, stay on the inside of turns. When the bulls go through turns, they can lose their footing and wind up sliding to the outside, pinning runners between bull and wall. If you stay on the inside of the turns, you'll not only save valuable ground distance, but avoid any slides of beef.

RIDE A BIKE WITH ZEBRAS AND WARTHOGS, THEN HIKE THROUGH THE SET OF *TOMB RAIDER*

I f you make the trip to Africa to see lions and elephants, make time in your schedule for Hell's Gate: Instead of riding in a safari van, it's a Kenyan National Park where you can bike through herds of zebras and warthogs past a face that inspired the *Lion King*'s Pride Rock, and then hike through a gorge with 30-foot walls where they filmed *Tomb Raider*.

All this *and* it's cheap. Bikes are about $6 to rent for the day (600 Kenyan shillings) and the park costs $30 to enter. You'll ride about 6 miles of bumpy terrain to the start of the hiking area. Once there, for another $20, you can get a local guide to take you on a 90-minute hike through the gorge—you'll climb ropes to get up to an area called the Devil's Bedroom, where a lion that terrorized local cowherds once lived (and looks a lot like the spot where Simba gets cornered by hyenas in the elephant graveyard).

You'll then tramp through the river past mineral-green waterfalls from hot springs so hot you can boil an egg, and up and down sheer faces using slippery ladders cut into the rocks. At the end of the hike, here's the payoff: a panoramic view of the gorge for a killer photo, a short walk back to the ranger station, and a well-deserved picnic lunch (that you bring). Just be careful: The vervet monkeys here are bold, and not afraid to steal your food!

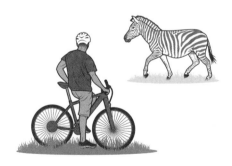

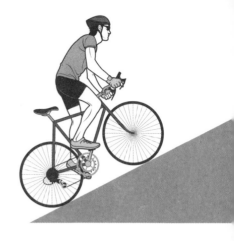

TACKLE THE MOUNTAINS OF THE TOUR DE FRANCE

The 2,000-mile route of the Tour de France is different each year, but one thing doesn't change: "a guy in a yellow jersey going up a big, bloody mountain," says Stephen Gallagher.

Gallagher is a 40-year-old pro cyclist and coach for Dig Deep Coaching, his own firm, and TrainingPeaks, a training app for endurance athletes. Many of his amateur clients dream of tackling one of the Tour's renowned climbs in the Pyrenees or the Alps. Here's a classic climb from each mountain range, with a favorite challenge route from Gallagher.

Zigzag through the Alps: Alp d'Huez

The Alp d'Huez isn't the Tour's tallest mountain, but its switchbacks capture that enduring image of the Tour—riders pumping their legs up a mountain ringed by thousands of screaming spectators. The Alp d'Huez has 21 switchbacks, zigzagging more than 8 miles at an 8 percent grade to 10,930 feet.

For a ride of the Tour Alps that includes Alp d'Huez, Gallagher suggests pairing it with the Tour's highest peak, the Col du Galibier. The 8,668-foot mountain is also one of the Tour's toughest because it's such a long climb: Approaching from the village of Saint-Michel-de-Maurienne in the north, the climb up Gabilier is more than 19 miles, at a near constant 5–6 percent grade. After summiting, you can ride down the other side of the valley to climb Alp d'Huez's switchbacks. To pair mountains like this, though, will take some serious fitness—see Gallagher's preparation tips below.

WORKOUT CONTINUES >>>

In the Pyrenees: The Col du Tourmalet

Gallagher used to live and train in the Pyrenees, and sounds a bit wistful when describing the low-slung mountains of France's southwest. "It's a lot greener. It's a lot more rural," he says, saying the spread-out population adds to its scenic look. Because the range is more temperate, Gallagher says, you can be more deliberate and planned about your ride—you're less likely to get an unscheduled snow dump in the warmer Pyrenees. The eastern and western approaches of the Pyrenees' pinnacle, the Col du Tourmalet, are the most-used climbs in the history of the Tour de France. Both grades are monsters. The eastern approach climbs over 10.7 miles, while the western climb ascends over 11.8 miles. Both are a grueling 7.4 percent grade.

For an epic Tourmalet ride, Gallagher again suggests pairing the climb with a nearby peak. This time, it's the Col d'Aspin, an "easier" climb to the east of the Tourmalet. From the village of Arreau, you'll approach the Col d'Aspin from the southeast, climbing 7.5 miles at a 6.5 percent grade to the summit. The surroundings, though, are divine—lush, green, and ringed by the rest of the Pyrenees. From the peak of Col d'Aspin, you'll continue west to the Col du Tourmalet.

DREAM OF THESE EPIC DOUBLES? HERE'S HOW TO TRAIN FOR THEM

To climb a single Tour mountain, "If you have a high pain threshold and your fitness is moderately good, it might take six hours, but you can get to the top," Gallagher says. But when you start to pair climbs together into a single ride, he says, you'll need to be able to climb hard for long, interrupted stretches: "A climb like the Tourmalet, for a moderately fit cyclist, could take two to two-and-a-half hours of climbing."

Here's a workout format he recommends to build the "aerobic par" needed to conquer these double rides. Since you probably don't have two-plus hours to put in on the trainer each day, this session is shorter—but harder.

Start by warming up thoroughly. Then work your way up to a rate of perceived exertion (RPE) of eight out of ten—at this level, you're on the lower end of some of the hardest work you can do. Once you've reached this level, pedal for one to two minutes, then maintain that effort level while changing your torque and cadence to slow down your legs—basically, climb a steeper grade while keeping the RPE around eight. Alternate between "flatter" sections and "steeper" sections for one to two minutes, trying to get to ten minutes. Over time, work to make this session last 40 minutes while maintaining this eight-level effort.

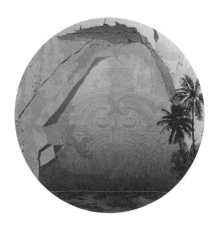

MAKE LIKE INDIANA JONES: PADDLE TO A 30-FOOT FACE CARVED INTO SHEER ROCK

In the middle of New Zealand's northern island, a 30-foot face stares out from granite, glaring across the waters of Lake Taupo. The three-story carving shows Ngatoroirangi, a legendary Maori navigator who guided his tribes to the lake more than a thousand years ago.

The giant face looks like it could have been carved centuries ago, but it's only about 40 years old . . . but that may make it even more interesting. The giant face was carved by Matahi Whakataka-Brightwell, a 27th-generation descendant of the navigator. He wasn't paid a cent to carve it: Whakataka-Brightwell says he "saw an image of a tattooed face" calling out to him from the rock and spent four summers carving the visage into the rock.

The best way to see this literally towering achievement is by kayak. For around $70, local companies like Taupo Kayaking Adventures (www.tka.co.nz) lead paddling tours from nearby Acacia Bay. The trip can be windy and is about 6 miles round trip, but, to glide straight up to this mammoth monument, hear its story from your guide, and envision the passion put into carving, every paddle stroke is worth it!

ROAD TRIP THROUGH SCOTLAND TO LIFT GIANT ROCKS

All over Scotland's lush green highlands (and lowlands), you'll find "clach cuid fir," or "manhood stones." Weighing 190, 250, 300 pounds, and more, these hunks of granite are more like small boulders than stones. And for hundreds of years, they've been the centerpiece of rites of passage: Young men would prove their might by lifting the local testing stone off the ground to waist height, and become a man.

Many of these stones, some from the fourteenth century, are still there, just waiting for you to test your own strength. They're sitting in gravel next to local hotels along the rugged coast, sticking up from clumped grass in an unassuming emerald field, or plopped next to the seventeenth hole of a golf course. They're a history lesson, a workout, and an excuse to road-trip around the windy landscape of Scotland, all rolled into one. Start planning your own clach cuid fir journey: There's a map of many of these stones at www.liftingstones.org/map.html, along with descriptions and instructions on finding them. Here are three historic hefts to start your checklist.

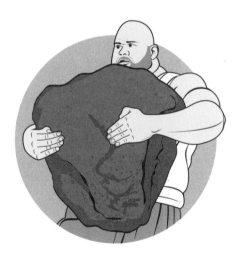

The Inver Stone

One of the most celebrated lifting stones in Scotland, this slippery, smooth ellipse is stamped with its weight—265 pounds. It sits across the road from the Inver Hotel in Crathie, Scotland, and those who attempt to lift it will attract a crowd: Pub patrons will follow you across the street, pints in hand, to watch your attempt to hoist this 300-year-old rock. But you'll need permission: Check with the folks at the hotel to help connect you to the Inver's owner.

The Puterach

If you've seen the *World's Strongest Man* on TV, you've probably seen an event called the "Atlas Stones," where competitors heft huge stone spheres up onto stands. The original Atlas Stones were actually Scottish proving stones and had the same challenge—not just to pick up the rock, but to place it on a pedestal. That's the deal with the Puterach, located near Balquhidder village. Since the 1600s, Scots have attempted to place the 207-pound stone onto its accompanying plinth.

The Dinnie Stones

They're probably the most famous lifting stones in Scotland, having been featured in *Sports Illustrated* and on the *World's Strongest Man*. But the Dinnie Stones weren't originally proving stones. The two giant rocks, weighing 435 and 340 pounds each, were originally for riders to tether their horses in place—that's why these behemoths outside the Potarch Hotel in the town of Banchory have chains and rings attached to them. But when legendary Scottish strongman Donald Dinnie carried them across the nearby Potarch Bridge in 1860, the Dinnie Stones got their reputation and their name. If you've trained for the challenge of a lifetime, you'll need an appointment to try to heft these storied boulders. Go to www.thedinniestones.com to learn more.

GET STRONG TO LIFT THOSE STONES

The list of Dinnie Stones lifters is short. And the list of women who have hoisted them is even shorter: Between 1979 and 2018, zero females successfully lifted them. Since that time, a handful of the world's strongest women have accomplished the feat. Twenty-four-year-old Chloe Brennan wanted to join their ranks: Allured by what she calls "the aura around the stones," she trained to become the lightest person to ever lift the Dinnies—and she did!

In October 2019, weighing just 140 pounds, Brennan lifted the 733-pound pair of Dinnies. Here's a workout she says can help you build the strength to lift your first proving stone—or just a really heavy bag of dirt in your garden.

EXERCISE 1: Barbell Front Squats (5 sets of 3 reps, resting about 2 minutes between sets)

EXERCISE 2: Atlas Stone Lift (3 to 4 sets of just 1 rep, resting 2 minutes between sets)
Work up from smaller weights to a decently heavy lift. If you don't have access to Atlas Stones at your gym, try swapping in Zercher Squats. To do them, set a barbell in a power rack at waist height. With a pad over your arms, place the bar in the crooks of your elbows. Perform squats with the bar in this position.

EXERCISE 3: Loaded Carry (65 feet [20 meters] each for 4 sets)
One challenge with many of the stones is not just to lift them, but to carry them for a distance. Work on heavy carries with dumbbells, and, when you can, a really heavy sandbag.

EXERCISES 4 AND 5: Gut Wrench Row and Incline Dumbbell Bench Press (4 sets of 8 reps of each exercise)
These two exercises are performed as a superset: Perform one set of the row, then move directly into a set of the press. Rest 90 seconds, then repeat.

The Gut Wrench Row mimics rowing the stone, but with a small pile of weight plates. With the plates stacked on the floor in front of you, push your hips back to bend over at the waist with a flat back and a slight bend in your knees. Get your hands beneath the plates and remain bent over with tension in the hamstrings. Pull the plates to your chest, hold for a beat, and return them to the floor.

WALK IN THE STEPS OF MAYANS AT RUINS YOU CAN ACTUALLY CLIMB

Mexico's Chichen Itza gets all the tourist love, but for a less crowded experience that lets you walk in the footsteps of Mayans by climbing their towering temples, head a little farther south to Caracol, the largest Mayan archaeological site in Belize.

Near the country's western border with Guatemala, the Caracol site covers more than 30 square miles. At its peak, this Mayan city was home to more than 180,000 people, but there's almost no one here now: Caracol is in the middle of the jungle, and only about a dozen tourists visit the site each day. When we visited, we had the place to ourselves.

That silence lets you take your time and take it all in—and there's a lot to take in. There are ruins everywhere, including three temples you can climb to get panoramic views of the jungle. Towering over them all is the Sky Palace, a 141-foot structure that's more than a thousand years old, but is still the tallest building in Belize. Scramble up its stairs and take in the same breathtaking views that Mayan residents would have seen before the year 1000 CE.

And it's not just temples! Walking the grounds around the ruins, the lack of other tourists means you'll see plenty of wildlife—howler monkeys, colorful birds, and, if you're lucky, a toucan.

The fee to enter is about $10. Tours are available from San Ignacio for about $100 per person. You can also rent a 4 x 4 and drive to the site.

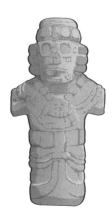

SWIM FROM ASIA TO EUROPE

For one July day each year, one of the world's busiest shipping lanes goes boat-free so thousands can cross from one continent to another. Turkey's Bosphorus Strait is home to one of the world's most epic open-water swims: In 4 miles, swimmers race between two continents.

Those 4 miles can be choppy, with strong currents pushing swimmers back toward shore into eddies, and even past the finishing point on the European side. But the really hard part is getting into the race at all: More than 24,000 swimmers from around the globe register, but just 1,200 non-Turkish entrants are allowed to take part in the two-hour swimming event.

If the title of "transcontinental swimmer" is just your bag, register early—the Turkish Olympic Committee, which handles applications, opens its registration gates online in January. You'll need your passport to sign up, of course, but also a swimming certificate or a letter from a swimming coach saying you're fit to swim the strait. Visit http://bogazici .olimpiyatkomitesi.org.tr, or try to get a spot through a combination vacation/trek company, like www.swimtrek.com.

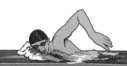

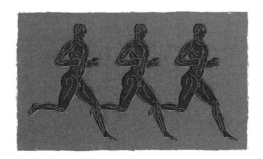

RUN THE ROUTE OF THE ORIGINAL MARATHON

The Athens Classic Marathon, known as the Authentic, traces the fabled route run by Pheidippides, an ancient Greek messenger sent from the Battle of Marathon to Athens to announce victory. The race finishes at the Panathenaic Stadium—the location of the original modern Olympics in 1896, and the same spot where ancient Greeks competed as far back as 500 BCE.

The race is loaded with history, but don't forget: Pheidippides dropped dead at the end of this run. That may be a legend, but the challenge is very real—the Authentic is the toughest major marathon on Earth, with an uphill section that lasts for 13 straight miles. So get some hill training in and join more than 40,000 other runners for this huge historic race, held in November each year. The race costs 100 euros—about $117. Visit www.athensauthenticmarathon.gr to register.

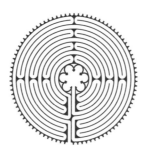

WALK AN 800-YEAR-OLD PATH OF MEDITATION IN A FRENCH CATHEDRAL

For 4,000 years, humans have walked the winding paths of circle- and square-shaped labyrinths, seeking enlightenment, forgiveness from sin, otherworldly power, or just peace and quiet. And at Chartres Cathedral, 56 miles southwest of Paris, you can walk one of the world's oldest labyrinths—it's been on the floor of the church's nave for 800 years.

Forget the Minotaur for a second. Labyrinths aren't mazes. "Real" labyrinths have only one route—you follow one path that leads you, circuitously, to the center and back out the other side. And these meandering paths, built of stone, hedges, or tile, are hiding in plain sight all over the world—there's probably one near you.

At the Chartres Cathedral labyrinth, you can walk the same floor tiles that pilgrims have walked since the 1200s, slowly twisting through the 42-foot-diameter ring and its 11 concentric circles. You might feel enlightenment, peace . . . or nothing. It's only about an 850-foot walk, so it's not a huge commitment if the experience doesn't move you—and you're still in France, so you can get some delicious pastries afterward.

The Chartres labyrinth isn't always open. It's traditionally available for walking on Fridays from 10 a.m. to 5 p.m., starting in Lent and continuing until November 1. Visit www.chartrescathedral.net for details.

VISIT A LABYRINTH CLOSER TO HOME

They're not just in France: Labyrinths are in parks, parking lots, gardens, and other locations throughout the US. Try one of these three or visit www.labyrinthlocator.com to find one near you.

Mazzariello Labyrinth, Oakland, California

Installed in secret by a psychic, Helena Mazzariello, this 50-foot-wide labyrinth of grass and rock has spiraled through the Sibley Volcanic Regional Preserve since 1989. It's a hike to get there, but amazing to behold—it looks as if it appeared in the old quarry as if by magic. Visit http://mazzariellolabyrinth.orgfree.com/ for directions on how to reach it.

Labyrinth of Lavender, Shelby, Michigan

Forget corn mazes. At Cherry Point Farm & Market in Shelby—about an hour from Grand Rapids—there's a labyrinth of lavender so large you can see it on Google Earth. In mid-July, the lavender is in full bloom, carpeting the winding path in purple and filling the air with incredible fragrance. The labyrinth is free and takes more than an hour to walk. Visit www.cherrypointmarket.net for details—or just to check out the pictures.

Audubon Park Labyrinth, New Orleans, Louisiana

At the end of a brick pathway in this Uptown park, there's an exact replica of the Chartres Cathedral labyrinth. But while scholars argue over the meaning and purpose of the French pathway, this one is clear: The stones were laid as a meditative journey to facilitate healing after the ravages of Hurricane Katrina in 2005. The park is big: To find the labyrinth, set Google Maps to the Tree of Life in Audubon Park, at Laurel Street off East Drive. Head north from the Tree, and you'll find it.

CLIMB EDMUND HILLARY'S TRAINING MOUNTAIN: SNOWDON

Summiting Everest costs more than $60,000—and that's to be on a mountain so crowded that multiple people have died in recent years due to logjams at the peak. Not quite the same as when Tenzing Norgay and Edmund Hillary completed the first summit in 1953.

If it's not already on your bucket list, save the 60 grand and still climb a Norgay/Hillary classic: Snowdon, near Llanberis in Wales, was where the pioneering mountaineers trained for their first ascent of Everest in 1953. And you can climb it in a day.

Snowdon is Wales' tallest mountain, but at 3,560 feet, it's less than one-eighth the height of Everest. Just because it isn't tall doesn't mean it's easy sledding: The Welsh mountain has tricky traverses and sheer cliffs that made it a perfect proving ground for Everest's pioneers.

You don't need crampons or an oxygen tank to reach the top, though. The Snowdon Horseshoe—the mountain's most trekked route—is a Class 1 scramble, meaning you can climb it with a sturdy pair of hiking boots.

From the Pen-y-Pass Car Park parking area (set your GPS there), follow the path west to the Col of Bwlch-y-Moch. Turn right there, and approach the East Ridge of Crib Goch—follow the knife-edge rock ridge to the summit. At the rocky top, you'll get views (if it's not too cloudy) of the area's other fun-to-say peaks, like Y Lliwedd and Garnedd Ugain.

The Pen-y-Pass Car Park fills up early, but a bus service—the Snowdon Sherpa—offers service from all over the area for £5 (about $7) per day. Visit www.traveline-cymru.org for bus information. And go to www.snowdonia-npa.gov.uk for maps of the mountain.

Finish your Hillary-and-Norgay-inspired day with a visit to their training headquarters—the charmingly antiquated Pen-y-Gwryd Hotel, near Llanberis, where you can enjoy a pint and see a small museum of items used by the Everest team.

TRACK A GORILLA THROUGH THE JUNGLE

If you get the chance to go on an African safari (and you should!), it's breathtaking to get so close to elephants, big cats, hyenas, and other incredible creatures. But tracking gorillas is, if you'll excuse the pun, a whole different animal. You'll hoof it through jungle humidity for hours, sometimes as your guide hacks through vegetation with a machete, just to spend an hour with our enormous evolutionary cousins.

Gorilla tracking is most popular in Rwanda, Uganda, and the Democratic Republic of Congo (DRC). Whichever country you choose, you'll need a permit—they're for a specific day, and only a set number are released for that day. And they're expensive: Rwanda's permit is $1,500; Uganda's is $600; and it's $400 in the DRC (you can tag-team this trip with a climb of Mount Nyiragongo, one of the world's most active lava lakes—see page 103).

Once inside, a guide will divide all the permit-holders into groups, and you'll head off into the forest. You could climb the mountains for an hour, or all day, as your guides are in contact with gorilla trackers who keep their eyes on the apes to help you find them. Once you do locate them, you'll have one hour to observe them feeding, nursing their young, and generally being enormous. The large male silverbacks weigh as much as 480 pounds but are gentle enough to pluck single leaves from the trees to eat.

It's sweaty, it's buggy, and it's pricey, but it's an adventure of a lifetime.

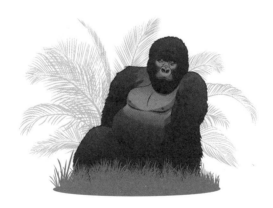

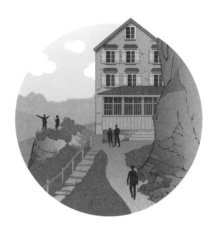

HIKE 2,800 FEET UP TO EAT AT A 170-YEAR-OLD RESTAURANT

M ost climbs end with munching on a protein bar or a bag of trail mix. But in the Swiss Alps town of Wasserauen, your hike can finish with a real meal at a centuries-old restaurant— and pass plenty more history along the way.

The Berggasthaus Aescher restaurant sits on the edge of a 330-foot-high ledge 2,800 feet above town, where it has served traditional Swiss cuisine—sausages, pastries, and other hearty fare—since the mid-1800s. A cable car will take you most of the way there, but to work up a real appetite, head to your table the way every diner did until the 1950s: Hike 4.5 miles from town.

Along the way, you'll climb to extraordinary Alpine heights, and take in sights that have been on the mountain longer than even the restaurant: Near the top, you'll hike through three 40,000-year-old caves used by prehistoric humans, see a small chapel that was carved into the rocks by 17th-century Capuchin monks, and visit a small museum in a hermit's house that's 200 years old.

When you've reached the restaurant, you're in for unobstructed views of the sur- rounding Alps on the outdoor patio. Marvel at the vistas, wonder at how they move all the food and water and other materials up to the restaurant, and then savor the ultimate treat: Instead of hiking down, you can ride a cable car back to the village.

Visit https://aescher.ch/en/ to see some beautiful photos and reserve a table.

RIDE YOUR BIKE ON THE MOON

In the Atacama Desert's *Valle de la Luna*, the "Valley of the Moon," breathtaking landscapes and otherworldly rock formations will make you feel like you've left Earth behind. The Chilean landscape is so alien that NASA has used the area to test rovers destined for Mars before their interplanetary journeys. The Atacama is extremely dry, like the surface of the Red Planet; even microbial life is driven underground or into rocks—the types of places rovers look for life on Mars.

You don't need a spacesuit to explore this alien world: Moon Valley is less than 8 miles west of the tourist town of San Pedro de Atacama in northern Chile and accessible by bike. The total round-trip ride is about 25 miles, so it's not for complete beginners. But the hills are gentle, and you'll want to take all day—jumping out of the saddle to scramble up dunes, snap photos in front of rocky outcroppings, and savor the views of the moonlike landscape.

Entrance into the park costs 3,000 Chilean pesos, or around $3.50. Tours are available, but you can also rent bikes from local hostels and they'll give you directions to the park entrance—as well as the unofficial circuit route to follow.

Things to Know
- The total ride can take up to seven hours. Start early! You'll miss the hottest weather that way.
- You're biking in the world's driest desert: Bring plenty of water, sunscreen, a hat, and snacks. Oh, and make sure your phone is fully charged—for photos and GPS!

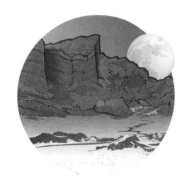

KAYAK THE MELTWATER OF A GLACIER

Each summer, the sun turns North America's glaciers into waters so turquoise they look Photoshopped—rivers of crystal blue, flowing through the sheets of ice that continue to shape our continent.

It ain't cheap, but you can paddle along these gorgeous rivers and get a close-up look at what our changing climate is doing to them. After a one-hour helicopter flight, guides from Compass Heli-tours in Abbotsford, British Columbia—about a two-hour drive north from Seattle—will outfit you with kayaks and lead a four-hour trip through the crystal rivers. The views are mind-blowing, as is the perspective the trip will give you on our changing climate: Each year, the glaciers melt a little more . . . and freeze a little less. Check this unbelievable trip off your bucket list before it's too late, then make a donation to your favorite environmental charity when you get home.

Tours cost $1,250 Canadian—about $920 US. Visit www.compasshelitours.com to book.

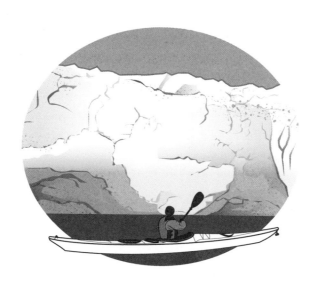

Cape Town is a must for any African trip: There's sobering history, but also great white sharks in the ocean, penguins running around a park, the windswept rocks of the Cape of Good Hope, and world-class wineries just a train ride away.

No trip to the cape is complete without climbing Table Mountain, the 3,558-foot plateau that towers over the city. But you can double your Cape Town climbing adventure—and make more room for wine and meat—by tackling two mountains in the same day.

Start with nearby Lion's Head. It's just 2,195 feet, and scalable in about an hour. But that can be a tough 60 minutes, as you navigate the metal ladders and brackets pounded into the mountain, known as a "via ferrata" (iron path). From the top's pointed peak, you'll have a nearly 360-degree view of the city, as well as the flat top of Table Mountain. Head there next.

From the base of Lion's Head, take a cab (or a short jog) to the base of Table Mountain. This climb is more of a hike—less scrambling, but the path is longer, akin to a steep, meandering staircase. You'll hoof it past waterfalls and proteas, South Africa's national bloom, until reaching the summit, where prairie dog–looking rock hyraxes mingle with tourists and munch on vegetation.

Grab ice cream (or a beer) at one of the cafes at the summit, and enjoy your well-earned view. You can ride a cable car back down the mountain, but you've already climbed two today—you've got a hike down left in you!

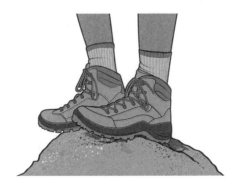

RUN AND PEDAL YOUR WAY TO THRILLS
AT ITALY'S HUMAN-POWERED AMUSEMENT PARK

All aboard the Bicycle of Death! Riders on this candy-colored contraption strap themselves into a cage to strain, struggle, and pedal themselves—and the cage—up the side of a 30-foot steel wheel. They then let themselves go, and the car spins around the wheel, looping around and daring passengers to lose their recently eaten lunch.

This thrilling, terrifying ride is one of more than 40 contraptions at Osteria Ai Pioppi, a restaurant and homemade amusement park in the foothills of Italy's Dolomite Mountains. For the price of a meal, visitors can climb up and careen down slides that are more than three stories tall, power a spinning "gravity wall" for others to stick to by running around in a circle, and take on the thigh-taxing Bicycle of Death.

Each ride is the brainchild of the restaurant's owner, a self-taught welder who started constructing the attractions to build buzz for his eatery more than 40 years ago. And their homemade, hand-welded nature makes the rides not only slightly intimidating, but unique: Almost all the attractions at Osteria Ai Pioppi are powered by human locomotion—you provide the power that makes each ride scream-worthy.

Admission is free: You've just got to buy something to eat at the Osteria, about an hour north of Venice. Visit www.aipioppi.com for more details.

ASCEND 999 STEPS TO THE "GATEWAY TO HEAVEN"

In the forests of Zhangjiajie, China, a 420-foot-high natural arch has beckoned travelers for centuries: With sunlight streaming through it, the Tianmen Shan, or Heaven's Gate, is said to be where the gods and the mortal world meet in Hunan Province legends. So you can go to heaven—you've just got to climb there.

It's 999 steps to the 180-foot-wide window in Tianmen Mountain, an ascent of 4,100 feet that takes most visitors around 30 minutes to complete.

Things to Know
- A visit to the Zhangjiajie will take all day, and you should get going early: The 999 steps begin at the middle station of the park's cable car, and tickets sell out quickly!
- Experts say the best months to visit—to avoid the biggest crowds—are April, October, and early November. If you choose October, though, make sure it's not the first week: October 1–8 is a national holiday week in China.

CLIMB AND CAMP IN THE GLOW OF BUBBLING LAVA

Bubbling, smoking, and casting an orange glow into the sky, the world's most active lava lake is mesmerizing—but you'll have to work to get there. On the shores of Lake Kivu in the Democratic Republic of Congo (DRC), Mount Nyiragongo rises 11,380 feet to a steaming crater. You can climb it—and camp at the top.

Fly to Kigali, Rwanda's capital, before driving through the small nation to Goma, the town nearest Nyiragongo in the DRC. The winding drive is breathtaking, with sweeping vistas of seemingly endless hills of bright green, dotted with fields so steep you'll wonder how it's possible to farm there.

After passing through the DRC border and arriving in Goma, you'll go to the Virunga National Park—also home to the some of the last mountain gorillas (which you can hike through the jungle to view—see page 97). Signs at the park entrance are peppered with rusty bullet holes, a reminder that this area wasn't always open to tourists—those signs were used for target practice by rebel fighters armed with AK-47s. It's a blessing that you can now trek here: The mountain is thick with vegetation, and, as you climb, the views of the lake below and other nearby volcanic calderas are worth every step.

But it's all about the lava lake at the top: After six or so hours of climbing with your group—including plenty of breaks—you'll reach the lip. When the smoke clears, you can watch the bright orange of the lava exploding below as you drink a well-earned cup of tea. The real treat comes at night, though: In the pitch-black, the lava glows bright, hypnotizing your whole group as you shiver on the mountain's peak.

You'll need a permit to climb the volcano (these are limited daily), and a tour company to get you there. The easiest way to schedule a tour is at www.visitvirunga.org.

WORKOUT CONTINUES >>>

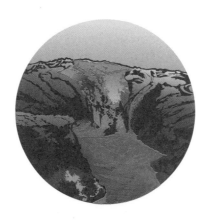

MORE VOLCANOES YOU CAN CLIMB

∞ **Roast marshmallows in the lava of Pacaya (Guatemala):** From the colonial town of Antigua, book a bus trip to climb Pacaya—the trip takes about an hour, and tickets are around $20. Your guide will lead you on a deceptively tough two-hour walk through forest and up rises of loose, volcanic rock to the top—well, as high as you can go, at least. Here, at the "fumaroles"—holes in the volcanic rock—you'll be given sticks and marshmallows to plunge into the holes, where magma beneath your feet roasts them for s'mores.

∞ **Gaze at glowing lava under starlight at Masaya (Nicaragua):** Masaya Volcano National Park, about 12.5 miles from Managua, has two active volcanoes and several extinct cones, nicknamed the Mouth of Hell by Spanish conquistadors. The big draw is the bubbling, massive Santiago crater. From the visitor center, you can hike to its edge during the day—but only stay for 15 minutes or so, lest the gases irritate your eyes and throat. At night, for an extra $10, you can return to the crater's edge via car to gaze into its bubbling maw.

∞ **Hike the world's most famous volcano, Vesuvius (Italy):** Its last eruption was more than 75 years ago so there's no lava to be seen, but the terror of Pompeii remains the world's most famous volcano. And it's a piece of history you'll definitely want to climb: Just 15 minutes from downtown Naples is Vesuvius National Park, offering nine different trails up the mountain. Trail 5 is the most popular, taking you to the edge of the volcano's three-mile-wide cone.

PART 2

WORKOUTS THAT LET YOU BE SOMEBODY

They say you don't know someone until you've walked a mile in their shoes. Do them one better: Run, lift, swim, bike, and hike in their shoes. You (probably) can't go back in time, play in the World Series, or perform before a sold-out crowd, but you can exercise the way the people from all those places did. Be somebody (else) with these workouts.

CHAPTER 7

TRAVEL THROUGH TIME

Where you're going, you don't need a DeLorean. You've already got a time machine: your body. With it, you can do battle with medieval knights, walk on the decks of the *Titanic*, play ball on the White House lawn, or play a round of tennis with Henry VIII.

This is how you *really* sweat to the oldies. Try these workouts from decades and centuries past to experience what it was like to live—and move—in the past.

YOUR HEART RATE WILL GO ON WITH THE *TITANIC* WORKOUT

The *Titanic* didn't just have lower-class stowaways sketching nudes and falling in love with first-class passengers—the unsinkable ship also had a 784-square-foot gymnasium.

Thanks to Jason King, who creates historically perfect models of the *Titanic*, we've got the plans to the mega-boat's swole center. It was filled with equipment you won't see in your gym 100 years later, including a "horse-riding" machine, a "stomach-massaging" machine, even a "camel hump"!

But there were some apparatuses you'd recognize. So do this workout that would have been possible on the *Titanic* to help build the barrel chest of a 1910s strongman, and, more important, the grip strength you'll need to hang on to a piece of driftwood until the rescue ships arrive.

SECTION 1: Warm Up on the Bicycle Race Machine
The *Titanic* was equipped with a "bicycle race machine"—basically a pair of stationary bikes with a giant clock in front. Hop on a stationary bike and warm up for five minutes.

SECTION 2: Build Strength on the High Cable Pulley Machine
The *Titanic*'s gym had a two-handle cable stack with the handles anchored high—basically a cable cross machine. Use it to perform these four exercises.

EXERCISE 1: Cable Fly (5 sets of 8 reps)
1. Begin in the "Jack, I'm flying" position: Stand tall, holding the cables out to the side, palms facing forward. Bend forward slightly into an athletic position.
2. Squeeze your chest to bring the cables down and in front of your chest, keeping your arms straight, until your fists touch.
3. Control the movement to return to start, and repeat. This exercise will give you the hugging strength you need so you won't let go of the driftwood door.

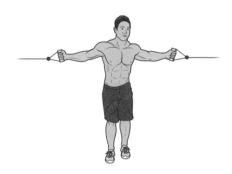

WORKOUT CONTINUES >>>

EXERCISE 2: Half-kneeling Single-Arm Lat Pull-Down (5 sets of 8 reps per side)

1. Kneel in front of the stack with your right knee down, your left foot flat on the floor. Both knees should be bent at a 90-degree angle. Reach up to grab the cable handle with your right hand.
2. Keeping your chest up and your torso and hips square, bend your elbow and pull the handle down toward your shoulder.
3. Return to start, and repeat. Do all your reps on one side, then switch your leg positions and perform reps with the left hand.

EXERCISE 3: Standing Cable Wood Chop (5 sets of 10 reps per side)

1. With the cable stack at your side, grab the handle with one hand and step away from the tower. You should be around an arm's length away from the pulley, with the tension of the weight on the cable.
2. In this position, set your feet shoulder-width apart and get into an athletic stance with knees slightly bent. Grab the cable with your other hand so you're now holding it with both hands in front of your body.
3. From this position, pull the handle down and across your body, past your front knee, as you rotate your torso. The motion should look as if you're chopping wood.
4. Return to the higher position, and repeat. Do all your reps on this side, then switch sides and repeat.

EXERCISE 4: Standing Cable Biceps Curl (4 sets of 12 reps)

1. Stand straight with the cable handles at each of your sides. Hold your arms in a "T" pose with a cable handle in each hand.
2. Keeping your chest out and your shoulders back, curl each handle until you're in a classic "muscle man" pose, with your fist at or near your bicep.
3. Return to start, and repeat.

SECTION 3: Forge Some Stamina on the Rowing Machine

The *Titanic*'s rowing machine looked imposing: big, long oars that resembled an Olympic sculling boat. But the rowing machine at your gym will do fine. By performing intervals—bursts of intense work alternated with rest—you can increase your stamina and burn more fat in less time than you would at a constant pace. Row hard for 1 minute, then rest for 1 minute. Repeat six to seven times.

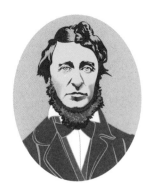

SWIM IN WALDEN POND

Sure, you could swim in a pool. Or you could make like Henry David Thoreau: "If you would get exercise, go in search of the springs of life."

Walden Pond isn't exactly a spring, but it inspired Thoreau to write an American classic. And for more than a century, the 103-foot-deep, glacier-scraped hole in Concord, Massachusetts, has been a destination where tourists can hike, swim, and camp. There's a trail around the pond that rambles through the woods for about an hour—much as Thoreau did on walks in search of enlightenment in the 1840s. Along the way, you can visit a replica of the one-room house he built on the property and see the original site of his homemade shack. In the water, there's a very un-Thoreau-like feature you'll welcome: Lifeguards patrol the roped-off swimming area to keep wisdom-seeking bathers safe.

Also not Thoreau-like: the people. With around 600,000 people visiting the Walden Pond Reservation each year, you shouldn't expect the type of solitude Henry David craved. But the area draws crowds because it's wonderful—still wild, mostly pristine, and an unmatched place to cool off while experiencing a bit of American history.

Parking is $8 for Massachusetts residents, and $30 for others. Walden Pond Reservation's hours change throughout the year. Visit https://www.mass.gov/locations/walden-pond-state-reservation for details.

DO A *GAME OF THRONES* WORKOUT

Whether you're a fantasy fan, a history buff, or just love Jon Snow, chances are you've imagined what it would be like to swing a real sword—and work up the kind of sweat that's worthy of a grail of mead. And, lucky for you, the Armored Combat League (ACL) makes it a reality.

Participants strap on 100-pound suits of armor to whale on each other—not with plastic swords, but with honest-to-goodness metal blades, axes, maces, and other Dark Ages–era weaponry in battles of up to 300. It's like a Renaissance Faire that got seriously real—and then invited you to party (and parry). Combatants usually come out relatively unscathed, but there's real risk—in past battles, one ACL competitor said he'd seen someone get their skull partially split by an ax.

You don't have to get your cranium crushed—or drop $3,000 on armor—to work up a sword-fighting sweat. ACL chapters across the country offer classes or other opportunities to get your knight on. At Sword Class NYC (www.swordclassnyc.com), a studio in Harlem, an intro class is just $10, and resembles a high-intensity interval training (HIIT) cardio class with sword and shield added in.

At an intro class I attended, competitors prepared for an upcoming international battle by working on conditioning—being weighed down by 100 pounds of chain mail and metal plate can be tiring, so knight cardio is key. We performed a high-knee run, mountain climbers, burpees, and squat jumps in a countdown style—performing each exercise for 1 minute, then for 45 seconds, then for 30 seconds, then 15.

After that, we did a four-station circuit: In station 1, we grabbed foam swords and shields to spar, trying to land a hit on the head or shoulders. In station 2, we practiced big strikes, slamming swords and wooden clubs into tires suspended from the ceiling. The other battlers taught me to push the tire with my shield to create space before smashing it. Stations 3 and 4 were more conditioning: ladder drills and rope slams.

For all the play violence, an ACL class was a pretty typical workout class that just happened to include swinging swords and wielding shields. Which is to say: You should go. Visit nycswordclass.com if you're going to be in the Big Apple, or try a knight-inspired workout right in your own gym: Find "Knight Fit" Tabata workouts at www.theknightshall.com.

WORK YOUR ABS LIKE BABE RUTH (YES, REALLY)

When you think abs, you probably don't think Babe Ruth. He wasn't considered the picture of health in his own day, either. The Yankees legend was so rotund that in one newsreel, called "Sultan of Swat Starts Battle on Fat," the announcer says, mockingly, that Ruth is "almost 40 and kind of fat" as his legs are pumped into his stomach by trainer Artie McGovern.

One of America's first prominent personal trainers, McGovern worked with celebrities like boxing champion Jack Dempsey, cartoonist Rube Goldberg, and department store magnate Marshall Field. But his most famous client was America's most famous man: the Bambino himself. And McGovern agreed that the Babe was fat—but thought that should inspire the average American.

Ruth would put in two hours of work each day to battle the bulge, working with medicine balls, dumbbells, and treadmills. But to ab acolyte McGovern, who advocated for ab work long before *Men's Health* made a six-pack trendy, it was work on the trunk that gave the Sultan more Swat: "I believe the intensive abdominal workouts we gave Babe in 1925 were as much responsible for the great showing he made during the 1926 season." [In the 1926 World Series, Babe Ruth hit three home runs in one game.]

In his book, McGovern outlined exercises he says he used with the original Home Run King. See if you can keep up with 1925's "fat and 40" super-athlete.

EXERCISE 1: Weighted Vacuum (40 reps)
1. Lie faceup in a classic sit-up position. Hold a book or weight against your abdomen.
2. Raise the weight by expanding your abdomen, then lower it by relaxing your stomach.

EXERCISE 2: Supine Alternating Toe Touches (6 reps for each side)
1. Lie faceup with your arms and legs extended.
2. Keeping your arms and legs straight, lift your right arm and left leg up, trying to touch your left toes with your right hand.
3. Return to start and repeat on the other side.

WORKOUT CONTINUES >>>

EXERCISE 3: Reverse Supine Alternating Toe Touches (6 reps for each side)

1. Reverse exercise 2: Start with your arms and legs lifted up as if you were trying to touch your toes.
2. Lower your left leg and right arm simultaneously, keeping your right leg and left arm lifted.
3. Return to the top and lower the right leg and left arm. Alternate.

EXERCISE 4: V-Up and Touch (6 reps)

1. McGovern calls this the "perfect abdominal exercise." Lie faceup with arms and legs fully extended.
2. Keeping both your arms and legs straight, raise your legs until they are perpendicular with your torso so your feet point at the ceiling. At the same time, raise your arms up and to the sides of your legs until your palms touch the floor next to your butt.
3. Return to start.

EXERCISE 5: Straight-Leg Sit-Up (6 reps)

1. Lie faceup with your arms and legs extended.
2. Keeping your legs on the ground, perform a sit-up, reaching for your toes.

EXERCISE 6: Arm and Leg Clap (6 reps)

1. Lie faceup with your arms extended straight in front of your chest, and your legs perpendicular to the floor so that your feet point toward the ceiling.
2. Place your hands together and your feet together.
3. Now simultaneously separate your arms and legs so both form "V" shapes.
4. Clap them back together.

EXERCISE 7: Arm and Leg Scissor (8 reps for each side)

1. Start in the same position as exercise 6, with hands touching each other and feet touching each other.
2. This time, cross your legs and arms simultaneously to one side, return to start, then cross the other way.

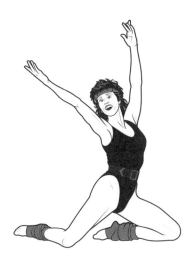

WORK YOUR BOOTY LIKE IT'S 1982

Before P90X, Tae Bo, 8-Minute Abs, and Sweatin' to the Oldies, there was Jane Fonda. Her 1982 tape, *Jane Fonda's Workout*, was a blockbuster: When fewer than 10 percent of American households had a VCR, it sold 200,000 copies in a year—more than *Star Trek 2*.

Almost 40 years later, it is just as groovy to watch. Fonda, dressed in leg warmers and a striped unitard, counts through the moves while the backup talent occasionally whoops over funky music. But it's not just a laugh: Some of the leg lift exercises have had staying power in the fitness world and have become known as "Jane Fondas." Well-known trainers use them in programs even today to help train the rear view, and they're a mainstay in barre studios.

But you don't have to pay studio fees to try them. Feel the original burn with this group of "Jane Fondas" inspired by her second tape, *Jane Fonda's Advanced Workout* (you can watch *that* video and the 1982 original on YouTube). Do all the moves on one side, then repeat on the other.

EXERCISE 1: Jane Fondas (16 reps)
1. Lie on your right side, propped up on your elbow. Your legs should be straight and stacked, with toes pointed.
2. Now lift your left leg up as high as you can, keeping it in line with your right leg.
3. Return to start.

WORKOUT CONTINUES > > >

EXERCISE 2: Alternating Knee Bend and Lift (8 reps for each side)

1. From the original starting position in exercise 1, bend your left knee and bring it toward your chest.
2. Return it to start, and then perform a lift as you did in exercise 1. Perform this alternating sequence—knee to chest, then lift.

EXERCISE 3: Forward Leg Drops (16 reps regular time; 32 reps double time)

1. Raise your left leg up to the top position from exercise 1. Hold it here.
2. Keeping your bottom thigh where it is, bend your bottom knee 90 degrees.
3. From this position, lower your left leg forward so it's perpendicular with your torso.
4. Return to the top and repeat. Then double your speed and double the reps!

EXERCISE 4: Forward Kick (8 reps each side)

1. Assume the bottom position of exercise 3—with your bottom knee bent 90 degrees, and your top leg lowered so it's perpendicular with your torso.
2. From this position, kick your top leg toward your head until it forms a 45-degree angle with your torso.
3. Return to the 90-degree position and repeat the kick.

EXERCISE 5: Prone Backward Lifts (32 reps)

1. Straighten both legs. Now roll forward onto the front of your right (bottom) hip. You shouldn't be quite turned over—your top hip should still be off the ground.
2. Keeping your legs straight, lift your top (left) leg up.

EXERCISE 6: Bottom Leg Lifts (32 reps per side)

1. Jane says this one is for the "wibble wobbles on the inner thigh." Lie on your right side again. Bend your left knee and bring your foot forward so it's flat on the floor in front of your right thigh—your legs should form a figure "4."
2. Keep the bottom leg straight, toes pointed. In this position, lift the right (bottom) leg up and down, repeating all moves on the other side.

PLAY HENRY VIII'S TENNIS GAME

I f you've watched *The Tudors*, you may remember Henry VIII and a courtier, played by Henry Cavill, playing a different kind of tennis—indoors, with lines on the floor, walls all around, and spectators in windows along one side. It's not just something the show made up. It's a real game—one that Henry VIII played, and one you can still play today—and it's a blast.

It's called court tennis—or sometimes "real tennis"—and it's actually even older than Henry. The game grew out of monasteries going back as far as the 1300s and has been played by other kings, including France's Louis XVI. In fact, one of the revolutionary votes for a French constitution was held inside a Paris "real" tennis court.

That court is much different from the outdoor version. Besides having windows for spectators and walls on three sides, there's a small, sloped roof along three sides. Players must serve so the ball hits this roof before coming down into play, and the rules get weirder: If you hit the ball into one of three window targets, you automatically score. You can bounce the ball off any of the court's 13 surfaces, and try to outwit your opponent with one of more than 50 serves, with names like the "giraffe" and the "backspin underarm twist."

That variety of surfaces, serve types, and scoring gives the game a combination of outdoor tennis-level aerobic challenge with strategy that borders on chess—meaning older, wily players can excel, too. The current world champion is 54 years old!

You can join the 6,000 worldwide players of this centuries-old game and get your own taste of its mind- and body-challenging rules and play—there are 11 court tennis clubs scattered throughout the United States, including in Boston; Philadelphia; New York; Aiken, South Carolina; Newport, Rhode Island; near Washington, DC; and in Chicago. Many offer free lessons and seminars and loaner equipment to players. At the Prince's Court in McLean, Virginia, where I've played, the club pro, Ivan Ronaldson, is the son of a former world champion and grew up living at Henry VIII's home court. Visit www.princescourt.com to learn more about him, or find one of the other clubs via Google.

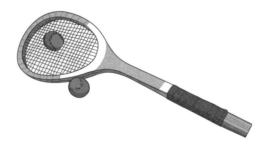

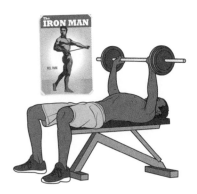

LIFT LIKE ARNOLD'S IDOL

R eg Park was Arnold before Arnold was Arnold: A three-time Mr. Universe bodybuilding champion in the 1950s and '60s, Park went on to star as Hercules on the silver screen and a young Schwarzenegger took notice. Park became Arnold's idol from the first time he saw the big Brit on a magazine cover.

A lot has changed in the 60 years since Park was a champion, but one of his signature training techniques—performing 5 sets of 5 repetitions of an exercise—has stood the test of time. Here's a 5x5 program inspired by the one Park prescribed for beginners in the 1960s.

Perform the following workout three times a week for 3 weeks. For each exercise, rest 3 to 5 minutes between the last 3 sets of the move.

EXERCISE 1: 45-Degree Back Extension (3 sets of 10 reps)

1. On a back extension bench, position your thighs on the upper pads and your lower legs under the lower pads to brace them. Cross your arms in front of your chest.
2. Lower your body by bending your waist.
3. Raise back up until your torso is in line with your legs. Repeat.

EXERCISE 2: Back Squat (5 sets of 5 reps)

1. Stand in a normal back squat position, barbell across your shoulders, feet between shoulder- and hip-width apart, toes slightly out.
2. Push your hips back to initiate the squat.
3. Bend your knees to descend until your thighs are at least parallel to the floor, keeping your chest up and your weight on your heels.
4. Keep your weight in your heels and press back to standing.

EXERCISE 3: Bench Press (5 sets of 5 reps)

1. Lie faceup on the bench and grab the bar with an overhand grip just wider than shoulder-width. Unrack the bar and hold it above your sternum with straight arms.
2. Brace your core and bend your elbows to lower the bar to your chest. Your elbows should stay close to your sides, forming a 45-degree angle.
3. Pause for a beat, then press back to start.

EXERCISE 4: Barbell Deadlift (5 sets of 5 reps)

1. Stand with the barbell at your shins.
2. Bend at your hips and knees to grab the barbell a little wider than shoulder-width: You can use an overhand grip, a mixed grip, or a hook grip. Your feet should be flat on the floor.
3. Keeping your weight in your heels and maintaining the natural curve of your spine, pull the bar up as you thrust your hips forward and stand. The bar should remain close to your body as it comes off the floor.
4. Reverse the maneuver to return to start. Repeat.

LEAVES OF KICKING ASS: WALT WHITMAN'S WORKOUT

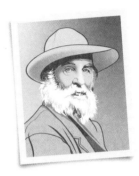

When you think of an active, "manly" author, Ernest Hemingway may pop to mind. But Papa's got nothing on Whitman. Like the ambulance-driving novelist, Whitman worked numerous jobs—as a teacher, a journalist, and a battlefield nurse in the Civil War—before becoming an author. And the *Leaves of Grass* poet was as much a proponent of a vigorous life as the amateur boxer Hemingway.

Even into his 60s, a decade after suffering a stroke that partially paralyzed him, Whitman would spend an hour each day exercising. At 66, the poet described his workout of wrestling with an oak tree "as thick as my wrist, 12 feet high—pushing and pulling." For cross training, he would shout "declamatory pieces, sentiments, sorrow, anger . . . or inflate my lungs and sing . . . I make the echoes ring, I tell you!"

Whitman says his reader should not "be afraid of . . . 'how it will look' to outsiders, or what they will say." Still, shouting and sapling-bending might make you self-conscious. Fret not! You can still get a Whitman-approved workout. In 1858, the poet wrote a series of newspaper columns, titled "Manly Health and Training."

"If you are a student," Whitman writes, "be also a student of the body . . . realizing that a broad chest, a muscular pair of arms, and two sinewy legs will be just as much credit to you, and stand you in hand through your future life, equally with your geometry, your history, your classics, your law, medicine, or divinity. Let nothing divert you from your duty to your body."

Now that's poetry. Try this workout derived from Whitman's advice from his column, and you don't need a gym to do it. Whitman was adamant that exercises be done in the open air.

WARM-UP
Dynamic Overhead Stretch (10 reps)
Whitman's instructions: "Throw forward the arms, with vigorous motion, and then extend them or lift them upward."

A little more detail: Stand with your arms at your sides, palms facing in. Forcefully bring your arms forward and up in an arc until they're over your head. As you get to the top, reach backward into a slight back bend, creating a crescent moon shape with your body.

Active Plank (8 reps)
Whitman's instructions: "Place the body in position occasionally, for a moment, with all the sinews of the arms and legs strained to their utmost tension . . ."

A little more detail: Assume the classic plank position, with your forearms on the floor, elbows beneath your shoulders, and your body forming a straight line from head to heels. Instead of just hanging out here, tense everything: Squeeze your thighs and glutes, grip the floor with your hands, and brace your abs as if you're about to take a punch. Do this all-over tensing for ten seconds, then pause and repeat.

GET MOVING
Lunges (8 reps for each side)
Whitman's instructions: "Take very long strides rapidly forward, and then, more slowly and carefully, backward."

A little more detail: Stand with your hands on your hips, feet shoulder-width apart. Take a long lunge step forward with your right leg, descending as you step until your knees both form 90-degree angles. Press through your front foot to return to standing in control. Repeat on the other side.

Single-Leg Deadlift (4 reps for each side)
Whitman's instructions: "The simple exercise of standing on one foot and lowering so as to touch the bent knee of the other leg to the ground, and then rising again on the first foot, is also a good one."

A little more detail: Stand next to a wall or chair so you can grab it for support if you need it. Stand on one foot, with the raised knee bent at a 90-degree angle. Keeping your torso upright, bend the knee of your planted leg to descend until your raised knee taps the floor. Press back to standing, then repeat. Then switch sides and repeat.

WORKOUT CONTINUES > > >

Fence or Bench Hops (10 reps for 4 sets)

Whitman's instructions: ". . . spring over a fence, and then back again, and then again and again . . ."

A little more detail: Stand on one side of a flat bench, with legs parallel to it, and grip the bench with one hand on each side. Hop over the bench as if it were a horse, landing with both feet on the other side. Repeat. Over time, try to increase the rate at which you jump over and back, then increase the number of total jumps in each set.

Shadowboxing (4 reps)

Whitman's instructions: ". . . pummel some imaginary foe, with stroke after stroke from the doubled fists, given with a will . . ."

A little more detail: Try this simple shadowboxing routine: Standing in a traditional boxing stance, perform three punches—for a right-handed fighter, think left-right-left. Then shuffle to your left in a circle, as if around a heavy bag. Then repeat: three punches, shuffle. Do this for a one-minute round. In the next round, shuffle right instead of left. Start by going for four one-minute rounds, working your way up to three-minute rounds.

BURN IT OUT

Jump Squats (number of reps varies)

Whitman's instructions: ". . . clap the palms of the hands on the hips and simply jump straight up, two or three minutes at a time . . ."

A little more detail: For many adults, jumping right back into jumping can be rough on the joints. If you haven't been jumping recently, do a full-body extension instead. To perform the move, stand with your feet shoulder-width apart, knees slightly bent. Keeping your chest up, drive your hands behind your glutes and bend your knees as if you were going to initiate a jump. Then explosively extend as if you were jumping straight up, bringing your hands up overhead into a full-body extension while coming up onto your toes—but without jumping. Return to start and repeat. Once you've done this for a few weeks, you can graduate to jumping.

GET PUMPED LIKE A POTUS

When they're not jetting around the world with a security detail to meet other world leaders . . . presidents: They're just like us!

That's probably why video of Barack Obama working out in a Polish hotel room went mega-viral in 2014: The 44th president was outed as a sweatpants-wearing doer of dad workouts.

Try this Barack Obama workout, inspired by that footage. It's 4 sets of six exercises—most of which are good for the lighter dumbbells you'll find in a hotel gym—followed by a little time on the elliptical. Then try these other workouts, inspired by POTUSes past.

Perform 4 sets of each exercise, resting 30 seconds between sets.

EXERCISE 1: Bent-Over Reverse Fly (8 reps per set)
1. Stand with your feet together, dumbbells hanging in front of your thighs, palms facing in.
2. Push your hips back to bend forward, keeping your back flat as your chest moves toward the floor. The weights should hang straight down from your shoulders.
3. Maintaining a flat back, raise the dumbbells out to the sides so that your body forms a bent-over "T" shape.
4. Return them to hanging and repeat.

EXERCISE 2: Seated Shoulder Press (6 reps per set)
1. Sit with your feet flat on the floor, back straight. Bring the dumbbells up to your shoulders, palms in.
2. Maintaining an upright posture, press the dumbbells overhead until your elbows are almost straight.
3. Return the weights to your shoulders and repeat.

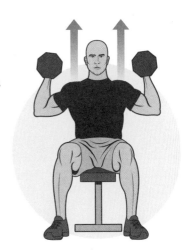

WORKOUT CONTINUES >>>

EXERCISE 3: Lateral Lunge (6 reps on each leg per set)
1. Stand with your feet together, toes pointed forward, with the weights in front of your legs.
2. Take a big step to the right, pushing your hips back and descending as you step by bending your right knee, keeping it tracking over your right toes. Keep your torso upright as you descend, maintaining the position of your arms in relation to your body.
3. Press back to start, and perform the move to the left.

EXERCISE 4: Step Up with Knee Drive (6 reps on each leg per set)
1. Stand with the bench in front of you, or in front of a flight of stairs. Hold the dumbbells at your sides, palms in.
2. Keep your torso upright as you place your right foot on the bench (or stair) and press through your heel to bring your left foot up so you're standing on the bench. Continue lifting your left foot up until your knee forms a 90-degree angle in front of you.
3. Return to the ground and repeat with the other leg.

EXERCISE 5: Lunge with Curl and Overhead Press (5 reps on each leg per set)
1. Stand with your feet shoulder-width apart, dumbbells at your sides.
2. Take a large lunge step forward with your right leg, descending as you step until your knees both form 90-degree angles.
3. At the bottom, curl the weights to your shoulders, then press them overhead.
4. Reverse the press and curl so the weights are back at your sides.
5. Press through your right foot to stand back up.
6. Repeat this entire sequence on the other leg.

EXERCISE 6: Lateral Raise (8 reps per set)
1. Stand with your feet together, dumbbells at your sides, palms in.
2. Keeping your torso upright, lift the dumbbells out to the sides until your torso and arms form a "T" shape.
3. Control the weights as they return to your sides and repeat.

Finish: Elliptical Intervals (8 reps)
Go slow for 60 seconds, then fast for 60 more. Repeat.

KEEP UP WITH JEFFERSON TO GET TO 10,000 STEPS

"If the body be feeble, the mind will not be strong," Thomas Jefferson wrote in a 1786 letter to his son-in-law. And while later in his life he often rode a horse, the younger Jefferson considered walking to be king—or, er, chief executive—of exercises: "The sovereign invigorator of the body is exercise, and of all the exercises, walking is best."

Jefferson encouraged his daughter Patsy—and anyone who would listen—to do two hours of exercise per day. His own regimen included daily walks at Monticello, especially a jaunt to and from a stone a mile away from his home. He even kept track of his pace and the number of steps it took to get there. In a 1787 memo, the future president recorded that he finished a "French mile" (which measures around 1.2 modern miles) in 17.5 minutes, covering the distance in 2,106 of his lanky steps.

You may not have two hours a day to devote to exercise, but declare your independence from your chair and try keeping up with Jefferson's morning pace: Go for a walk that covers 2.4 miles in 35 minutes.

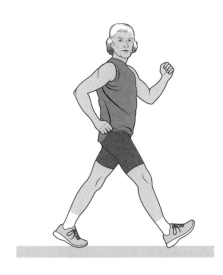

ANSWER JFK'S CHALLENGE: MARCH 50 MILES

"The harsh fact of the matter is that there is also an increasingly large number of young Americans who are neglecting their bodies—whose physical fitness is not what it should be—who are getting soft. And such softness on the part of individual citizens can help to strip and destroy the vitality of a nation."

John F. Kennedy wrote these words in *Sports Illustrated* a month before he took the oath of office in 1961. Two years later, the White House unearthed a 1908 executive order from Theodore Roosevelt decreeing that all Marines should be able to hike 50 miles in three days. JFK upped the ante, asking that his own Marine Corps be ready to hump the half-century in a single day, and, perhaps jokingly, challenged his staff to do the same.

If it was a joke, Robert Kennedy didn't get it. He strapped on a pair of Oxfords, grabbed four staffers, and started walking, hiking 17.5 hours from Great Falls, Virginia, outside DC, to Harper's Ferry, West Virginia. The president's call to action—and his brother's acceptance of that challenge—inspired a brief fad of long-distance walking in America.

Decades later, Paul Kiczek, now 60 years old, started a long-distance walking organization called FreeWalkers. With the JFK/RFK challenge still lingering in Kiczek's mind from his childhood, he organized an event to trace the younger Kennedy's exact steps along the Potomac River to Harper's Ferry. In 2013, the Kennedy 50 was born.

In the 2019 edition, 134 walkers from 20 states and four countries braved the February cold to make their own trek. Want to join? Register in advance at Kennedy50.org, as it's capped at 200 participants. Registration starts at $100.

TEST YOUR ENDURANCE AGAINST JOHN QUINCY ADAMS

Your mental image of John Quincy Adams is probably . . . round. But POTUS #6 was obsessed with fitness, timing his daily walks to Congress, and aiming for new records in marathon skinny-dipping sessions in the Potomac River.

At age 55, JQA wrote in his journal that he'd swum in the DC river for 50 minutes without touching bottom. The next year, he smashed his own record, staying afloat for an hour and 20 minutes. His wife and doctor begged him to stop, so 80 minutes became his high-water mark.

Find a safe pool and see how long you can stay off the bottom while swimming around. Can you beat 50 minutes? Or are you going to be beaten by a rotund, 55-year-old man from the 1820s?

THE PRESIDENTIAL WORKOUT GAME THAT INSPIRED AN NFL LINEBACKER

Hate cardio? Here's your solution: Play volleyball with a medicine ball.

You may have seen videos of former Steelers linebacker James Harrison and his teammates playing this game—they called it Danneyball after the trainer who taught them the game.

But the game's roots go deeper: The original name was Hooverball, named for Herbert Hoover. Our 31st POTUS hated exercising. To keep him trim, his doctor devised this game, and the president loved it. Hoover played it so much, in fact, that his cabinet was nicknamed the "medicine ball cabinet."

You can play the same game he played on the White House lawn—the official rules are available online.

YOU'LL NEED:
- A volleyball court
- A soft-sided medicine ball (the official rules call for 9 pounds)
- Three friends

HOW TO PLAY:
- One team serves the entire game.
- Throw the ball over the net to the other team. If they drop it, you score.
- Score the game like tennis: 15, 30, 40, and then game. The president played seven-game sets, alternating serving teams each game.

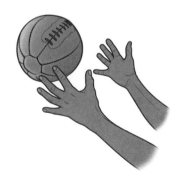

FOLLOW THE FOOTSTEPS—AND PACE—OF PRESIDENT BILL CLINTON

An invitation to jog with Bill Clinton was a bigger deal than getting to meet him in the Oval Office: The 43rd president would hoof it around DC three days a week, with Secret Service, aides, reporters, and some choice donors in tow. His regular runs were a media sensation and were even lampooned on *Saturday Night Live*.

They caused a bit of a stir for the Secret Service, too. The presidential protectors wanted POTUS to run at a track that was installed on the White House grounds, but Clinton wasn't interested—he wanted to be seen running out among the people. So the Secret Service mapped a few jogging routes they felt they could secure, and Bill was off and running—sometimes joined by regular DC joggers.

"When he would encounter people, sometimes he would stop and say hello," says Dan Emmett, then a member of the president's personal protection unit in the Secret Service. Emmett wrote a book about his time protecting presidents, *Within Arm's Length*. "They were all potential voters."

Clinton reportedly kept around a nine-minute-per-mile pace. You won't have a Secret Service detail in tow, but you can follow some of his exact routes—courtesy of Emmett—on your next visit to DC.

ROUTE 1: Around the Lincoln Memorial Reflecting Pool
1.   Start on 17th Street NW, just outside the World War II Memorial.
2.   Run three laps around the Lincoln Memorial reflecting pool's inner walkway. One lap is about 0.85 miles, so try to finish each lap in 7:39 to match Clinton's pace.
3.   At the end of your third lap, run across 17th Street toward the Washington Monument—run up the hill past the monument, around its backside on 15th Street NW, and back to your starting point.
4.   Run one more lap of the pool and you're done—ready to head into your National Security Council meeting.

ROUTE 2: FDR Memorial Loop
1.   Start at the FDR Memorial on the DC Tidal Basin. There's a trail here by the water.
2.   Head southeast on the trail (toward baseball field #1), then cross before the Ohio River Bridge onto the Rock Creek Park trail, to the Potomac River.
3.   Head back up and make a right on West Basin Drive SW.
4.   Return to the start. Run this loop two or three times.

Route 1

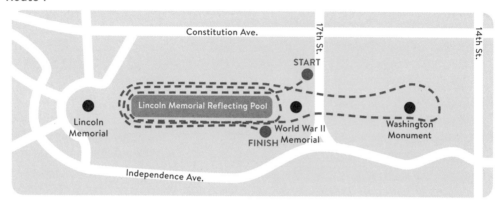

Route 2

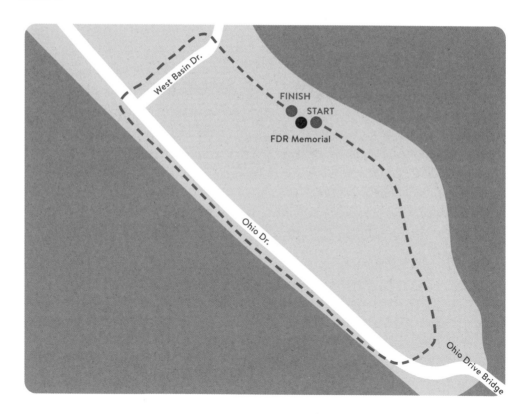

CONQUER MAINE'S TALLEST MOUNTAIN LIKE TEDDY ROOSEVELT

When you think of an active president, you think Teddy. The 26th president's motto was "Get action," and he did—on horseback with the Rough Riders, in the ring with heavyweight champions in the White House, and especially outdoors. Roosevelt's love of nature led him on marathon rowing trips across the ponds near his Long Island home, and on breakneck-paced walks through DC's Rock Creek Park.

At 20, Roosevelt tackled an outdoor challenge he'd dreamed of since his early teens—climbing Mount Katahdin, the imposing granite edifice that towers 5,268 feet above northern Maine. The future president endured slick conditions on the mountain's stone scrambles, hefting a 45-pound pack to the summit in 1879.

Almost 150 years later, Katahdin remains a daunting challenge. It's the northern terminus of the Appalachian Trail, finishing off northbound through-hikers' months-long journeys from Georgia with an intense flourish: The 5-mile climb is characterized by high winds, unpredictable weather, and much strenuous scrambling—at times, nearly bouldering—over granite stones the size of a Subaru.

The bigger challenge, though, may be getting onto the mountain itself. If you're not hiking the AT or camping in Baxter State Park, you'll need to register for one of a limited number of day-use parking passes to climb the mountain in summer. Maine residents can register for a pass for any day starting on April 1, but for visitors from other states, registration doesn't open until two weeks before the date of your hike—and spots go fast. Plan to stay up to register starting at midnight, when new registration opens, and even then, you might not get a spot. Camping reservations can be made four months in advance. Visit www.baxterstatepark.org for details.

ROGER BANNISTER'S FOUR-MINUTE-MILE WORKOUT

If you've ever said, "I don't have enough time to work out," meet Roger Bannister: The man who broke the four-minute barrier in the mile did almost all of his training for that feat during half-hour lunch breaks as a medical student in 1953 and 1954.

Given: Bannister was already pretty fast. He'd finished fourth in the 1,500 meters at the 1952 Olympics, but he pushed himself to the four-minute record with just a few short workouts per week. In his autobiography, *Twin Tracks*, Bannister described the regimen he followed with training partner Chris Brasher:

"In December 1953, we started a new intensive course of training and ran several times a week a series of ten consecutive quarter-miles, each in 66 seconds. Through January and February we gradually speeded them up, keeping to an interval of two minutes between each. By April we could manage them in 61 seconds, but however hard we tried it did not seem possible to reach our target of 60 seconds."

Bannister did reach that target when he set the record on May 6, 1954. Use his interval program to go for your own mile record, or just go out and see how quickly you can do his running regimen—and be amazed at how much faster a medical student was eating up the same distance 65 years ago.

HOW TO DO IT: A standard track is a quarter-mile for one loop. After warming up, run a lap as fast as you can, then rest for two minutes. Repeat ten times.

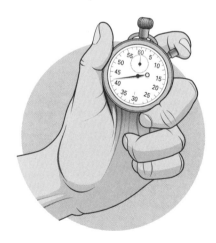

TRAIN LIKE THE GREATEST RUNNER OF ALL TIME

When Emil Zatopek toed the starting line at the 1952 Olympic marathon, he'd already won the 5K and 10K, setting Olympic records in both events. The Czechoslovakian army officer had never raced a marathon before, though. He just decided to run it . . . and broke the tape at the end, setting another Olympic record.

The results were beautiful, but Zatopek ran ugly: One sportswriter, in describing his form, said he looked like "he'd just been stabbed through the heart."

But Zatopek was having the time of his life—he loved to run, and happily chatted with other runners as he flew past them. When he finished his gold medal–winning marathon, he was hoisted onto the shoulders . . . of the Jamaican track team, who had fallen in love with him. Another competitor said, "His enthusiasm, his friendliness, his love of life, shone through every movement."

His training theory, said Fred Wilt in his book *How They Train*, was to work so hard in training that the race seemed comparatively easy: "Before Zatopek, nobody realized it was humanly possible to train this hard."

That training was merciless—described by Zatopek himself as "horse dosage, every day"—and it made him *Runner's World*'s "Greatest Runner of All Time." See if you can keep up with *half* of a Zatopek workout—and keep the kind of smile that would make other teams want to hoist you on their shoulders.

THE WORKOUT: Run at a track, or at a place where you can mark off 200 meters and 400 meters.

1. Warm up. Jog for 10 minutes, then do a few 100-meter sections at a slightly faster, but still controlled, pace.
2. Run 10 intervals of 200 meters each (Zatopek would do 20). Run 200 meters fast, and then jog 200 meters more slowly, taking about double the time of your fast run. Zatopek's times for these intervals: 34 seconds for the fast ones, 60 seconds for the recovery run.
3. Run 20 intervals of 400 meters each (Zatopek would do 40). Run 400 meters fast, followed by 200 meters of jogging at a much slower pace. Zatopek's times for these intervals: 75–90 seconds for the fast ones, 60 seconds for the recovery run.
4. Repeat step 2, doing 10 intervals of 200 meters (Zatopek did another 20 here).

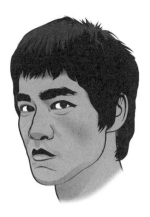

BRUCE LEE'S 1,300-REP "LETHAL PHYSIQUE" PUNCHING PROTOCOL

The feats Bruce Lee could perform with his body are the stuff of legend: He once sent a man flying across a room using a punch that started just an inch away. He could leap to the ceiling to shatter a light bulb with a flying kick.

The ripped, lean muscle he used to accomplish these feats is equally legendary. The wife of the director of *Enter the Dragon* once grabbed his bicep on set and exclaimed that his upper arm was "like feeling warm marble." Chuck Norris said that Lee had "muscles on muscles," and claimed that "no other human being had ever trained the way Bruce trained—fanatically."

His training between 1965 and 1970 included a three-day-a-week lifting program nicknamed "lethal physique." After a six-move lift, he'd finish with a weighted punching pyramid: Use your gym's small weights and see if you can do Lee's 1,300-repetition finisher.

How to do it: Perform 100 punches holding a 1-pound weight in each hand. Then repeat with weights of 2, 3, 5, 7, and 10 pounds. Then come back down: Do 100-rep sets with 10-, 7-, 5-, 3-, 2-, and 1-pound weights. Finish with 100 punches without weights in your hands.

CHISEL YOUR ABS LIKE JESUS

In classical art, you know what you're getting from the body of Christ: Golden halo, crown of thorns . . . and rippling, six-pack abs. If you're going to defeat death and crush Satan—not to mention being hung shirtless for all Jerusalem to see—the divine strength needed starts in the core.

I'm joking, of course, but for performers who appear as JC, it's no laughing matter.

"I believe that the audience wants to see someone who looks strong enough to overcome death," says Dylan Barnes, who was crucified three times a day for several years at the Holy Land Experience, a religious theme park that held theatrical performances of biblical events until closing in 2020. "Since muscles and a lean stomach help convey this on a basic level, I maintained this look on a regular basis."

Barnes says he usually maintained a solid four-pack as the Redeemer, but the audience never criticized him for the missing pair of abs—one spectator was more worried that he was a green-eyed Jesus. So what he was doing to impress the crowd was working. Here's the daily ab routine he used to maintain that miraculous midsection.

Perform 2 rounds of the following exercises, resting as little as possible between moves.

EXERCISE 1: Elbow-to-Knee Crunch (20 reps for each side)
1. Start by performing these on the left: On each crunch, bring your right elbow to your left knee.
2. Switch and repeat.

EXERCISE 2: Bicycle Crunch (20 reps for each side)
1. Lie faceup with your legs extended and your hands clasped behind your head.
2. Bend your left knee toward your chest as you crunch up and bring your right elbow to touch your left knee.
3. Switch your legs so your right knee is now at your chest, and twist your torso so your left elbow touches your right knee.
4. Continue exchanging in this way.

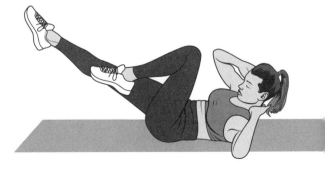

EXERCISE 3: V-Up Sit-Up (20 reps)

1. Lie faceup with arms and legs fully extended. Keeping both your arms and your legs straight, raise your arms and legs until they touch.
2. Return to the floor and repeat.

EXERCISE 4: Hollow Hold (2 reps)

1. Start in the same position as the V-up, with arms and legs fully extended. Lift your arms and legs slightly off the ground, brace your core, and hold for 10 seconds.
2. Perform 2 holds of 10 seconds each, with lower legs hovering 6 inches from the ground.

EXERCISE 5: Flutter Kick (15 reps)

In the Hollow Hold position (exercise 4), perform small scissor kicks, keeping your legs close to the ground.

EXERCISE 6: Bicycle Crunch Again (15 reps)

EXERCISE 7: Mountain Climber (15 reps)

1. Assume the classic push-up position: Your hands should be directly beneath your shoulders, your body forming a straight line from head to heels.
2. Maintaining this body line and keeping your hips parallel to the floor, lift your right foot off the ground and bend your knee so that it comes up toward your chest.
3. Return your right foot to the start position, and repeat with the left leg. Move your legs rapidly back and forth, as if you were climbing a mountain.

WORK OUT LIKE HOLLYWOOD'S ORIGINAL HERCULES

If you've ever torn down a wall in an old house, you know what you were hoping to find: a bundle of cash, a priceless work of art, or even bars of gold. Owners of one Oakland, California house had something no less historic behind their garage walls—the workout of a golden-age bodybuilder.

Before there was Arnold or The Rock, there was Steve Reeves: The 1950 Mr. Universe's physique—considered the most aesthetic of all time—helped him become the biggest box office draw in 25 different countries by the late 1950s, playing classical heroes like Hercules and Aeneas.

The workout that built his mythic body remained hidden behind the walls of his childhood home until George Helmer, the founder of the Steve Reeves International Society, unearthed it like a gym rat Indiana Jones. Peeling back the drywall, he found 15 exercises scrawled in black pencil on the underlying wood. Try this workout—Reeves's original—and chisel your own legendary physique. Perform 3 sets of each exercise.

EXERCISE 1: Barbell Cleans (7 reps per set)

EXERCISE 2: Overhead Press (10 reps per set)

EXERCISE 3: Barbell Curl (15 reps per set)

EXERCISE 4: Bench Curl (15 reps per set)

EXERCISE 5: Bent-Over Row (10 reps per set)

EXERCISE 6: Bench Press (10 reps per set)

EXERCISE 7: Squat (20 reps per set)

EXERCISE 8: Barbell Pullover (40 reps per set)

EXERCISE 9: Good Morning (20 reps per set)

EXERCISE 10: Lateral Raise (30 reps per set)

EXERCISE 11: Upright Row (10 reps per set)

EXERCISE 12: Front Raise (10 reps per set)

EXERCISE 13: Dumbbell Bench Press (10 reps per set)

EXERCISE 14: Barbell Triceps Extension [Skull Crusher]
(15 reps per set)

EXERCISE 15: Sit-Ups (20 reps per set)

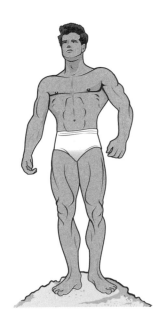

GET STRONGER WITH THE ONE-MINUTE, MUSCLE-BUILDING MIRACLE OF 1961

More strength and muscle in just one minute a day? Sounds like magic, but it's really just modern science!

Well, modern in the 1960s, anyway—and the science was isometrics, a term for exercise where the muscles don't move. Instead, they strain against an immovable object—or each other—for a short period. If you've ever done a plank, you've done an isometric exercise.

Thanks to studies by German scientists, isometrics was all the rage in the early '60s—the World Series–winning Pittsburgh Pirates, Notre Dame's football team, and Olympians began to swear by these "don't move a muscle" workouts. Then they spread to everyone. The Navy suggested a nine-move isometric routine for deskbound personnel in 1963. *Sports Illustrated* published isometrics articles three times in 1961. *American Weekly* told women in 1962 that it would make their muscles "less bulgy, more firm."

Put a modern twist on this swinging '60s strength sensation with a three-exercise isometrics session that takes less than five minutes. Add this to your workout as often as five times a week.

EXERCISE 1: Isometric Power Rack Squat

The 1960s craze led to isometric-specific equipment, like a static squat rack that could hold the bar at different heights for all-out, no-movement pressing. Your gym's power rack can do the same thing with a move called a "pin press."

1. Set the bar on one set of pins that would be about halfway through the squat movement. Place another set of pins just above this set.
2. Assume a normal back squat position, with your feet slightly wider than shoulder-width apart and the barbell over your shoulders.
3. Push your hips back to assume a mid-squat position.
4. Now drive up through your heels to push the bar up into the higher set of pins. Press the bar against these pins as hard as you can for six to eight seconds.
5. Rest, then repeat two more times. Over time, perform this exercise at various positions through the squat pattern—at the bottom, at 20 percent of the way up, etc.

WORKOUT CONTINUES >>>

EXERCISE 2: Isometric Power Rack Bench Press

In one of the *SI* articles, an athlete named Bill March said he used isos to set four North American records in powerlifting in just a year. It's done the same way as the squat.

1. Set the bar on one set of pins that would be about halfway through the bench press movement. Place another set of pins just above this set.
2. Keeping your elbows tucked near your sides and without shrugging your shoulders, press the bar up against the top set of pins with as much force as you can. Hold there for six to eight seconds.
3. Rest, then repeat two more times. Over time, perform this exercise at various positions through the movement pattern.

EXERCISE 3: Isometric Deadlift

You can do this exercise on the power rack, as with the other moves, or, for a bit more fun, just load up a bar—using way more weight than you can actually lift.

1. Stand with the barbell at your shins. Bend at your hips and knees to grab the barbell a little wider than shoulder width with an overhand grip. Your feet should be flat on the floor.
2. Keeping your weight in your heels and maintaining the natural curve of your spine, pull the bar up, straining to try to lift it from the ground. Pull for six to eight seconds.
3. Rest, and repeat two more times.

CHAPTER 8

TRAIN LIKE A CHAMPION

You may not ever strap on NFL pads, touch gloves in the Octagon, or mount an Olympic podium. But you can work out like a linebacker, jump rope like a contender, and get higher, faster, and stronger like Team USA.

These are real workouts from real champions that you can really do. You may not get to hear the roar of the crowd, but so what? Even if it's just for a single session, trying these workouts will give you a taste of what it takes to become a champion.

BUT FIRST . . . LET'S GET LOOSE LIKE A THREE-TIME STANLEY CUP WINNER

Star athletes warm up. Chances are, you don't.

Yeah, yeah, you know you should. Warming up can reduce your risk of injury during a workout and reduce how sore you are in the days after. But for most exercisers I talk to, if they're short on time, a warm-up is the first thing to go. Why? Because . . . *yawn*. Warming up is boring.

It could also be the key to enjoying *all* your workouts as you age: Chicago Blackhawks right-winger Patrick Kane had the best season of his career at age 30—playing more minutes and scoring more points than he had in any of his first 12 NHL seasons. That's in large part thanks to Ian Mack, and a specific bodyweight warm-up.

"[Patrick] was *healthy* overall, but was restricted, tight, and putting himself in a compromised position . . . he didn't have the full range of motion," says Mack, founder of Tomahawk Science in Chicago. He says Kane "has a V8 or V10 engine, and he only had access to four of those cylinders."

That's not just a problem for hockey players. Thanks to all the sitting we do, few of us are firing on all cylinders. But Mack says many of the same bodyweight movements he focuses on with Kane can help us all access a little more horsepower. Try this lunge sequence from Kane's routine before your next workout, or just to start your day moving with a little more fluidity.

Perform each of the following lunge variations for 15 yards.

Lunge 1: Lunge and Overhead Backbend
1. Stand with your feet shoulder-width apart.
2. Take a big step forward with your right leg, descending as you step, until both knees form 90-degree angles.
3. At the bottom, reach your arms up and back, stretching the front of your body.
4. Come out of the stretch, stand back up, and lunge again, this time with your left leg.

Lunge 2: Lunge and Twist, Lunging Side
1. Stand with your feet shoulder-width apart, hands on your hips.
2. Take a big lunge step forward with your right leg, descending as you step, until both knees form 90-degree angles.
3. At the bottom, keep your hips squared forward and twist your torso to the right, so your left shoulder goes toward your right leg.
4. Untwist, stand up, and lunge again with your left leg, this time twisting to the left.

Lunge 3: Lunge and Twist, Opposite Side
Perform just as above, but twist away from your lunging leg each time.

Lunge 4: Crossover Lunge
1. Imagine that your feet are both facing 12 o'clock.
2. Instead of lunging straight forward to 12, lunge across your body with your right leg so that your right foot lands on 10 o'clock.
3. Stand back up, and lunge with your left leg so that your left foot lands on 2 o'clock. Continue alternating in this way.

Lunge 5: Lateral Lunge
1. Stand tall with your feet together.
2. Keeping your feet facing forward, take a big step to the right, descending as you step so you drop into a squat position on the right, your weight in your heels.
3. Press back up to start, and repeat on the left side.

WORKOUT CONTINUES >>>

Lunge 6: Spider-Man Climb with Rotation

1. Get in a classic push-up position.
2. Bring your right foot up so it's planted outside your right hand, knee bent 90 degrees.
3. Now press into the floor with your right hand and rotate your torso so your left hand goes up toward the ceiling. In this position, your upper body will have a "T" shape.
4. Bring your hand back down, and repeat on the other side.

Lunge 7: 45-Degree Lunge

1. Stand with your feet hip-width apart, arms at your sides.
2. Take a big lunge step forward and 45 degrees from your body to the right with your right foot, descending until both of your knees form 90-degree angles. Your right foot steps to 2 o'clock here. Keep your hips facing forward throughout the move.
3. Press through your right foot to return to start, and repeat on your left side, stepping to 10 o'clock.

Lunge 8: Airplane Lunge

1. Stand with your feet together.
2. Step about 3 feet forward with your right leg, planting your foot flat on the floor.
3. Lean forward so your left leg comes off the ground and goes behind you as you balance your body over your right leg. Your arms should be out to the sides, forming a "T."
4. In this position, keep your hips level and twist your torso to the left so your left hand goes down to your right foot, and your right hand points toward the ceiling.
5. Untwist, stand up, and take the next step forward with your left leg. Repeat.

Lunge 9: Airplane Lunge, Reverse Twist

Same as the previous lunge, but twist in the other direction—on a right-footed step forward, your right hand will come down to your right foot.

Lunge 10: Curtsy Lunge with Reach

1. Stand with your feet hip-width apart, hands on your hips.
2. Take a big step backward and to the left with your right leg so that your right foot crosses over your left foot as if you were going to curtsy. Descend as you step until both knees are bent 90 degrees, or as deep as you can go. Reach your right hand up high, and your left hand low as you lunge.
3. Press through the heel of your left foot back to start, and repeat the move on the other side, this time stepping back with your left foot and reaching up with your right hand.

THE 21-MINUTE WORKOUT THAT BUILDS WORLD CUP WINNERS

The US Women's National Soccer Team has dominated the last two World Cups because they've got Megan Rapinoe and Alex Morgan netting goals, midfielder Rose Lavelle patrolling the entire field, and defenders like Kelley O'Hara locking down their opponents' best scorers. But the USWNT also wins because all those amazing athletes are so *prepared*. And when they're gunning for another World Cup victory, the USWNT have to prepare not just to play championship soccer, but to play a lot of it.

"We're preparing for the most world-renowned tournaments, and they're on condensed schedules—with the goal of seven games in under a month for the World Cup," compared to just one or two games per week on their club teams, says Ellie Maybury, head of performance for the USWNT. "The intensity and the game schedule [are] that much more elevated."

To help prepare the team for back-to-back games, Maybury and her team put the US superstars through batteries of conditioning drills that would leave lesser athletes gasping. Some, like this 21-minute Pitch Widths workout, are deceptively simple . . . but brutally efficient. Head to a local soccer field to see if you can keep up with the world's best.

How to do it:
1. After warming up thoroughly, stand on the sideline of a soccer field.
2. Run the width of the field and back in 25 seconds or less.
3. Rest for 25 seconds.
4. Repeat 5 times.
5. Jog 2 minutes to recover.
6. Repeat 2 more rounds of 5 pitch widths, jogging for 2 minutes in between.

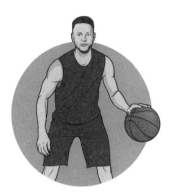

DRIBBLE AND SWEAT WITH STEPH CURRY'S DRILLS

Steph Curry's so slick with his dribbling that Allen Iverson—who broke Michael Jordan's ankles!—said that Curry has a better handle than a young AI.

To warm up that ball-handling, Curry does this two-basketball drill before games. It takes the Golden State great just three minutes—but for us normals, it'll take much longer, and could prove to be a workout in and of itself.

1. Holding one ball in each hand, toss them lightly from the sides over your head so they bump together. Catch and repeat 6 times.
2. Push your hips back to bend down so you're dribbling the balls with both hands. Bounce them at the same time 20 times.
3. Same position: Alternate the bounce for 20 bounces.
4. Same position: Cross the balls in front of you 10 times.
5. Same position: Bounce them so they cross between your legs (!). Do this 10 times.
6. Same position: Simultaneously bounce them left and right. Repeat 20 times.
7. Same position: Now alternate the left-and-right bounce: Both balls come in, then both go back out. Repeat 20 times.
8. Bring your feet together, and perform double-bounces front to back 20 times.
9. Same position: Alternate front-to-back bounces 20 times.
10. Stand up. Dribble one ball normally, while dribbling the other ball between your legs, catching it with the same hand. Do this 10 times with each arm.
11. Dribble the left ball between your legs, then the right ball, then cross both. Do this 10 times.

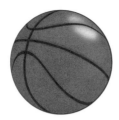

THE 30-MINUTE, SHIRT-SOAKING WORKOUT THAT WILL FINALLY TEACH YOU TO DRIBBLE WITH YOUR LEFT HAND

We can't all handle like Curry. If you're a pickup regular who can only dribble to your strong side, you're not alone—even some NBA players have this problem. When Jeremy Lin sparked "Linsanity" in 2012, the knock on the former Harvard guard was that he couldn't go left.

"[Players] always want to go to the strong side because that's where they feel most comfortable," and that can lead to an even greater disparity between the skills in the hands, says Mike Allen, a high school, college, and Junior NBA coach at Mike Allen Sports. Improving off-hand dribbling is a big part of what Allen does with hundreds of players each year. It takes practice, though—you're not going to improve it during a game, he says, since you'll go back to your most comfortable moves.

If you're a typical adult, though, you don't have time for basketball practice, but you *do* need cardio. With this 30-minute ball-handling workout from Allen, you can do double duty—get your heart-pumping cardio while helping your handle. You'll need two basketballs, two cones (or empty water bottles), and a bouncy medicine ball—a 6-, 8-, or 10-pounder. Swap this workout in for one of your cardio workouts each week.

WORKOUT CONTINUES >>>

Do each of these drills twice, resting 30 seconds between drills.

Drill 1: Double Dribbles
In a wide, athletic stance, dribble two balls—one in each hand. Continue for one minute.

Drill 2: Double V-Dribbles
In the same position, dribble the balls in "V" shapes in front of you, keeping the balls going no higher than knee level. Continue for one minute.

Drill 3: Double Dribbles with Single Passes
1. Stand 6 to 8 feet in front of a wall. Dribble both balls in front of you in an athletic position.
2. After a few dribbles, use your right hand to bounce pass the right ball against the wall while continuing to dribble with your left.
3. Retrieve the right-hand ball, get your bearings, then bounce pass the left ball toward the wall. Continue alternating in this way for three minutes.

Drill 4: Cone in One Hand Drill
1. Hold a cone in your stronger hand and dribble with your weak hand. Do three dribbles as you move around the court.
2. Put the cone down, then do three crossovers.
3. Pick the cone back up with your strong hand, still dribbling with your weak hand. Continue for 3 rounds of 1 minute each, resting 30 seconds between rounds.

Drill 5: Medicine Ball Double Dribble and Push-Up
1. Dribble a medicine ball with your weaker hand for eight bounces.
2. Then put the ball on the floor and perform two push-ups with your weaker hand elevated on the ball.
3. Stand up, and repeat on the other side, dribbling eight times with your strong hand, then doing two push-ups with your strong hand on the ball. Repeat for 8 rounds.

Drill 6: Medicine Ball Dribble, Slam, Dribble
1. Do three dribbles with the medicine ball with your weak hand, then grab the ball with both hands, bring it overhead, and slam it down onto the ground.
2. Dribble three times with your strong hand, then slam again. Continue for 8 rounds.

THE TREADMILL WORKOUT OF THE NFL'S TOUGHEST TAILBACK

Since blasting onto the scene as a freshman at the University of Oklahoma, Adrian Peterson (aka All Day, or AD) has run over more than 11 billion unsuspecting defenders in his 15 NFL seasons. More than half of his career yards have come after contact because AD's legs just keep churning. He shared the superhuman treadmill workout he uses to train for that endurance on Twitter in 2018. Peterson's tip: "Pray and ask for strength before starting!"

Here's a halfway-there AD challenge: Are you half as tough as the NFL's toughest tailback?

The workout (you'll run for a total of 3.5 miles):
Mile 0–0.5: Run at 6 mph.
Mile 0.5–1: Run at 9 mph.
Miles 1–3.5: Alternate one-eighth-mile "laps" on the treadmill: Odd-number laps should be run between 5 and 6.5 mph, and even-number laps at 12 mph. Repeat for 20 laps to run the remaining 2.5 miles.

BURN IT LIKE BECKHAM

David Beckham isn't just really, really ridiculously good-looking. In his prime, he was one of the best on the planet—and his training helps explain why. This treadmill challenge helped keep him fit for the pitch and kept his body fat microscopic. Beckham revealed it to Adam Bornstein, author of *Engineering the Alpha*, in 2012.

To do it, start by calculating your max heart rate by subtracting your age from 220. (So if you're 40, your max is 180.) Wearing a heart rate monitor, you'll then run for two minutes at 95 percent of that heart rate. Rest for a minute, then repeat eight times.

Yes: *Eight.* No wonder Bornstein labeled this one of the "Hardest Workouts in the World!"

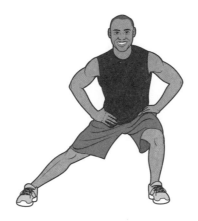

SEE IF YOU CAN TACKLE AN NFL SACKMASTER'S RETIREMENT WORKOUT

DeMarcus Ware looks like he could step back onto an NFL field at any moment—and go right back to slamming quarterbacks to the turf. Since retiring in 2016, the nine-time Pro Bowl linebacker has stayed in game-ready shape—and shared his fitness challenges with social media followers and clients at 3Volt Fitness, his gym in Trophy Club, Texas.

This two-dumbbell interval challenge is a favorite of Ware's—and is often done at his gym. Perform each exercise combination for 6 sets of 30 seconds each, resting 15 seconds between exercises.

EXERCISE Combo 1: Half-Squat Dumbbell Curls with Squat Thrust

1. Assume the classic push-up position, but with your hands on the dumbbells: Your hands should be about shoulder-width apart, your body forming a straight line from head to heels.
2. Jump your feet forward and outside the dumbbells so you're halfway into a wide squat.
3. Curl the dumbbells off the floor up to your shoulders, then return them to the ground.
4. Jump back to the top of the push-up position. Repeat: Jump up, curl, jump back.

EXERCISE Combo 2: Modified Push-Up and Row

1. Assume the starting position from exercise combo 1, but bring your feet closer to the dumbbells—in this position, your knees will be bent and slightly off the ground, your upper body forming a tabletop.
2. Keeping your back straight, bend your elbows to lower your chest between the dumbbells, then press back up.
3. At the top, row the right dumbbell to the side of your chest. Return the dumbbell to the floor, do another push-up, and row the left dumbbell.
4. Repeat this sequence: push-up, row, push-up, row.

EXERCISE Combo 3: Thruster

1. Curl the dumbbells up onto your shoulders and stand with your feet slightly wider than shoulder-width apart, toes pointed slightly out.
2. Keep your weight in your heels and push your hips back to squat, descending until your thighs are at least parallel to the floor.
3. Press through your heels back to standing, and press the dumbbells overhead until your elbows are by your ears.
4. Bring the dumbbells back to your shoulders and squat again.

EXERCISE 4: Lateral Squat

1. Stand with your feet wide, toes pointed forward, holding one dumbbell in front of you with both hands.
2. Push your hips back and descend to your right by bending your right knee, keeping it tracking over your right toes.
3. Press back to start and perform the move to the left.

TRY THE BOXING FINISHER OF ONE OF THE NFL'S YOUNGEST SACK ARTISTS

Chase Young was already lightning-quick and thunderously strong when he came out of Ohio State in 2020. But the defensive end got an extra boost by training for another sport: boxing.

"Coming off the line, players have to use their hands a lot. Boxing makes their hands faster, their reaction time quicker," says CJ Hammond, owner of Fit Legend and the trainer who introduced Young to the heavy bag as part of his pre-draft routine.

"An average football play is three to four seconds, and you're going all-out. You need to train the way you're going to play—all-out, then rest," Hammond says. Hitting the bag intensely, then resting briefly and repeating, trains Chase—and you—to be able to do this kind of effort repeatedly, whether it's at the line of scrimmage or in a pickup basketball game.

Build some draft pick–worthy, explosive endurance of your own with these heavy bag intervals Hammond uses with Young. Add this as a finisher to the end of a workout where your shoulders, hips, and core are already warmed up.

To do the finisher, you'll do a series of one-two punches on the heavy bag—a jab and a cross. (Not sure how to jab and cross? See instructions on page 297.) Set a timer, and punch as hard and fast as you can—all-out—for 15 seconds. Then punch slower and lighter for 15 seconds. Repeat this—15 seconds hard, 15 seconds easy—for 3 minutes. Rest 35 seconds, then do another 3-minute round.

Start with 2 or 3 rounds, and gradually work your way up to 8 rounds, adding 1 per week.

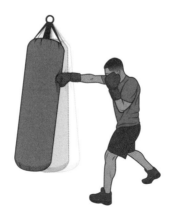

DO SPEED WORK LIKE A KENYAN MARATHONER

Almost every Kenyan marathon champion comes from one ethnic group, the Nandi, who number fewer than 1 million people. There's something special about the Nandi. But Kenneth Mungara is *not* a Nandi—and he's still really fast.

Mungara previously held the world record for marathoners age 40 to 44, at 2 hours, 8 minutes. He's won 11 of the 17 marathons he's ever raced in, and he got started late: Until he was 35, Mungara was a barber. Some of his clients were runners, and when they talked about their training and racing, he thought, *I can beat these guys*. He was right.

Here's the speed workout Mungara performs weekly to get so fast. It's easiest to do at a track, where two laps equal 800 meters, the distance of Mungara's intervals.

After warming up for 5 minutes, run 800 meters at a pace faster than your race pace (Mungara's goal is 2 minutes, 27 seconds). Jog for 100 meters to rest. Repeat this sequence 8 to 10 times.

TRY THE INSANE WORKOUT WATER POLO PLAYERS DO TO STAY FIT

Water polo is "like Greco-Roman wrestling in the water," according to Shea Buckner, a US Olympian–turned–Hollywood actor. Water polo players have to tread water, throw a ball, and wrestle beneath the surface with opponents weighing over 200 pounds.

Their workouts are nuts: four hours of pool time, often fighting against resistance bands tethering them to the pool wall or with weight belts pulling them down.

To get a taste of how they train, Buckner shared this "simpler" workout. If you're a strong swimmer, it's one you've got to try.

To start, tread water near (but not touching) the wall of the pool.

1. Sprint to the other end of the pool as fast as you can, but don't touch the wall.
2. Tread water near the wall with your hands overhead for 10 seconds.
3. Sprint back to the starting wall, but don't touch it. Tread water with arms overhead for another 10 seconds.
4. Rest for 15 seconds.
5. Repeat steps 1 to 4 for 20 rounds.

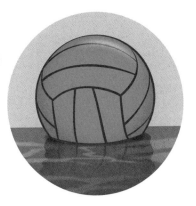

SHRED YOUR CORE LIKE A PING-PONG CHAMP

Olympic table tennis players can burn as many as 500 calories per match, hitting those lightning-fast, long-distance rallies you've seen on YouTube. The points usually only last three to five seconds, but they're blasting shots at 60 mph—with the ball crossing the table in less than a quarter-second.

"You have to put so much power into the ball in such a short time," says Kanak Jha, a two-time Olympian for Team USA. "It takes a lot of explosive power."

To build it, Jha doesn't just spend hours at the table. He also puts in 30 to 90 minutes in the gym daily. But not for his arms and shoulders—table tennis practice covers that. Instead, he's focused on building power in his legs and core—he's rotating his entire torso on each shot. Jha does this 24-minute core workout two to three times a week to build a powerful midsection.

Perform each exercise for 30 seconds. Then, during the next 30 seconds, perform 10 push-ups. Continue in this way—core exercise, 10 push-ups, core exercise, 10 push-ups—until you've completed all eight moves. Repeat the entire sequence three times for a 24-minute workout.

EXERCISE 1: Russian Twist

1. Sit on the floor with your heels on the ground. Your torso should be at a 45-degree angle from the floor, and should be straight from your butt to your head. Place your arms in front of you as a guide.
2. From this position, twist to the left, twisting your whole torso, not just your arms, until your hands point out to 9 o'clock. To use your hands as a guide, your shoulders and chest should remain in the same position relative to your hands as you twist.
3. Twist back to start, and then go to the right, twisting until your shoulders, chest, and hands point toward 3 o'clock. That's 1 repetition.

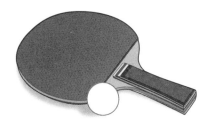

EXERCISE 2: Hanging Knee Raise

1. Hang from a bar with an overhand or neutral grip.
2. Use your core to pull your knees up to your chest. Try not to feel it in your back.
3. Return to hanging and repeat.

EXERCISE 3: Pulse-Up ("Butt Up")

1. Lie on your back with your legs straight up, perpendicular to the floor.
2. Use your core to lift your butt up, moving your feet toward the ceiling.
3. Return to start and repeat.

EXERCISE 4: Side Plank with Rotation: Left Side

1. Assume a side plank position on your left side: Prop yourself up on your left elbow and stack your feet. Your body should form a straight line from head to heels. Point your right arm perpendicular to your torso so it's pointed toward the ceiling.
2. Maintaining your plank, bring your right arm down and under, threading the needle under your left arm.
3. Return back to start, and repeat.

EXERCISE 5: Side Plank with Rotation: Right Side

Do the move on the opposite side.

EXERCISE 6: V-Up

1. Lie on your back with your legs straight and your arms overhead.
2. Without bending your elbows or knees, contract your abdominal muscles. Fold your body up by lifting your legs off the floor and stretch your arms toward your toes. Keep your back straight.
3. Pause, then return to the starting position.

EXERCISE 7: Traditional Crunch

EXERCISE 8: Hollow Body Hold

Start in the same position as the V-up, with your arms and legs fully extended. Lift your arms and legs slightly off the ground, brace your core, and hold.

BECOME KING OF THE CABLE MACHINE WITH THIS LEBRON-INSPIRED WORKOUT

Whether or not you're a fan of LeBron James on the court, he's undeniably the NBA's king of Instagram fitness videos. When he's not jacking you up with fist-pumping dances or plastering sweaty selfies with inspirational quotes, the King is posting snippets of the intense workouts that enable him to continue to dominate his sport in his late 30s.

One piece of equipment gets lots of LeBron love: the cable machine. Get your pull on with pulleys and this 6-move workout, inspired by moves in James's online workouts.

Perform 3 sets of 8 to 12 reps of each move, resting 1 minute between sets.

EXERCISE 1: Lateral Cable Reverse Fly

1. Stand with your feet shoulder-width apart in front of a cable cross machine or a two-cable stack with the handles set at shoulder level. Grab the handles with the opposite hand—right handle in your left hand, left handle in your right hand—so that your arms form an "X."
2. Pull your shoulder blades back and down, squeeze your butt, and tighten your core.
3. Keeping a slight bend in your elbows, pull the cables out until your arms form a "T" shape. Return to the "X" and repeat.

EXERCISE 2: Standing Cable Chest Press

1. Stand with your feet shoulder-width apart with the stack behind your right shoulder. Hold one handle of the cable machine with your right hand next to your right nipple line, elbow bent.
2. Keeping your shoulders square, press your right hand forward until your elbow is nearly straight.
3. Control the cable as you move it back to the starting position. Repeat for all reps. Then switch sides and repeat.

EXERCISE 3: Cable Rotational Chop

1. Stand next to a cable station with a rope attached, cable set low. Kneel on your right knee (closest to the base of the cable), your left knee bent 90 degrees.
2. Grab the rope with both hands and stretch it taut, holding it down below your right hip.
3. Keeping your arms straight, twist and pull the rope up and across your body until it's past your left shoulder. Return to start, repeat for all reps, and then switch sides.

EXERCISE 4: Standing Single-Arm Row

1. Stand in a quarter-squat with your feet about hip-width apart, holding one handle of the cable stack in front of you with an extended arm. Pull your shoulder blades together and down.
2. Maintaining a flat back, bend your elbow to row the handle to the side of your body. Your knuckle should be around your nipple line.
3. Return the cable to start and repeat for all reps. Then switch sides and repeat.

EXERCISE 5: Half-Kneeling Pallof Press

1. Kneel on your left knee (with your right knee at 90 degrees, foot flat on the floor), with a cable stack at around chest level on your right.
2. Pull the cable out and hold it against the front of your chest with both hands. The cable should be taut. Hold your core tight.
3. Maintaining this body position, press the cable straight out away from your chest— the cable will try to rotate you toward the station. Resist this rotation. Return the handle to your chest and repeat.
4. After 12 reps, switch your knees—put your right knee down, with the cable stack still on your right. Repeat, then repeat both positions with the stack to your left.

EXERCISE 6: Side Plank Cable Row

1. Lie on your left side in a side plank position, facing a low cable pulley. Prop yourself up on your left elbow, with your feet stacked and your body forming a straight line from head to heels.
2. Maintaining this body position, row the handle of the cable machine with your right arm until your hand is in line with your torso.
3. Return the cable to start and repeat for all reps. Then switch sides and repeat.

DO THE 20-MINUTE AB WORKOUT OF A WORLD CHAMPION

Chris Algieri may be the smartest man in boxing—between bouts, the WBO international junior welterweight champion has earned a master's degree in clinical nutrition, and has future plans to attend medical school. He's used those brains to help him build and maintain brawn into his mid-30s.

"I would take time off when I was younger with my strength and conditioning . . . now, I have to do it year-round" to stay healthy and in fighting shape, he says. He has fewer sparring sessions, but they're more intense in terms of building strength and power.

Algieri's nutrition has changed, too. He's added a focus on vasodilators, foods that dilate blood vessels so more blood flows to recovering muscles. Algieri provides this and more nutrition advice to other fighters as a consultant, and in his book, *The Fighter's Diet*. Incorporating vasodilating foods, like beets and fatty fishes, he says, has helped with his recovery from twice-daily training sessions.

One thing he hasn't cut back on as he's aged: ab work. Like any fighter worth his spit bucket, Algieri has built a midsection that can take a punch—well, lots of punches. Build your own championship core with this two-part, 20-minute session from the smartest fighter in the business.

PART 1: 400 REPS

Algieri does 400 consecutive repetitions of ab exercises during each workout. To reach that number, he performs 50-rep sets each of moves for his upper abs, lower abs, rotational core muscles, and lower back. Use one of the sample exercises below, or choose a different move for each category. Do 2 rounds of 50 reps of each move.

Upper Abs: Slant Board Sit-Up
1. Lie faceup with your legs under the pads of a slant board with your knees bent. Cross your arms over your chest.
2. Maintain a flat back as you sit up until your arms touch your thighs.
3. Return to start. Repeat.

Lower Abs: Hanging Leg Raise
1. Hang from a bar with a shoulder-width, overhand grip.
2. Keep your legs straight and together as you use your core to lift your legs up in front of you until your body forms a 90-degree angle.
3. Lower your legs back to start, and repeat.

Rotational Core: Seated Russian Twist

1. Sit on the floor with your heels on the ground. Your torso should be at a 45-degree angle from the ground, and should be straight from your butt to your head. Place your arms in front of you as a guide.
2. From this position, twist to the left, twisting your whole torso, not just your arms, until your hands point out to 9 o'clock. To use your hands as a guide, your shoulders and chest should remain in the same position relative to your hands as you twist.
3. Twist back to start and then go to the right, twisting until your shoulders, chest, and hands point toward 3 o'clock. That's one repetition.

Lower Back: Superman

1. Lie facedown on the floor with arms and legs extended.
2. Lift your arms, legs, and head up off the floor. You'll look like you're flying like Superman. Hold for a beat.
3. Return to the floor. Repeat.

PART 2: PLANKS

Algieri finishes his ab session with 12 minutes of planks—not in one straight hold, though. He performs 4 rounds of 3-minute planks, resting 30 seconds between each plank.

Round 1: Forearm Plank

1. Assume the classic forearm plank position: Your elbows should be directly beneath your shoulders, your body forming a straight line from head to heels.
2. Squeeze your core and hold this position for 3 minutes, then rest 30 seconds.

Round 2: Side Plank, Left Side

1. Prop yourself up on your left elbow, with feet stacked and body forming a straight line from head to heels.
2. Brace your core and hold this position for 3 minutes. Then rest 30 seconds.

Round 3: Side Plank, Right Side

1. Prop yourself up on your right elbow, with feet stacked and body forming a straight line from head to heels.
2. Brace your core and hold this position for 3 minutes. Then rest 30 seconds.

Round 4: Forearm Plank

Perform for 3 minutes, then rest 30 seconds.

HOW MODERN BOXERS JUMP ROPE LIKE ALI

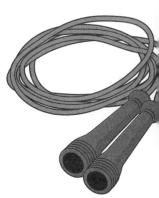

They may not chase chickens, but pro boxers like Algieri definitely have one training method in common with Rocky: They skip rope. A lot.

"I use it as a warm-up and a cooldown around my boxing sessions," Algieri says. And he takes his cues on how to jump rope from the Greatest.

Muhammad Ali used to say that when you're jumping rope, try not to step in the same place twice, Algieri says. Algieri moves between double-foot jumping, skips from foot to foot, changes his pace . . . but always moves his feet to new spots. "It's to help your footwork, and help your movement in the ring."

Try Algieri's Ali-inspired jump-rope session for yourself. Do 5 rounds of 3 minutes of jumping, mixing your pace and style of jumping, but always landing in new places. Just like a fight, rest 30 seconds between rounds.

KURT ANGLE'S RIDICULOUSLY ANGLED PITTSBURGH CLIMB

Long before he was jumping from the top ropes in WWE, Kurt Angle trained for the 1996 Olympics with punishing, daylong workouts around his native Pittsburgh. News footage at the time would show Angle with neck veins bulging, screaming as he sprinted up one of the city's steepest hills, Sycamore Street—while carrying a training partner on his back.

Even without a piggyback, this hill is a gasser: Its grade is more than 20 percent, and it serves as one of the Steel City's toughest challenges for riders in the annual Dirty Dozen bike race (see page 10), which climbs the city's steepest slopes.

Point your GPS to the intersection of Sycamore Street and Lava Street, then look for a place to park farther up the hill. Pick out a steep 200-yard stretch to sprint between here and the peak of Mount Washington—Angle says he would do 200s like this as many as 30 times in a row after a 6- to 7-mile run through the city. For a less Olympian-level workout, try starting with five sprints . . . then head to the top for amazing views of the skyline.

DO A UFC FIGHTER'S CONFIDENCE-BOOSTING CARDIO WORKOUT

A five-minute round in an MMA ring feels as long as a marathon, but a fight is really like a series of short, all-out sprints—sprints you're doing while being punched, kicked, and strangled.

"You could be in the best shape of your life . . . but you're getting hit. You're taking damage," says UFC bantamweight Rob Font. That damage makes fighters tired, makes every move hurt, and makes it more difficult to execute skills they've practiced thousands of times.

At Skill of Strength, the Massachusetts gym where the 32-year-old fighter trains, "We just go through hell" to be ready to execute through the pain: "The better shape you're in, the more you can think clearly and feel more confident that you can get the job done."

Skill of Strength's Mike Perry puts Font through a battery of workouts to build that confidence, and "They all suck," but this interval conditioning routine is the fighter's favorite. Using an assault bike—the type with simultaneous arm-and-leg movement, and a fan—Font does all-out sprints with brief periods of rest.

To do Font's workout, start by warming up for 5 minutes. Then perform all-out intervals in one of two ways: In option 1, sprint all-out for 10 seconds, then rest for 20 seconds. Repeat this 15 times. Sprinting for 10 seconds is "easier" than longer bouts like 30 seconds, because you're less likely to dog it. You can really go all-out.

Once you feel like you can really push, try Font's longer option: Sprint for 30 to 35 seconds, again going as fast and hard as possible. Rest for 90 seconds between sprints. Repeat five times.

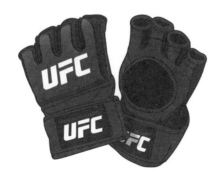

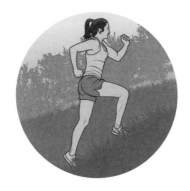

SPRINT HILLS LIKE A HALL OF FAMER

Hill sprints are simple: Get to the top . . . fast! They work, too: One study found that sprinting for just 2.5 total minutes burns up to 200 calories during the day. And hills help: Running uphill shortens your stride so you're less likely to pull your hamstrings.

Another study, conducted by me, found that when you get to the top, you'll feel awesome. Gaze down on what you just climbed, breathe heavily, and know you're doing the same workout that helped build power for some of the most legendary athletes in history. Here are two of their favorite hills you've got to visit.

Sweetness's Slope

Walter Payton (aka Sweetness) credited hills for his legendary lasting power: 13 NFL seasons, and power that seemed to increase as games wore on. From his childhood, Payton would find a hill and sprint up over and over until he was worn out, trying to do one more with each workout. Sweetness called his last hill—a dirt pile in a landfill in Chicago's Arlington Heights suburb—a "will-maker."

Today, the landfill is a park, but the hill is still there. It's surprisingly easy to find and surprising to run: It doesn't look like much, but by the fifth or sixth sprint, you're gassed. Take a breather at the top and check out Payton's plaque, commemorating the site where the Bears' GOAT built those legendary legs.

The hill is at Nickol Knoll Golf Club in Arlington Heights. It's free to visit. Just put the course in your GPS or visit https://www.ahpd.org/golf/nickol-knoll-golf-club/.

Jerry Rice's Redwood City Run-Up

For more than two decades, Jerry Rice made defenders look silly—jumping over defenders and outrunning the opposition to score 197 career touchdowns. And he credits his own hill, south of San Francisco, with giving him the conditioning to stay so great for so long.

Rice's hill is a tree-lined trail through the woods of Edgewood Park & Nature Preserve, an unassuming park in Emerald Hills, California. Like Payton's place, Rice's hill is deceptive—it's not a super-steep grade, but it just never stops climbing; for 2.5 miles, you're almost always running uphill. For Rice-like results, take those grades with gusto: Try sprinting or running hard up each rise and switchback.

Point your GPS to "'The Hill' Starting Point, Old Stage Coach Road." Go to the back of the parking lot, to a dirt and grass area that runs parallel to a private road. Look for the sign marked "Sylvan Trail Exercise Loop." Start here.

Getting to the top: It's not crystal-clear how to get to the top from here, so bring these directions along. From the starting post, start running. Make the first left to stay on the Sylvan Trail, heading up into the woods. There's one fork along this path in the first mile—take the upper route. You'll reach a clearing with another sign; stay left to head up the Live Oak Trail, which ironically, doesn't have many trees. Climb up those switchbacks.

There's another sign at the midway point up this hill face—follow it right toward SCENIC VIEW. You'll see one more sign: Turn left toward SCENIC VIEW and hit the top—you know you're there when you see a memorial bench. The bench's plaque includes the quote, "What are we doing that's fun today?" Your answer: Climbing like the NFL's greatest receiver!

TRY THE 500-REPETITION WORKOUT OF A CHAMPION NATURAL BODYBUILDER

Building muscle size worth showing off takes volume—the total amount of weight you lift in a workout. And packing on that size is even harder when you're all-natural, like Brandon Lirio. The owner of Battleground Fitness in Newington, Connecticut, Lirio was the 2019 Mr. Natural Olympia in Classic Physique—meaning he was tested to be sure he's drug-free.

To get in a ton of volume fast, Lirio's go-to workout is his Centurion workout strategy. It's a minimal-rest, maximum-rep strategy to get in 500 repetitions in about 15 minutes.

To create a Centurion workout, pick four to five exercises that can be done using a single apparatus—one or two of the same dumbbells, or one cable attachment. You'll then do 100 repetitions of each exercise, taking breaks of three to five seconds—but no longer—as needed.

For a sample Centurion, try these moves on a single cable pulley station. Do 100 reps of the first exercise, resting minimally, then move to the next exercise without resting.

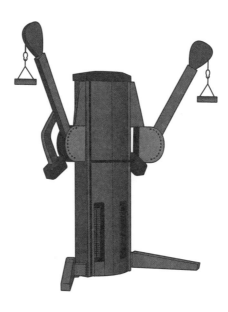

EXERCISE 1: Rope Tricep Pushdown (100 reps)

1. Stand in front of a cable stack with the pulley set high and the rope attachment clipped onto the cable. Grab each side of the rope with one hand in front of your chest, palms facing in.
2. Keeping your shoulders back and torso upright, push the rope down by straightening your arms so your fists are by your thighs.
3. Return to start. Repeat.

EXERCISE 2: Rope Face Pull (100 reps)

1. With the pulley still set high, grab each side of the rope with one hand in an overhand grip, palms facing forward. Take a big step back so the rope and cable are taut, with your arms straight out from your shoulders at or above eye level, the points of your elbows out. You should be in a staggered stance.
2. Keeping your elbows at shoulder height, pull the rope so the center comes toward your face.
3. Straighten your arms to return to start. Repeat.

EXERCISE 3: Rope Hammer Curl (100 reps)

1. Set the cable stack's pulley in a low position. Grab each end of the rope with an underhand grip. Begin with your hands next to your thighs.
2. Keeping an upright torso, bend your elbows to curl your hands up to your shoulders.
3. Return to start. Repeat.

EXERCISE 4: Rope Standing Row (100 reps)

1. With the pulley still set low, hold the rope with an overhand grip at your thighs.
2. Pull your elbows up so your hands come up next to your neck, palms facing down. At the top, your elbows will be higher than your hands.
3. Return to start. Repeat.

EXERCISE 5: Rope Cable Crunch (100 reps)

1. Set the pulley up high again. Stand facing away from the cable stack. Place the center of the rope behind your neck, and hold the ends of the rope against your chest. The cable should be taut in this position.
2. Flex your waist so your torso pulls the rope down and forward—the same move as when doing a crunch on the floor, but while standing.
3. Return to start. Repeat.

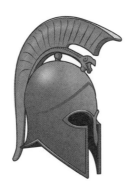

CRUSH THAT OBSTACLE RACE LIKE A SPARTAN-RACING PRO

Rose Wetzel has always liked to run, and run fast: Long before she was an *American Ninja Warrior* star, a professional Spartan racer, or an all-American at Georgetown, she had a paper route. And she *ran* her paper route—fast.

"I always liked running fast. I liked being explosive and powerful," she says. And her high-energy pursuit of that childlike thrill has led the 38-year-old to some serious achievements: Besides her feats as a Ninja and a college runner, Wetzel has run a sub-five-minute mile, ridden a 200-mile bike race, and won 26 Spartan races.

"I didn't make [the Olympic] trials . . . so [I thought] let's go run in the woods and jump over things," she says. "It felt like play!"

To get to that play, she still does serious training. Here's a workout Wetzel has used to get ready for Spartan's 5K and 10K distance races. Head to a local track to try it.

Throughout the workout, you'll run at about an 8-out-of-10 effort—one lap if you're training for a 5K obstacle race, or two laps if you're training for a 10K. You'll then perform an exercise for 30 seconds or one lap. You'll rest briefly, run again, then do another exercise. The workout continues in this way for six exercises, doing 2 rounds of each.

Here's a sample workout to try, following this formula:

RUN 1: 400 meters (one lap) at a medium-hard pace. (If training for a 10K, do two laps.)
OBSTACLE 1: Burpees: 30 seconds.
REST: 30 seconds (Over time, reduce the rest period, eventually eliminating it.)

....

RUN 2: 400 meters
OBSTACLE 2: Alternating Lunge: 30 seconds.
REST: 30 seconds.

....

RUN 3: 400 meters
OBSTACLE 3: Bear Crawl: One lap.
REST: 30 seconds.

....

RUN 4: 400 meters
OBSTACLE 4: Sandbag Carry: Jog one lap carrying a sandbag on your shoulders.
REST: 30 seconds.

....

RUN 5: 400 meters
OBSTACLE 5: Push-Ups: 30 seconds.
REST: 30 seconds.

....

RUN 6: 400 meters
OBSTACLE 6: Jump-Squat: 30 seconds.
REST: 30 seconds.

....

REPEAT: Repeat the runs and obstacles for 1 more round.

HOW AMERICA'S FASTEST MARATHONER GOT SUPER SWOLE

Ryan Hall is the only US-born runner to run a marathon in less than two hours, five minutes (at the 2011 Boston Marathon) and he was the first American to run a half-marathon in less than an hour (in 2007). And when he was breaking those records, he was thinner than the walls of your first apartment.

Just after retirement in 2016, though, Hall got swole, adding 38 pounds of muscle four months after hanging up his distance shoes. He's built serious strength since then as he's launched his coaching company, Run Free: Hall can deadlift and squat more than 400 pounds.

So choose your own gym-venture: Run like the marathon champion with his skinny-era tempo workout, or lift like the buff coach with one of the workouts he's used to add size.

Running Ryan's Tempo

Tempo run is runner-speak for a workout consisting of a warm-up, then a bout of running at a hard, consistent pace—usually their goal race pace. When Hall was competing, he said that tempo runs were the most important part of his training. But instead of running a single hard effort, he'd break the tempo into multiple parts—three hard efforts of 4 miles each instead of a single, 12-mile effort.

To do a run like this, start by warming up for five to ten minutes, then run your chosen chunk of mileage at your goal race pace. Slow down to catch your breath for a few minutes, then repeat two more times.

Swole Ryan's Supersets

Just because he started lifting doesn't mean Hall lost his endurance. His muscle-building routines require some serious wind. Here's a chest and back routine Hall did on Monday and Thursday each week as he added those 35 pounds. Tuesdays and Fridays, Hall lifted arms. Wednesdays and Saturdays were leg days.

For all supersets, perform exercise A, then move to exercise B without resting. After finishing exercise B, rest 45 seconds, then repeat for as many sets as listed.

SUPERSET 1

EXERCISE A: Incline Dumbbell Bench Press (10 sets of 4 to 10 reps)

1. Lie faceup on an incline bench and hold dumbbells over your chest with an overhand grip.
2. Bend your elbows to lower the weights to the sides of your chest. Your elbows should stay close to your sides, forming a 45-degree angle.
3. Pause for a beat, then press back to start.

EXERCISE B: Chin-Up (10 sets, each to failure)

1. Hang from the bar with an underhand grip with your hands about shoulder-width apart.
2. Pull your chin toward the bar by bending your elbows. To help engage your back, concentrate on bringing your elbows down to touch your lats instead of thinking about bringing your chin over the bar.
3. Return to the start position, and repeat.

SUPERSET 2

EXERCISE A: Barbell Bench Press (8 sets of 4 to 10 reps)

1. Lie faceup on the bench and grab the bar with an overhand grip just wider than shoulder-width. Push your heels into the floor and unrack it, holding the bar above your sternum with straight arms.
2. Brace your core and bend your elbows to lower the bar to your chest. Your elbows should stay close to your sides, forming a 45-degree angle.
3. Pause for a beat, then press back to start.

EXERCISE B: Dumbbell Single-Arm Bent-Over Row (8 sets of 4 to 10 reps)

1. Stand with a firm bench on your left side.
2. Place your left knee on the bench, then bend your torso forward and place your left hand on the bench to support your body. In this position, your upper body should be parallel to the floor.
3. Reach down and grab the dumbbell with your right hand, returning to this position where your body is parallel to the floor, with the weight hanging straight down from your right shoulder.
4. Maintaining that upper body position, pull your right arm straight up until your hand reaches the side of your chest.
5. Lower the weight back to the starting position, and repeat. Do all your reps on this side, then switch sides and repeat.

WORKOUT CONTINUES >>>

SUPERSET 3

EXERCISE A: Dumbbell Fly (5 sets of 4 to 10 reps)

1. Lie faceup on a bench holding light dumbbells over your chest with palms in, elbows slightly bent.
2. Separate your arms to the sides until your body forms a "T" shape and you feel a stretch in your chest.
3. Hug the weights back together. Repeat.

EXERCISE B: Dumbbell Pullover (5 sets of 4 to 10 reps)

1. Lie perpendicular to a bench, with your upper back on the bench, knees bent 90 degrees. In this position, hold a dumbbell by one end over your chest with slightly bent elbows and an overhand grip.
2. Lower the weight over your head until your arms are even with your shoulders—as if they're overhead when you're standing.
3. Bring the weight back to start.

FINISHER

EXERCISE A: Diamond Push-Ups (100 reps)

1. Assume a modified push-up position, with your hands together beneath your sternum, and your feet slightly wider than normal. Your body should still form a straight line from head to heels.
2. Maintaining this rigid body position, bend your elbows to lower your chest to your hands.
3. Press back to start. Repeat.

EXERCISE B: Ab Work

Perform 10 minutes of ab exercises, alternating 1 minute of work, 1 minute of rest.

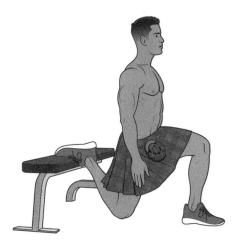

BE WORTHY OF A KILT: TRAIN LIKE A SCOTTISH GAMES PRO

Burly men in kilts flipping 200-pound logs, heaving 56-pound stones, and using a pitchfork to toss a filled burlap sack over a bar . . . what's not to love about Scottish Highland Games?

To get ready for all that throwing—in all, more than 400 pounds of implements are tossed, scooped, and flipped—Highland Games athletes have to be not only strong, but agile and explosive.

The key is moving the weight *fast*, according to Beau Fay, a professional Highland Games competitor who has competed for 18 years. Whether they're throwing a 16-pound stone for distance or flipping a 200-pound log in the caber toss, "The name of the game is to speed that thing up as fast as possible."

To stay competitive—and to continue to do so into his late 30s—Fay performs explosive movements and concentrates on the speed of the weight in his other exercises. Try this session to get a feel for how Fay stays powerful as he approaches 40.

EXERCISE 1: Power Snatch (5 sets of 3 reps each)

1. Stand over the barbell with your feet hip-width apart.
2. Squat down and grab the bar with a wide, overhand grip. Keep your torso upright.
3. Pull the bar off the floor by extending your hips and knees. As it passes your knees, raise your shoulders so the bar comes up over your head. The barbell should move in a straight line from the floor to overhead.
4. Return the bar to your shoulders, then to the floor. After warming up, perform 5 sets. This is an exercise best coached by a trainer at first.

WORKOUT CONTINUES >>>

EXERCISE 2: Bulgarian Split Squat (5 sets of 5 reps on each leg)

1. With a bar on your shoulders or dumbbells in your hands, place one foot behind you on the bench, with your other foot in front so you're in a position similar to a lunge.
2. Keeping your torso upright, push your hips back and bend your front knee to descend into a split squat.
3. Press through your front heel to return to the starting position.

EXERCISE 3: Romanian Deadlift (5 sets of 8 reps)

1. Unrack the barbell in front of you, palms facing the front of your thighs.
2. Push your hips back to bend at the waist and lower your body until your back is parallel to the floor. Let the weight hang down as you bend, and maintain a flat back.
3. Thrust your hips forward to return to standing to complete 1 rep.

EXERCISE 4: Push Press (5 sets of 5 reps)

1. Grasp a barbell from a rack at chest height with an overhand grip. Unrack it and hold it in front of you in rack position, your feet slightly wider than shoulder-width apart.
2. Bend your knees slightly, dip your hips, and explode up, pressing the bar overhead.
3. Return the bar to your chest and repeat.

WANT TO GET HIGH(LAND)?

Lifting weights is great, but let's talk about the fun stuff—throwing stones and hammers and giant logs! If you want to try out the implements for Highland Games, you may find a Celtic or Scottish festival that lets bystanders give these events a shot with lighter weights, but Fay says that's rare.

If you're serious about training to potentially compete, he says, look for local training groups on Facebook and other social media: These Scottish Games competitors are friendly and welcoming, and have the hammers, stones, and cabers needed to learn the techniques.

CHAPTER 9

BE A HERO

They pull us away from danger, push us toward justice, lift us up to our highest potential, and inspire us when we're at our deepest depths. Our heroes give us a better world—and better versions of ourselves—because they've got guts.

Well, actually, thanks to exercise, most of them don't have guts—they're trim and fighting-fit, thanks to grueling runs, intense lifts, and tests of their will that make sure they're ready when we need their helping hands.

Time to feel heroic: Try their workouts to appreciate what these amazing people go through to keep our world safe . . . and see if they make you a little more gutsy, too.

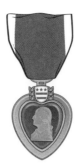

DO 101 REPS LIKE A HERO

....

When a roadside bomb took his left arm and left leg, Noah Galloway thought he was "done"—done with the Army career he loved and done with the workouts that had helped him excel.

Galloway was depressed, unhappy, and felt as if he couldn't do anything without being stared at. But one day, he decided he wanted to be happy again. And for him, part of feeling happy was exercising.

His love of working out had blossomed at age 12, and continued into adulthood and into his service—and, he says, it helped him become himself again after his injury. Since then, he's inspired millions of people as a motivational speaker, fitness cover model, contestant on *Dancing with the Stars*, and as the author of *Living with No Excuses*.

Thirteen years after his injury, Galloway is still in the gym and his favorite workout is simple but no joke: 101 repetitions of whatever exercise he's chosen, in as many sets as it takes to get there, resting as little as possible.

Why 101? Well, it's a lot, so Galloway knows he'll really tax his muscles. But that extra one honors his service: Noah was in the 101st Airborne Division.

On a leg day, for example, Noah will perform his 101s with two exercises: A leg extension and a lying leg curl. For each move, he's using a relatively light weight—probably around 50–60 percent of the amount he could lift for just one repetition.

"The first set may be 30 reps," he says. But as the workout wears on, the sets get shorter and shorter—your last sets may be 3, 4, or 5 repetitions. Choose two exercises for one body part, and complete 101 of each.

DO LEG DAY LIKE AMERICA'S TOUGHEST FIREFIGHTER

When Trisha Jozwiak joined the Denver Fire Department, she felt she had something to prove: "In order for the guys to be comfortable with me, they had to know I would work harder than anyone else," she says.

Sixteen years later, there's no question that Jozwiak is one of the toughest firefighters anywhere—man or woman. The 40-year-old has built a physique that can help her team save lives, and one she's proud to show off: In 2019, she appeared in the Colorado Firefighter Calendar.

Even more amazing: She's done all this with one eye. After losing an eye to cancer as a baby, Jozwiak joined the fire department while wearing a glass eye. Her testers had no idea she was passing the examinations with half the vision of her competitors—and when they found out during her medical exam, she'd already shown that she could make it through! How could you not want to try out the workout of this incredible woman?

Here's her favorite: No surprise, it's leg day. Perform all sets of each exercise before moving to the next exercise. Rest two minutes between sets.

EXERCISE 1: Deadlift
Perform 4 sets of 3 reps of the maximum you can lift for that amount.
1. Stand with the barbell at your shins.
2. Bend at your hips and knees to grab the barbell a little wider than shoulder width. You can use an overhand grip, a mixed grip, or a hook grip. Your feet should be flat on the floor.
3. Keeping your weight in your heels and maintaining the natural curve of your spine, pull the bar up as you thrust your hips forward and stand. The bar should remain close to your body as it comes off the floor.
4. Reverse the maneuver to return to start. Repeat.

EXERCISE 2: Barbell Squat
Perform 4 sets of 3 reps of the maximum you can lift for that amount.
1. Stand in a normal back squat position, barbell across your shoulders, feet between shoulder- and hip-width apart, toes pointing slightly out.
2. Push your hips back to initiate the squat.
3. Bend your knees to descend until your thighs are at least parallel to the floor, keeping your chest up and your weight on your heels.
4. Keep the weight of your body in your heels and press back to standing.

EXERCISE 3: Leg Press
Perform 4 sets of 12 reps. Use the leg press machine and keep the weight pretty heavy,
Jozwiak says.

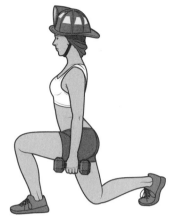

EXERCISE 4: Dumbbell Forward Lunge
Perform 4 sets of 25 to 30 reps on each leg.
1. Stand with your feet shoulder-width apart, dumbbells at your sides, palms facing in.
2. Take a large lunge step forward with your right leg, descending as you step until your knees both form 90-degree angles.
3. Press through your right foot to stand back up.
4. Repeat, this time stepping with your left leg.

EXERCISE 5: Leg Extension
Perform 4 sets of 10 reps. Choose a weight that doesn't burn you out, but is still a fairly heavy lift.

EXERCISE 6: Lying Leg Curl
Perform 4 sets of 10 reps. Choose a weight that doesn't burn you out, but is still a fairly heavy lift.

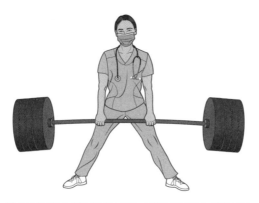

MAX OUT LIKE THIS POWERLIFTING NURSE

When 31-year-old nurse Kelsey Horton works with patients, she brings care, skill, smiles, and another superpower: super strength.

Horton is a mother of two, a surgical nurse, and a competitive powerlifter who can squat and dead-lift more than 400 pounds. And she does all her training to pick up that heavy stuff after finishing her nursing and mom shifts. Then she heads to the gym from 8 to 10 p.m.

Horton says she hopes "to have one mother challenge her own status quo at home and want to take time for herself." Through her training videos on Instagram (@kelseyhorton1989) and her appearance on the athletic game show *The Titan Games*, that's happened. "Mothers have reached out and said I inspired them to actually get to the gym, or even take time to go run."

Horton challenges her status quo in every workout, gunning for new personal records. Here's how this uplifting, powerlifting nurse does squat day.

Squats (2 to 3 working sets of 3 to 5 reps)
1. After warming up, Horton performs a set of three squats with a comfortable weight.
2. Increasing the weight each time, she continues performing sets until she's reached a weight she can only lift once. Between each set, she rests fully.
3. After her max set, she backs the weight off to 80 to 85 percent of her max weight to perform the remaining working sets.

Other Leg Exercises (3 sets of 10 to 12 reps)
1. Leg extensions
2. Lying leg curls
3. Walking barbell lunges

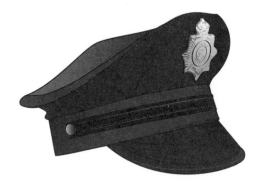

AMERICA'S FITTEST COP HONORS OTHER HEROES WITH THESE WORKOUTS

Casey McAllister fell in love with Crossfit the way many of its devotees do: doing "Murph." Named in honor of Congressional Medal of Honor recipient Michael Patrick Murphy, the workout is the most famous of Crossfit's "Hero" workouts, performed in honor of military members, law enforcement officers, and firefighters who have died in the line of duty. Murph is done by thousands each Memorial Day.

A fellow SWAT officer at the police department in Norman, Oklahoma, invited McAllister to do the workout, and he was hooked. McAllister did hero workouts every day for a year: "Not only was I doing a workout trying to challenge myself, but every day . . . I would read the story of whoever it was [named] for," he says. "There was a deeper meaning to it, and that forced me to work that much harder."

Within a few years, the former "anti-Crossfit" officer had won Crossfit's title of America's Fittest Cop, an honor he earned in 2016 and 2017.

McAllister left his career in law enforcement in late 2018, moving from Oklahoma to Lafayette, Colorado, to start his own box, named Koda CrossFit Iron View—but he's continued doing hero workouts. Here are two of his favorites.

Zachary Tellier

Army sergeant Tellier's unit ran over an explosive device while on patrol in Afghanistan in 2007. Tellier, then 31, pulled two paratroopers from the burning vehicle, burning his hands, before manning the turret to return fire against enemy combatants. He died from wounds sustained in the battle and was posthumously awarded the Bronze Star.

Tellier's memorial workout consists of five sections of bodyweight exercises, completed for time.

1. 10 burpees
2. 10 burpees, 25 push-ups
3. 10 burpees, 25 push-ups, 50 lunges (each leg)
4. 10 burpees, 25 push-ups, 50 lunges, 100 sit-ups
5. 10 burpees, 25 push-ups, 50 lunges, 100 sit-ups, 150 air squats

Murph

Lieutenant Michael Patrick Murphy was scouting in the mountains of Afghanistan in 2005 when more than 50 Taliban militia attacked his four-man SEAL team from three sides, driving the Navy men into a ravine. Stepping into the open to get the reception needed to place a distress call to headquarters, Murphy was shot in the back but still completed the call. Thanks to his efforts, one of Murphy's teammates survived the two-hour gunfight, but he and 18 others were killed. Murphy was posthumously awarded the Congressional Medal of Honor.

The workout named in his honor was one of Murphy's personal favorites, nicknamed Body Armor. Today, it's performed across the country on Memorial Day.

Wearing a 20-pound vest, complete the following events for time, resting as necessary:

1. One-mile run
2. 100 pull-ups
3. 200 push-ups
4. 300 air squats
5. One-mile run

A "beginner" time for completion is around 70 minutes. Elite Crossfit competitors take a little more than a half-hour to finish the event. For an easier version of the workout, perform half of each of these numbers without the vest.

HOW AN ULTRAMARATHON-ING SKI PATROLLER TRAINS HIS MIND FOR 100 MILES

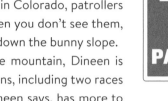

You don't notice heroes like the ski patrol until you really need them—but when you have an accident in a remote corner of a snow-covered mountain, those red-coated super-skiers are there almost instantly. At resorts like Breckenridge in Colorado, patrollers like Ryan Dineen are protecting you even when you don't see them, making sure avalanches don't crush your run down the bunny slope.

When he's not protecting people on the mountain, Dineen is running . . . far. He's run a dozen ultramarathons, including two races over 100 miles. Traversing all those miles, Dineen says, has more to do with his mind than his body.

"There's a lot of intrigue and mystery to it, dealing with, 'Why are you here? Why are you doing this?'" he says. "You've got to answer that with every step."

While Dineen logs lots of miles for long races, he also trains his mind with shorter workouts, including "every minute on the minute," or EMOM training. Every time the clock hits a new minute, you do a new set. When it's done, you rest until the next minute. Dineen does EMOM with weight-lifting exercises, but he says the rowing machine really tests his mettle.

Here's how he does it:
1. Warm up! This is a near-max effort workout, so you should be loose and warm.
2. When your watch hits the start of a new minute, row hard for 30 seconds. You're trying to reach complete exhaustion, so really push yourself.
3. At the 30-second mark, rest.
4. When a new minute starts, row again for 30 seconds. Continue this pattern for 10 to 15 minutes, or until your mind tells you to quit—and you give in.

A WORKOUT INSPIRED BY THE NAVY SEALS

In November 1943, as the US Navy steamed into the Gilbert Islands' Tarawa Atoll, disaster struck for 18,000 Marines: Their landing crafts got hung up on the reef in unexpected places, leaving them to be pounded by Japanese guns on the island—more than 1,000 Marines were killed.

This disaster led to the creation of the Navy's Underwater Demolitions Team, or UDT. Among other underwater duties, these "frogmen"—precursors of the Navy SEALs—would swim in before battles and place explosives on reef areas to clear the way for landing crafts, including at Omaha Beach on D-Day.

This workout from Steve Madden is inspired by Tarawa and the work of the UDT. Madden is the author of *Embrace the Suck*, a memoir about Crossfit, and an avid swimmer and coach.

Consider yourself warned about this session, adapted from a Navy SEALs workout: "If you're not in shape or not comfortable in the water, you're going to kill yourself doing this," Madden says.

You'll need an empty lane in the pool for the lap-swimming portions.

1. Begin in the deep end of a pool with a weight—Madden uses a 25-pound plate.
2. Tread water holding the weight. Or you could do as Steve does: Go down to the bottom of the pool holding it, wait a beat, then push back up for a breath. Whichever you choose, do this for one minute.
3. After 60 seconds, drop the weight and swim the length (or width) of the pool and back.
4. When you get back to where you started, swim down and get your weight. Repeat steps 2 to 4 for as many rounds as you can in 45 minutes.

NOT ALL HEROES WEAR CAPES . . .
OR BADGES OR UNIFORMS . . .

. . . but they're heroes all the same. They can inspire a nation to freedom, teach us to be kind, or just let someone know they should be included, too.

THE WORKOUT THAT SHAPED THE BOSTON MARATHON'S FIRST FEMALE RUNNER

Kathrine Switzer just wanted to do what she loved: run. And it made her a hero.

The running establishment said marathons were dangerous for women's health. Even Switzer's coach initially told her the distance was too long for "fragile women." But the Boston Marathon didn't have a gender line on the application in 1967, and Switzer wanted to run it. So she applied, signing her name as she always did—K. V. Switzer.

Just like that, Switzer became the first woman to officially race Boston. Well, not *just* like that: During the run, race director Jock Semple tried to physically stop Switzer and remove her race number. But she persisted.

"I knew if I quit, nobody would ever believe that women had the capability to run 26-plus miles . . . it would set women's sports back," she wrote in her book, *Marathon Woman*. "If I quit, Jock Semple and all those like him would win."

But she didn't set the sport back: She finished the race and pushed it forward, inspiring thousands of female—and male—runners. At 73, she still inspires . . . and runs, albeit a little slower than she used to: "Let's say I've got 45 minutes in the morning. Now I cover maybe 4.5 miles," she said. "Back in the day . . . I'd knock off a 10K, easy."

Back in the day, she told me, she also did this workout in the run-up to the 1967 Boston: a series of quarter-mile repeats that Switzer says "was torture." You might not have the weight of the entire women's sports world on your shoulders, but you can do the interval workout that trained Switzer in her quest.

Start by warming up: Stretch, jog, and move your body until it's nice and warm. Then run 400 meters—one lap on a regulation track—at your goal marathon pace or better. Jog or walk for 200 meters to recover, then do it again. Repeat this sequence 20 times.

In 1967, Switzer says she ran her 400s in 85 seconds each, jogging her 200s for recovery.

SWIM A MILE IN MR. ROGERS'S SNEAKERS

Some heroes wear cardigans. Mr. Rogers's kindness, gentle teaching, and lessons in dealing with emotion were as heroic as any superhero's acts of derring-do. And he built all those days of singing and sharing with you around a daily workout, as he described in 1982. Each day, he swam a mile.

"I like to swim. But there are days I don't feel much like doing it," he told his neighbors in an episode on discipline. "But I do it anyway. I know it's good for me, and I promised myself I'd do it every day. I try to keep my promises."

And that is one more way we could all stand to be a little more like Fred Rogers. You may not instantly become the kindest person to ever live, but you can hit the pool. Be like Mr. Rogers. Swim a mile.

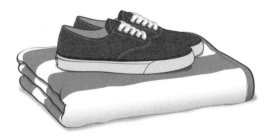

THE WORKOUT OF AN INDIAN WRESTLER WHO INSPIRED INDEPENDENCE

The stereotypical image of an Indian male presented by the media is a skinny IT guy in Bangalore, or even Dev Patel's slight character in *Slumdog Millionaire*. And that stereotype has colonial roots: The British popularized the idea of Indians as "effeminate, weak-kneed, and generally lacking in Victorian masculine virtues," writes historian Joseph Alter. "Although stereotypes such as this were ascribed to Indians by Englishmen, over time it became a pejorative self-image."

But for centuries, Indians revered physical strength—in texts dating back to the 1500s, Indian wrestlers are talked about in mythical terms: eight-foot behemoths eating mountains of almonds and swinging cannons around to get stronger, in addition to doing thousands of push-ups and squats each day as part of 15-hour workouts.

They weren't all myths, though: Gama, a poor, illiterate man born around 1882, walked into London, the belly of the ruling empire, and flipped the stereotype of the "weakling" Indian man onto its back.

When he tried to enter a 1910 world championship wrestling tournament held in London, the organizers wouldn't let Gama in: They said the 5-foot-6, 216-pound Indian was too small to take on the world-beating athletes assembled there. So Gama set up his own show, offering £5 to anyone who would come to a local theater and defeat him. In two days, he'd thrown 13 English wrestlers to the floor, and capped off his performance by trouncing the world champion, who weighed 55 pounds more than Gama.

Physical culture came to be associated with active protest against imperial authority. Gama—known now as the Great Gama—became an icon of the "Freedom Struggle" in India, and helped some on the subcontinent feel nationalism about India, a place that had not existed before colonization, as a contiguous nation.

Gama's strength, stamina, and skill were described as simply incomparable, and the daily workouts his biographers detail would explain why: By the age of 20, Gama is said to have been doing 5,000 bethaks (a type of squat) and 3,000 dandas (a type of push-up) every day, many of them while wearing a 200-pound stone ring around his neck. If you want a taste of this hero's world champion–building workout, start with one from his childhood—a mere 500 bethaks and dandas.

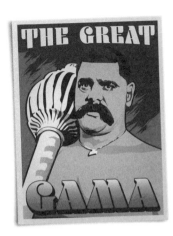

Here's how to do them.

EXERCISE 1: Bethaks, aka "Hindu Squats"
1. Stand with your feet hip-width apart and your arms extended straight in front of you.
2. Bend your knees to squat, keeping the weight on the balls of your feet—your heels will lift up off the ground, unlike in a regular squat.
3. As you lower down, bring your arms down so they're at your sides, keep your head facing forward, and maintain a straight back.
4. At the bottom of the movement, your butt should nearly touch your heels and your fingers should graze the ground. Swing your arms forward as you rise back up to the starting position.
   Unlike regular squats, bethaks push your knees far out in front of your toes, so if you've got knee issues, start with just a few, or skip them completely. If you're going for childhood Gama, though, work your way up to 500.

EXERCISE 2: Dandas, aka "Hindu Push-Ups"
1. Begin in the classic push-up position but bring your feet forward and raise your hips so that your body forms a "V" shape.
2. Keep your hips up as you bend your elbows to drop your chin toward the floor.
3. As your chin approaches the floor, swoop your hips under so they almost touch the floor, swinging your chest up as you raise your head and straighten your arms.
4. Reverse the move to return to start. If you're hoping for Gama levels of intensity, work your way up to 500.

SOME HEROES DO WEAR CAPES— AND THEY WORK OUT, TOO

All these real-life heroes can make all the princess-saving, villain-smashing stars of our favorite movies and cartoons seem a little silly. But they inspire kids—and some kidlike adults—to know the difference between right and wrong. And even they have to get in shape to beat the bad guys. See how you measure up to these mythical heroes.

BUILD MAXIMUM POWER LIKE ANIME'S STRONGEST HERO

The One-Punch Man may be the most powerful superhero in any comic book or movie— he can defeat any foe with a single punch. But in his fictional world, he didn't get these powers by getting bitten by a nuclear spider or zooming in from an alien world. He just did a lot of push-ups—and you can do his workout in about an hour.

Saitama (that's his name) did the following workout every day for three years. As a result, he "broke his 'limit'" so he could effortlessly destroy monsters and other threats to his planet.

His daily routine:
- 100 push-ups
- 100 sit-ups
- 100 bodyweight squats
- 10-kilometer run

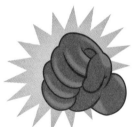

That's it. Really.

Will this workout give you one-punch power? Probably not. But it's a simple routine that can work if you're in a pinch without access to equipment or a gym—if you're traveling for work, or if a giant sea monster has flooded your fitness center temporarily. When YouTuber FinancialJoyTV worked his way up to the One-Punch workout over 100 days, he lost 15 pounds, dropped his body fat from 21 percent to 11 percent, and wound up with a six-pack. Pretty super!

RUN A MARIO

Sure, the world's most famous Italian plumber jumps, fireballs, and flies around to make his way to Bowser's castles, but one thing's been true since World 1-1: If he's going to save the princess, Mario's got to run.

But how far? Using maps from the first Super Mario Bros. game, one estimate has Mario running and swimming just 3.4 miles to save Princess Toadstool. The iconic World 1-1, in this case, is just 426 feet long—only 142 yards. Speedrunners, who compete to play video games as quickly as possible, can finish this level in about 21 seconds. So run a Mario! Head to a local football field and run 140 yards—70 yards down and back—in less than 21 seconds. For a full sprint workout, repeat this effort four to five times, resting for a few minutes between rounds.

Or, if you're feeling really heroic, turn your long run into an effort to save the princess: Run a 5K, then hit the pool for 7.5 laps—almost the same distance Mario swims on his way to fight Bowser in the original Super Mario Bros.

GET IN THE (HUNGER) GAME

With the sport of archery tag, you can work up a sweat slinging arrows like Katniss—but without the risk of actual death or going hungry in fictional woods. Using arrows topped with foam marshmallows, players run, dive, and sneak around trying to pelt each other in a game that's a mix between dodgeball and paintball. Unlike the gun game, though, archery tag doesn't really hurt, won't cover your clothes in paint dots, and, in my experience, involves a lot more laughing than being chased around by a gun-wielding 12-year-old.

It's also a lot more active. Unlike in paintball, where you're hiding (or cowering), there's more running, jumping, and dodging in archery tag. In the group of 30-somethings I played with, we were sweaty, out of breath, and needed some stretching afterward. The bow is really easy to learn, too: At most facilities, instructors give you a quick pregame lesson, with a recommended sideways shooting style that makes firing the foam-tipped arrows easier, quicker, and more accurate.

A session can cost around $25 per hour. Search ARCHERY TAG or COMBAT ARCHERY to find a location near you.

BUILD YOUR POWER LEVEL OVER 9,000 WITH THE *DRAGONBALL Z* WORKOUT

Get ready to get pumped and go Super Saiyan: We're doing a *Dragon Ball Z* workout. The story of Goku, who trains and trains (and eats) to do flying martial arts battles and morph into a glowing, yellow-haired "Super Saiyan," is probably the best-known anime series in the US not starring Pikachu. But *DBZ* didn't just help kids rack up screen time. Huge online communities of anime-loving fitness fanatics say they were once bullied, chubby kids before Goku's relentless training inspired them to hit the gym and go Super themselves.

In one of his most intense training sequences, Goku subjects himself to a "gravity room" as he hurtles through space. There, the ship's gravity is set 20, 50, and even 100 times higher than on Earth, so his exercises are tougher and more effective than ever. You may not be able to replicate the gravity boost, but you can mimic Goku's workout from the gravity room to build your own strength and stamina.

How to do this workout: Goku performs each exercise for 10,000 repetitions. Unless you've got a month on your hands, that's probably not going to work, so let's do a circuit to get to 100 repetitions of each. Perform 10 repetitions of each exercise, then move to the next exercise in the circuit with minimal rest. After you've done all six moves, rest briefly, and repeat for 10 total rounds.

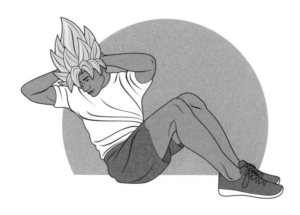

EXERCISE 1: Sit-Up with Twist

1. Perform a classic sit-up, but at the top, twist your torso to the right.
2. Return to start, and twist left on the next rep.

EXERCISE 2: Push-Ups

1. Get in the classic push-up position, hands directly beneath your shoulders, body forming a straight line from head to heels.
2. Maintaining this rigid body line, bend your elbows to lower your chest to the floor.
3. Press back to start.

EXERCISE 3: Walking Lunges

1. Stand with your feet shoulder-width apart.
2. Take a large lunge step forward with your right leg, descending as you step until your knees both form 90-degree angles.
3. Press through your right foot to stand back up and bring your left foot forward to transition into the next lunge.
4. Continue walking forward in this way.

EXERCISE 4: Shoulder Press Push-Ups

1. Place your feet on a step, bench, or chair, and form a 90-degree angle with your body—your upper body will form a vertical line beneath your hips, with your hands about shoulder-width apart. Your legs should be straight from hips to heels.
2. From this position, bend your elbows to lower your head toward the floor, maintaining straight lines in your legs and upper body.
3. Press back to start.

EXERCISE 5: Weighted Punches

Holding light dumbbells in each hand, alternate controlled punches for 10 reps on each hand.

EXERCISE 6: Shadowboxing

Perform a jab, jab, cross, jab combination. Repeat ten times in each round.

DO THE BODYWEIGHT CIRCUIT OF HOLLYWOOD'S REAL SUPERHERO

When heroes flip, fly, and soar across the screen, we know it's not our favorite stars doing that amazing stuff. It's either CGI or the blockbusters' real heroes: stunt performers. And if you've seen heroics on the big screen in the last dozen years, chances are you've seen Bobby Holland Hanton.

The British stuntman swings the hammer of Thor doubling for Chris Hemsworth. He's tussled with Tom Cruise in *Mission Impossible: Fallout*. But one of his scariest stunts, Hanton says, was on his first movie, *Quantum of Solace*. Doubling for Daniel Craig as James Bond, he jumped 21 feet between two buildings with no wires, no harnesses, and no safety equipment down below.

"As I jumped across, the camera followed me, and then looked down," showing that there was nothing beneath Bond, Hanton says. So he had to make it across for real.

To defy death like that, Hanton trains like an athlete—and still looks like a Greek god. To do *that* stunt, he always goes back to this bodyweight circuit.

Perform a set of 12 to 15 reps of each exercise (except the treadmill sprint), then move to the next exercise with as little rest as possible. Aim for 6 total rounds of the workout. Hanton says he can finish this in 20 to 30 minutes; it *might* take you a little longer.

EXERCISE 1: Treadmill Sprint
Sprint for 30 seconds at an incline.

EXERCISE 2: Chin-Ups
1. Hang from the bar with an underhand grip with your hands about shoulder-width apart.
2. Pull your chin toward the bar by bending your elbows. To help engage your back, concentrate on bringing your elbows down to touch your lats instead of thinking about bringing your chin over the bar.
3. Return to the start position, and repeat.

EXERCISE 3: Dips
1. Place your hands on a dip bench or parallel bars with your palms facing each other, and your arms straight.
2. Keep your torso upright—only leaning forward slightly—as you bend your elbows until they are at 90 degrees. For shoulder safety, don't go all the way down.
3. Press through your hands to return to start.

EXERCISE 4: Push-Ups

1. Get in the classic push-up position, hands directly beneath your shoulders, body forming a straight line from head to heels.
2. Maintaining this rigid body line, bend your elbows to lower your chest to the floor.
3. Press back to start.

EXERCISE 5: Scissor Lunges

1. Stand with your feet shoulder-width apart.
2. Take a large lunge step forward with your right leg, descending as you step until your knees both form 90-degree angles.
3. Now press through your right foot so explosively that you jump into the air, scissoring your legs so that you land in the opposite lunge—left foot forward, right foot back.
4. Repeat on the other side. That's one rep.

EXERCISE 6: Jump Squats

1. Stand with your feet slightly wider than shoulder-width. Push your hips back to squat while swinging your arms back.
2. Now drive up through your heels so forcefully that your feet leave the ground. Land softly, rest, reset, and repeat.

EXERCISE 7: Calf Raises

1. Stand on the edge of a step with your toes on the step, your heels hanging over the edge.
2. Let your heels hang down so you feel a stretch, then press into the balls of your feet until your calves are flexed and you're on your toes.
3. Return to start. Repeat.

Movie scenes of military fitness are famous for endless push-ups and grueling runs. While service members do both of those things, there's more to the fitness regimens that keep our military in fighting shape. Try out their tests so you can have a new appreciation for what our service members do. Maybe next time you'll say "thank you" not just for their service, but for their sweat, too.

US ARMY

Are you Army Strong? In 2020, the test of that standard changed. The old test: push-ups, sit-ups, and a 2-mile run. The new test: six events testing strength, endurance, power, and more.

See if you're strong (and fit!) enough for the US Army. The test requires some space and equipment, but can be completed in an hour and is scored out of 500 total points. Use the guide below to see if you can pass the minimum requirement—or reach the maximum possible points. After each of the first four events, rest for 2 minutes. Rest 5 minutes before the 2-mile run.

Event 1: Barbell Deadlift
Perform at least 3 reps in a 5-minute period.
Minimum passing weight: 140 pounds
Maximum points: 340 pounds

Event 2: Power Throw
Holding a 10-pound medicine ball, toss the ball over your head and backward. You get a practice throw, then two tries in 3 minutes. Longest throw counts.
Minimum passing distance: 4.5 meters
Maximum points: 13.5 meters

Event 3: HRT Push-Ups
To perform this push-up, lower your chest to the floor and then, at the bottom, spread your arms out on the ground in a "T" shape. Bring your hands back underneath and continue. You've got two minutes to do as many as you can.
Minimum passing reps: 10
Maximum points: 60

Event 4: Sprint-Drag-Carry

This event requires you to go 25 meters and come back five times. Each round involves a different activity: Sprint, then drag a sled (90 pounds), perform a lateral shuffle, carry two 40-pound kettlebells, and sprint again. Scored on total time.
Minimum passing time: 3 minutes
Maximum points awarded for: 1 minute, 33 seconds

Event 5: Hanging Leg Tuck

Hang from a bar at arm's length with a neutral grip. Pull your knees up to your elbows and return to start. Perform as many reps as you can in 2 minutes.
Minimum passing reps: 1
Maximum points: 20

Event 6: 2-Mile Run

Minimum passing time: 21 minutes
Maximum points awarded for: 13 minutes, 30 seconds

US NAVY

The Navy's Physical Readiness Test, or PRT, has three events. Each is done consecutively, with up to 15 minutes of rest between events.

Event 1: Plank

A forearm plank replaced sit-ups starting in 2020. You can wobble, but you must maintain a rigid body line from head to heels.
PASSING SCORE: An "excellent" rating is awarded for planking 3 minutes, 40 seconds. Aim for that.

Event 2: Push-Ups

Two minutes of push-ups. You can rest, but you must stay in the push-up position, not letting anything but your hands or feet touch the floor.
PASSING SCORE: To get an "excellent" rating, a male between ages 25 and 29 needs to perform 67 push-ups. For a female of the same age, "excellent" is awarded for 37 push-ups.

Event 3: 1.5-Mile Run

PASSING SCORE: A passing score for male recruits is 16:10. For female recruits, the passing score is 18:07. An "excellent" score for a male aged 25 to 29 is 10:52. For a female of the same age, it's 13:23.

US MARINE CORPS

The Marines have two tests: The Physical Fitness Test, or PFT, and the Combat Fitness Test, or CFT (the military loves acronyms). The PFT is similar to other tests on this list, but the CFT is an extra test designed to measure a Marine's "functional" fitness needed in a combat environment. The star of the CFT is the Maneuver under Fire event, or MANUF—a zigzagging course of sprinting, crawling, dragging, carrying, and throwing that's famous for leaving people gassed.

Check out the diagram to see how you can set it up for yourself. One tip: If you don't have a friend who wants to be dragged 65 yards and then carried for another 65, check a local thrift store or used sporting goods store for a cheap, used heavy bag.

1. Start by lying on your stomach, then spring up and sprint 25 yards to a cone.
2. Do a clockwise turn around the cone.
3. Drop and low-crawl for 10 yards.
4. High-crawl on your hands and knees for 10 yards.
5. Zigzag through cones spaced 5 yards apart for the next 25 yards.
6. Drag a "casualty" at the 75-yard mark in an arc to the 100-yard mark and back.
7. Drag the casualty through two cones spaced to cover 10 total yards.
8. Pick up the casualty in a "fireman's carry" with their torso over your shoulders. Run 65 yards back to the starting line. Drop the casualty.
9. Pick up two 30-pound weights. Run 50 yards, then zigzag through cones for 25 more yards.
10. Drop the weights at the 75-yard marker. Throw a grenade (or a softball) 22.5 yards.
11. Do three push-ups.
12. Pick up the weights and reverse: Zigzag through the cones for 25 yards, then sprint the remaining 50 yards to the original starting line.

For a 26- to 30-year-old male Marine, the minimum passing time is 3:22. For a female Marine of the same age, a passing time is 4:40.

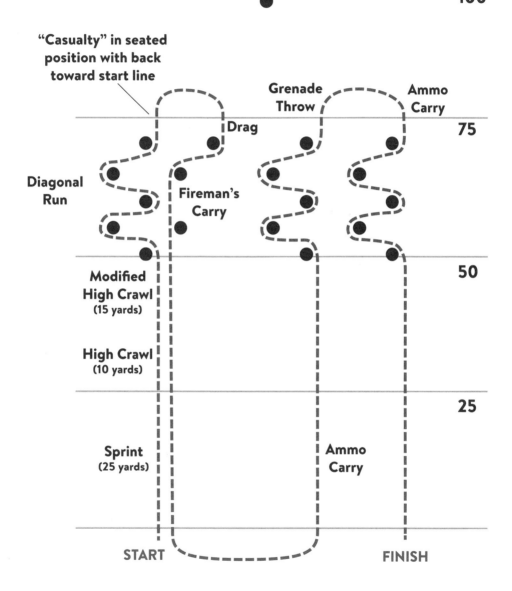

Grenade
Target

100

"Casualty" in seated
position with back
toward start line

Grenade
Throw

Ammo
Carry

75

Drag

Diagonal
Run

Fireman's
Carry

Modified
High Crawl
(15 yards)

50

High Crawl
(10 yards)

25

Sprint
(25 yards)

Ammo
Carry

START

FINISH

US AIR FORCE

Starting in 2019, airmen (both men and women are called "airmen" in USAF) in specific jobs, like those in bomb disposal, started taking a tougher Tier 2 test. In addition to push-ups, sit-ups, and running, this exam now includes running, lunges, crunches, deadlifts, pull-ups, farmer's carries, and a grip-strength exam. But its most notorious—and brutal—test is the Gruseter.

Named for now-retired Master Sergeant Matthew Gruse, who helped create the test, it's designed to simulate what it's like to be an Explosive Ordinance Disposal airman: These specialists wear a vest ranging from 77 to 82 pounds and have to move around—think Jeremy Renner in *The Hurt Locker*. For this test, airmen wear a 30-pound vest and carry a 50-pound sandbag. If you can get your hands on a vest and a sandbag, try this brutal test:

1. Pick up the sandbag and place it on your shoulder.
2. Drop to the ground while holding the sandbag, and roll over.
3. Stand back up. Run 15 meters, still holding the sandbag.
4. Repeat step 2. Drop to the ground while holding the sandbag, and roll over.
5. Run back to the start. Drop the bag.
6. Sprint to the 15-meter marker and back.
7. Repeat steps 1 to 6 nine more times.

US COAST GUARD

It's no surprise that the Coast Guard's fitness standards include a bit of swimming—in addition to push-ups, sit-ups, and a half-mile run, Coast Guard members must also perform a 100-meter swim, followed by a five-minute water tread.

But if you're looking for a bigger challenge, try the weekly fitness test administered to Coast Guard Rescue Swimmers. These elite rescuers jump off boats and out of airplanes to make daring rescues in dangerous seas. Their weekly fitness exam is comprised of seven events. One of the water events, the "buddy tow," may not be practical at your local pool or beach—it might make the lifeguards think someone's in trouble. So maybe skip that.

Event 1: Push-Ups
Perform 50.

Event 2: Bent Knee Sit-Ups
Perform 60.

Event 3: Pull-Ups (overhand grip)
Perform 5.

Event 4: Chin-Ups (underhand grip)
Perform 5.

Event 5: 500-Yard Swim with "Crawl" or Freestyle Stroke
Complete in 12 minutes or less. In an Olympic pool, this is about 10 lengths.

Event 6: 25-Yard Underwater Swim
Perform 4 times by swimming half the length of the pool underwater, pop up, and repeat 3 more times.

Event 7: 200-Yard "Buddy Tow"
Using a "cross-chest carry," where one arm is under the arm and chest of the person being rescued, swim while towing a "casualty" for 200 yards. Again, make sure you clear this with someone or skip it at the pool or beach: If not, it may look like you're in trouble!

CHAPTER 10

SWEAT LIKE A STAR

Your favorite celebrities are athletes, too: To build the types of bodies that can fill arenas with song, punch bad guys on-screen, and hot-step across stages for our entertainment, these stars challenge themselves to give us their very best. See if you're tough enough to give your body the star treatment with these workouts.

A WORKOUT THAT EVEN IMPRESSES THE ROCK

If you're running around shirtless on the beach, you need one hell of a physique to take the people's eyeballs off The Rock. But in 2017's *Baywatch*, Zac Efron did just that. Swinging around a beachside obstacle course, Efron was so lean that his costar, Alexandra Daddario, said he looked "like something Michelangelo carved."

To chisel Efron's impressive look, trainer Patrick Murphy put Zac through workouts six days a week for more than eight months. Murphy kept Efron's workouts intense by constantly changing the number of repetitions Zac did in his sets—one day, he might do 10 sets of an exercise, counting down from 10 reps to 1. Another day, he might do 5 sets, all with different rep numbers. Changing up these repetition numbers let Murphy turn a single workout into hundreds of different sessions that constantly challenged Efron.

Unlike other trade secrets of the movie biz, though, you can actually do Efron's complete program: Murphy sells the workout at www.murphyfitness.com. Here's a sample upper body workout in the *Baywatch* style that's composed of five exercise pairs.

Use the same weight for both moves in each pair, and alternate back and forth—without resting—until you've done all your sets. To do the workout with Murphy's "10-1/1-10" rep scheme, you'll do 10 sets of each exercise. Choose a weight that is 40 percent of your 1-repetition maximum. In set 1, you'll do 10 repetitions of Exercise A, and 1 repetition of Exercise B. You'll then do 9 reps of Exercise A and 2 reps of Exercise B. Continue counting down Exercise A and counting up Exercise B until you're doing a set of 1 repetition of Exercise B and 10 reps of Exercise A.

EXERCISE **PAIR 1**

EXERCISE A: Front Raise

1. Stand with your feet together, holding dumbbells in front of your thighs with an overhand grip. Pull your shoulder blades back and down, and brace your core and butt.
2. Raise the dumbbells up and forward until your hands are at shoulder level.
3. Return to start, and repeat.

EXERCISE B: Lateral Raise

1. Stand with your feet together, dumbbells at your sides, palms in.
2. Keeping your torso upright, lift the dumbbells out to the sides until your torso and arms form a "T" shape.
3. Control the weights as they return to your sides, and repeat.

WORKOUT CONTINUES >>>

EXERCISE **PAIR 2**

EXERCISE A: Dumbbell Floor Press

1. Lie faceup on the floor with your knees bent and feet flat on the floor. Hold dumbbells next to your chest. Your elbows should stay close to your sides, forming a 45-degree angle.
2. Pressing your mid- and upper back into the floor, press the weights straight up over your chest.
3. Once your arms are straight, bend your elbows to return to start.

EXERCISE B: Chin-Up

1. Hang from the bar with an underhand grip and your hands about shoulder-width apart.
2. Pull your chin over the bar by bending your elbows.
3. Return to the start position.

EXERCISE **PAIR 3**

EXERCISE A: Dumbbell Overhead Press

1. Sit with your feet flat on the floor, back straight. Bring the dumbbells up to your shoulders, palms in.
2. Maintaining an upright posture, press the dumbbells overhead until your elbows are almost straight.
3. Return the weights to your shoulders, and repeat.

EXERCISE B: Straight-Arm Pull-Down

1. Stand with the cable stack in front of you. Grab the handle with your right hand and hold it so it's just above and in front of your shoulder.
2. Keeping your core braced and your elbow straight, use your back to pull the weight down until the handle is in front of your right hip.
3. Return to start, and repeat. Do all your reps on this side, then switch sides and repeat.

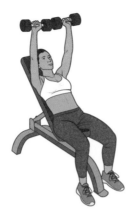

EXERCISE **PAIR 4**
EXERCISE A: Dumbbell Incline Bench Press
1. Lie faceup on an incline bench and hold dumbbells over your chest with an overhand grip.
2. Bend your elbows to lower the weights to the sides of your chest. Your elbows should stay close to your sides, forming a 45-degree angle.
3. Pause, then press back to start.

EXERCISE B: Chest-Supported Dumbbell Row
1. Lie facedown on an incline bench and hold dumbbells at arm's length, palms in.
2. Squeeze your shoulder blades together and row the dumbbells up to your sides.
3. Pause, then return to start.

EXERCISE **PAIR 5**
EXERCISE A: Cable Press
1. With cables slightly behind you, hold the handles with bent elbows at your nipple line. Stand in a staggered stance.
2. Squeeze your chest and press your arms forward and together until your elbows are straight.
3. Control the cables back to the start.

EXERCISE B: Standing Cable Horizontal Row
1. Stand in front of the cable stack with a V-handle in front of your chest. Set your shoulder blades back and down, and bend your knees slightly.
2. Pull the handle to your sternum with both hands.
3. Pause, then return to start.

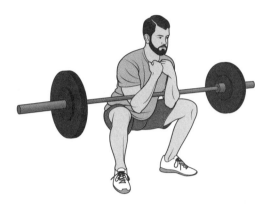

THEN TRY TO KEEP UP WITH THE *ACTUAL* ROCK WITH A *FAST*-INSPIRED LEG DAY

The best part about America's biggest movie star is that Dwayne Johnson doesn't hide the secrets to building his beef: If you want to try what The Rock is cooking, just pull up his Instagram account to find the recipes. Johnson posts full details of his workouts, so you can try to train like The Rock.

Or, in the case of this workout, like Hobbs, Johnson's character in the *Fast and the Furious* series. This routine is inspired by the leg workouts The Rock shared as he prepared for *Hobbs and Shaw*.

Perform one set of each exercise, then move to the next without resting. Take a breather after doing all four exercises, then repeat the circuit two more times.

EXERCISE 1: Barbell Hip Thrust (8 reps per set)

1. This move will give you a Rock-hard rear view: It's the mother of all butt exercises. Sit in front of the bench with it touching your back, your butt on the ground, and your legs straight out in front of you. Roll the weighted barbell onto your hips, and bend your knees so your feet are flat on the floor (you may want a pad around the bar at your waist).
2. Squeeze your butt and press your feet into the floor to thrust the barbell up so your body forms a tabletop from shoulders to knees.
3. Return the bar to the floor, and repeat.

EXERCISE 2: Zercher Squat (8 reps per set)

1. Set a barbell up on a squat rack at about waist height. Bend your elbows 90 degrees and put the bar so it rests at the top of your forearms, right below the elbow (you may want a pad).
2. Without using your hands, lift the bar—you'll use your arms in a 90-degree position to hold the bar.
3. In this position, perform a normal squat: Push your hips back to initiate the movement, keeping the weight in your heels, and descend until your thighs are at least parallel to the floor.
4. Press through your heels to return to standing.

EXERCISE 3: Leg Press (8 reps per set)

The Rock uses 450 pounds for this exercise—which seems like a *ton*, but the leg press is usually a move where people load on tons of plates. Take his lead and go a little lighter than you think you can max.

EXERCISE 4: Back Squat (25 reps per set)

1. Twenty-five reps is punishing, so go lighter than normal! Stand in a normal back squat position, barbell across your shoulders, feet between shoulder- and hip-width apart, toes slightly out.
2. Push your hips back to initiate the squat.
3. Bend your knees to descend until your thighs are at least parallel to the floor, keeping your chest up and your weight on your heels.
4. Keep the weight of your body in your heels and press back to standing.

GET LEAN LIKE HALLE BERRY

Halle Berry is timeless. Seemingly ageless, too: In *John Wick 3*, Berry was kicking ass and firing rifles at 52—a year *older* than Rue McClanahan was when she played Blanche on *The Golden Girls*!

The star stays that way with the help of Peter Lee Thomas, whose mixed martial arts training style is called "Combat Shape"—a boot-camp approach that combines elements of Muay Thai, jiujitsu, and MMA techniques with HIIT-style conditioning. Thomas and Berry share their fitness secrets on Instagram every week, posting ab-carving, fat-burning, age-defying moves that anyone can try. Try this 7-move workout, inspired by their #FitnessFriday posts.

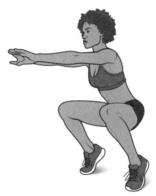

EXERCISE 1: Hindu Squat

1. Stand with your feet hip-width apart and your arms extended straight in front of you.
2. Bend your knees to squat, keeping the weight on the balls of your feet—your heels will lift up off the ground, unlike in a regular squat. As you lower down, bring your arms down so they're at your sides, keep your head facing forward, and maintain a straight back.
3. At the bottom of the movement, your butt should nearly touch your heels, and your fingers should graze the ground.
4. Swing your arms forward as you stand back to the starting position. Do 30 squats.

EXERCISE 2: Weighted Squat Jump

1. Holding dumbbells at your sides, push your hips back to squat, descending until your thighs are at least parallel to the floor.
2. Keeping the weight in your heels, press into the floor to stand back up so forcefully that you come off the floor, jumping.
3. Land, quickly reset, and repeat. Do 30 reps.

EXERCISE 3: Archer Squat

1.   Get in an extra-wide stance, with your feet as wide as they'd be for a lateral lunge, feet facing forward.
2.   Push your hips back and descend to your right by bending your right knee, keeping it tracking over your right toes. Keep your torso upright as you descend, continuing to descend until your butt is above your right foot, and your left foot has spun up onto the heel.
3.   Return your left foot to the ground and press back to start. Then perform the move to the left. Do 12 reps on each side.

EXERCISE 4: Weighted High-Knee Run and Punch

Holding dumbbells in your hands, do a high-knee run in place while punching with the dumbbells. Do 40 total punches.

EXERCISE 5: Leg Raise Toe Touch

1.   Lie on your back and raise your legs so they're straight and perpendicular to the floor. Crunch up and reach for your toes.
2.   Pulse up, reaching for your toes 15 more times.

EXERCISE 6: Hindu Push-Up

1.   Begin in the classic push-up position, but bring your feet forward and raise your hips so that your body almost forms an inverted "V" shape.
2.   Keep your hips up as you bend your elbows to drop your chin toward the floor.
3.   As your chin approaches the floor, swoop your hips under so they almost touch the floor, swinging your chest up as you raise your head and straighten your arms.
4.   Reverse the move to return to start, and repeat. Try for 30.

EXERCISE 7: Muay Thai Sit-Up

1.   Lie faceup with your legs straight out in front of you.
2.   Perform sit-ups with your legs straight out, coming all the way up to bring your chest close to your thighs. Go for 30 seconds.

THE FIVE-MINUTE CIRQUE DU SOLEIL ABS WORKOUT

When *Cirque du Soleil* performers fly through the air, it's part physics, part magic, and a lot of ab strength.

"I always start from the core," says Elizabeth Cauchois, a ten-year veteran of the high-flying shows.

She finishes with it, too. After flying around the tent of *Totem*, Cauchois would come offstage and do an ab workout. Set to the tune of the show's next act, a series of unicycle stunts, the five-minute routine was dubbed "unicycle abs" by her castmates. When the routine was posted to YouTube, it went viral: More than 1.8 million people have watched it.

"It was just something I was doing every day on my own—me and a friend," she says. "And it blew up into this *thing*."

That thing has turned into Cauchois hosting *Cirque It Out*, a 16-episode YouTube fitness series produced by Cirque du Soleil, and launching her own fitness brand, Cut 2 the Core Fitness, with her husband, also a Cirque performer. Here's the workout that started it all: Cauchois's unicycle abs routine (you can also see the full, original video on the YouTube channel, CirqueLife).

Each exercise is performed for a count of 8, or for 8 reps. Transition from one move to the next without rest. Throughout this sequence, Elizabeth suggests focusing on keeping your belly button pulled toward your spine.

EXERCISE 1: Traditional Crunch
Lie faceup with your knees bent, feet flat on the floor. Crunch up, then drop back down and repeat.

EXERCISE 2: Crunch with Legs in Tabletop Position
Knees should be bent 90 degrees, with lower legs parallel to the floor.

EXERCISE 3: Pilates March
From the tabletop position, with your upper body holding a crunch, lower your right leg to the ground to touch, then return to the tabletop. Repeat with your left side. Do 8 touches with each foot.

EXERCISE 4: Toe Touch
With your upper body still crunched up, straighten your legs so they're straight up, heels toward the ceiling. Reach up and touch your toes 8 times.

EXERCISE 5: Toe Touch, Alternate Reach
Same as Exercise 4, but reach across and touch the opposite foot. Do 8 on each side.

EXERCISE 6: Pulse-Up

In the same position, lift your butt up off the ground to push your feet toward the ceiling.

EXERCISE 7: Slow Bicycle Crunch

In the same position, bring your opposite elbow to your opposite knee, taking a count of 4 to do each rep. Do 8 total reps.

EXERCISE 8: Elbow-to-Knee Hold

Hold the elbow-to-knee position from a bicycle crunch for an 8-count.

EXERCISE 9: Reach Past Elbow-to-Knee

From the elbow-to-knee position in Exercise 8, straighten your arm and pulse past your leg 8 times. Then repeat Exercises 8 and 9 on the other side.

EXERCISE 10: Upper Body Circle

With your legs straight and flat on the ground, perform a rolling crunch with your upper body, making a circle to the right as your left shoulder comes off the ground, then both shoulders, then just your right shoulder. Circle 8 times, then switch directions.

EXERCISE 11: Oblique V-Up

Lying on your left side, with legs stacked, raise your legs and your torso up to the side simultaneously, forming a V.

EXERCISE 12: Oblique Elbow-to-Knee

On the same side, bring your knee up and over your waist as you bring your elbow up to touch it. After 8 reps, repeat Exercises 11 and 12, lying on your right side.

EXERCISE 13: Hollow Body Hold

Start in the same position as a V-up, with arms and legs fully extended. Lift your arms and legs slightly off the ground, brace your core, and hold.

EXERCISE 14: Hollow Body Ankle Cross

In the same position, with your legs straight, cross one ankle over the other, then switch. You'll do this for three counts of 8: For the first, hold the hollow body position. On the second 8, keep crossing as you raise your legs straight up. For the third 8, keep crossing as you return to the hollow body position.

EXERCISE 15: Boat Pose with V-Ups

Strike a boat pose—your torso and legs should form a "V," balanced on your sit bones. Hold for 32 total counts. On each count of 8, lower yourself flat and then perform a V-up back to the boat pose position.

THIS 30-MINUTE WORKOUT MAKES T.I. STAGE-READY

When hip-hop stars go on tour, they've got to look stage-ready—with rippling abs and boulder shoulders. But their bodies also need to be road-ready with stamina to perform show after show, and the ability to bounce back on limited sleep—both from traveling and partying.

CJ Hammond, owner of Fit Legend, and trainer to such stars as T.I. and Shad Moss, has one other challenge: He has to build these tour-ready bodies fast. Performers who are about to launch a global tour don't have hours to spend in the gym.

Even if you're not a platinum-selling artist, that probably sounds familiar—less time in the gym than you'd planned for, but still hoping to get the results your body needs to perform *your* world tour. Get it done! Try this lower-body-pushing and upper-body-pulling workout that Hammond uses with his performers—in the next session, they'd do a lower-body pull and upper-body push to complete the split workout.

Get loose, get warm, and get ready for a giant set: It's a series of exercises performed back to back, with minimal rest in between. In this workout, the giant set consists of four exercises. Do it four times, resting 60 seconds between each "set." Then do the finisher—two exercises that will burn you out so you can leave it all in the gym and get back to your life.

CJ'S GIANT SET

Perform 1 set of each exercise, then move to the next exercise without resting. When you've finished all 4 moves, rest for 60 seconds. Repeat this sequence four times.

EXERCISE 1: Goblet Squat (8 to 10 reps per set)
1. Stand with your feet hip-width apart, toes pointed slightly out from parallel. Cup one end of a dumbbell in both hands in front of your chest with your elbows pointing down.
2. Push your hips back to initiate the squat. Bend your knees to descend until your thighs are at least parallel to the floor, keeping your weight on your heels.
3. Press back to standing.

EXERCISE 2: Chin-Up (8 reps per set)
1. Hang from the bar with an underhand grip and your hands about shoulder-width apart.
2. Pull your chin toward the bar by bending your elbows. To help engage your back, concentrate on bringing your elbows down to touch your lats instead of thinking about bringing your chin over the bar.
3. Return to the start position, and repeat.

EXERCISE 3: Dumbbell Rear-Foot-Elevated Split Squat (8 reps on each leg per set)

1. With dumbbells in your hands, place one foot behind you on the bench, with your other foot in front so you're in a position similar to a lunge.
2. Keeping your torso upright, push your hips back and bend your front knee to descend into a split squat.
3. Press through your front heel to return to start.

EXERCISE 4: Dumbbell Bent-Over Row (8 to 10 reps per set)

1. Stand with a firm bench on your left side.
2. Place your left knee on the bench, then bend your torso forward and place your left hand on the bench to support your body. In this position, your upper body should be parallel to the floor.
3. Reach down and grab the dumbbell with your right hand, returning to this position where your body is parallel to the floor, with the weight hanging straight down from your right shoulder.
4. Maintaining that upper body position, pull your right arm straight up until your hand reaches the side of your chest.
5. Lower the weight back to the starting position, and repeat. Do all your reps on this side, then switch sides and repeat.

FINISHER

EXERCISE 1: Banded Hamstring Curl (1 set of 100 reps on each leg)

1. Lie facedown with one end of a band looped around your foot, the other end secured to a bench or pole.
2. Keeping your hips level, bend your knee to bring it to your butt, making the band go taut.

EXERCISE 2: Decline Sit-Up (3 sets of 15 reps)

Perform sit-ups on a decline slant board. Rest 45 seconds between sets.

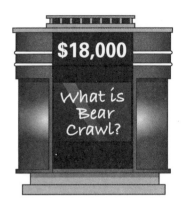

$18,000

What is Bear Crawl?

BE BETTER UNDER PRESSURE. DO THE *JEOPARDY!* CHAMPION WORKOUT

It's not just standing and pressing a button: Being on *Jeopardy!* is a physical challenge.

"If you start winning, you're playing back-to-back games. You're stressed and tense in that time," Buzzy Cohen says of his nine-win streak. The high-stress environment can make it tough to recall facts. "No matter how well you know something, when you're in that brain space, it's really hard to access it."

To simulate that high-stress environment for his appearance on the *Jeopardy!* Tournament of Champions (which he won), Cohen's trainer, Kasey Esser of Essers of Los Angeles, would quiz Buzzy while he performed exercises like planks and sled pushes.

"If you're holding a flexed-arm hang, around second 20, you probably couldn't spell your name, no less having to come up with the capital of Brunei," Cohen says. And it worked: "There were a couple moments in the Tournament of Champions where . . . there were answers where this really helped me. Even under a ton of cortisol, I could still access those parts of my brain. I felt pressure-tested in the gym."

Maybe you're not about to wager on a Daily Double, but if you've got an important presentation coming up or a wedding toast to give, this Buzzy workout could help train your brain to remember what you need to under pressure.

Perform Exercise A in each pair, then move to Exercise B without resting. Rest briefly, then repeat the pair two more times. While you're doing your sets, ask a friend to quiz you—on state capitals or some other fact—or try to recite your presentation.

EXERCISE **PAIR 1**

EXERCISE A: Prisoner Squat (3 sets of 8 reps)

1. Stand with your feet hip-width apart, toes pointed slightly out from parallel and your hands behind your head.
2. Push your hips back to initiate the squat. Bend your knees to descend until your thighs are at least parallel to the floor, keeping your chest up and your weight on your heels.
3. Keep the weight of your body in your heels and press back to standing.

EXERCISE B: Bear Crawl (3 sets of 10 to 15 yards)

Crawl on your hands and feet as fast as you can.

EXERCISE **PAIR 2**

EXERCISE A: Chest-Supported Dumbbell Row (3 sets of 10 reps)

1. Lie facedown on an incline bench and hold dumbbells at arm's length, palms in.
2. Squeeze your shoulder blades together and row the dumbbells up to your sides.
3. Pause, then return to start.

EXERCISE B: Single-Leg Glute Bridge (3 sets of 8 reps on each leg)

1. Lie faceup on the ground with your knees bent and your feet flat on the floor. Place your arms at your sides, palms up.
2. Straighten your right leg so your thighs are still parallel.
3. Keeping your left foot flat on the floor and your hips level, squeeze your glutes to raise your hips off the floor until your body forms a straight line from your knees to your shoulders.
4. Pause for a second at the top of the exercise, and then slowly return to the start position. Do all your reps on this side, then switch legs and repeat.

FINISHER

Jump Rope

Keep being quizzed while you work and rest! Perform 6 rounds of 30 seconds each, resting 60 to 75 seconds between rounds.

ARE YOU TOUGH ENOUGH FOR THE BROADWAY DANCER WORKOUT?

Imagine if your favorite NBA player had to sprint and jump all over the court while also singing loudly and clearly enough to be heard in the back row. That's what it's like to be in a Broadway musical.

"Cardiovascular stamina is the number one thing," says Beth Nicely, an actress who has appeared in *Chicago*, *42nd Street*, and more. In most of those shows, Nicely has been a member of the ensemble cast, meaning she's rushing offstage between songs to quickly change costumes.

In addition to her onstage work, Nicely is a certified personal trainer, and a master trainer at Body by Simone studio in New York, where she works with numerous other stage performers to help them stay in shape for these backstage cardio-and-strength challenges. Try this workout to get a taste of how she trains for—and performs in—these heart-pumping shows.

You'll alternate between a bout of treadmill work and 3 rounds of an exercise pair. In the exercise pairs, you'll perform one set of Exercise A, then move to Exercise B without resting. Do each pair three times, then hop back on the treadmill. The entire workout will take around 45 minutes.

Treadmill
Perform 5 rounds of the following sequence: Run 1 minute at 8.0, 30 seconds at 8.5, and 30 seconds at 9.0.

STRENGTH PAIR 1: Do 3 rounds.
EXERCISE A: Dumbbell Bent-Over Row (12 to 20 reps per set)

EXERCISE B: Overhead Press (12 to 20 reps per set)

Treadmill
Repeat the above sequence five more times.

STRENGTH PAIR 2: Do 3 rounds.
EXERCISE A: Goblet Squat (12 to 20 reps per set)

EXERCISE B: Dumbbell Step-Up (12 to 20 reps per set)

Treadmill
Repeat the above sequence five more times.

STRENGTH PAIR 3: Do 3 rounds.
EXERCISE A: Box Jump (10 per round)
Use a low box.

EXERCISE B: Jump Rope Double-Unders (40 per round)

For shots from her life onstage and more workouts—and to see how to take a class with her—follow Nicely on Instagram @bethjnicely.

THEN KICK IT LIKE A RADIO CITY ROCKETTE

Those famous kicks don't just look good onstage: They'll kick your butt, says Beth Nicely, and they're a workout unto themselves—and even tougher than they look.

"They have to be parallel—the tip of your toe is fixed to your eye level, and pointed," she says. "You have to make sure you snap them down faster than you want to."

They're so challenging that Nicely incorporates them into high-intensity interval circuits in her workout classes . . . and this HIIT circuit. Perform each exercise for the prescribed number of reps, rest for ten seconds, then move to the next exercise. Do the entire series three times.

Exercise 1: Chorus Kicks
Keep your chest up and your leg as straight as possible. Place your hands on your hips, thumbs forward. Try to kick up to eye level, and snap the kick back down. Do 16 kicks per round.

Exercise 2: Jumping Jack Pat-Downs
Do a jumping jack, then bend your knees to squat down and touch the ground next to your feet. Get back up and do another jumping jack. Do 8 total repetitions per round.

Exercise 3: High-Knee Run
Pump your knees high for 32 reps.

Exercise 4: Burpees
Do 8 per round.

GET A CHEST PUMP LIKE *DRAG RACE'S* "BODYBUILDER BARBIE"

When Kameron Michaels returned to drag shows after a few years of bodybuilding, her newly muscular physique wasn't celebrated—other performers criticized it.

That didn't stop Michaels: "Drag has no boundaries," she says. "And I could do anything I wanted."

That included performing *and* lifting. And it's clearly worked: Michaels wound up competing on *RuPaul's Drag Race*, coming in second overall and earning the nickname "Bodybuilder Barbie." Now this "muscle queen" tours, performing her single, "Freedom," at shows around the country six nights a week. And she still finds time to lift. Here's Kameron's favorite workout—a nine-move chest and shoulder routine.

Perform each exercise for 3 sets of 12 to 15 reps. Rest 30 seconds between sets and exercises.

EXERCISE 1: Dumbbell Bench Press
1. Lie faceup on a bench and hold dumbbells over your chest with an overhand grip.
2. Bend your elbows to lower the weights to the sides of your chest. Your elbows should stay close to your sides, forming a 45-degree angle.
3. Pause, then press back to start.

EXERCISE 2: Push-Up (between sets of the Dumbbell Bench Press)
1. Assume a classic push-up position, with hands directly beneath your shoulders, your body forming a straight line from head to heels.
2. Maintain this rigid body line as you bend your elbows to lower your chest toward the floor.
3. Press back to start, maintaining the straight body line.

EXERCISE 3: Incline Dumbbell Press
1. Lie faceup on an incline bench and hold dumbbells over your chest with an overhand grip.
2. Bend your elbows to lower the weights to the sides of your chest. Your elbows should stay close to your sides, forming a 45-degree angle.
3. Pause, then press back to start.

EXERCISE 4: Dumbbell Fly

1. Lie faceup on a bench holding two dumbbells over your chest, palms facing in.
2. With slightly bent elbows, lower the dumbbells to the sides of your chest until your chest is stretched.
3. Bring the dumbbells back together using a wide, hugging motion. Repeat.

EXERCISE 5: Low Cable Fly

1. With the cables anchored low, stand between them, holding the cables out to the side with palms facing forward. Bend forward slightly into an athletic position.
2. Squeeze your chest to bring the cables up and in front of your chest, keeping your arms straight, until your fists touch.
3. Control the movement to return to start, and repeat.

EXERCISE 6: High Cable Fly

Same as Exercise 5, but anchor the cables high.

EXERCISE 7: Dumbbell Shoulder Press

1. Sit with your feet flat on the floor, back straight. Bring the dumbbells up to your shoulders, palms in.
2. Maintaining an upright posture, press the dumbbells overhead until your elbows are almost straight.
3. Return the weights to your shoulders, and repeat.

EXERCISE 8: Alternating Front Raise

1. Hold dumbbells in front of your thighs with an overhand grip. Pull your shoulder blades back and down, and brace your core and butt.
2. Raise the right dumbbell up and forward until your hand is at shoulder level.
3. Return to start. Repeat on the other side.

EXERCISE 9: Dumbbell Lateral Raise

1. Stand with your feet together, dumbbells at your sides, palms in.
2. Keeping your torso upright, lift the dumbbells out to the sides until your torso and arms form a "T" shape.
3. Control the weights as they return to your sides, and repeat.

Diamond Dallas Page is not your typical yoga teacher: He's a WWE Hall of Famer who spent more than 20 years in the squared circle. Take that kind of punishment, and you could use some time on the yoga mat to recover—and for more than a decade, he's been selling his program, DDP Yoga, on DVDs and in online subscriptions.

DDP's yoga workout uses traditional yoga poses, but with some pro wrestling–style branding and attitude twists. The main sequence of poses, the "Diamond Dozen," is composed mostly of traditional yoga poses, but with the names given some extra edge: The "warrior" sequence is now called the "road warrior" and "child's pose" is your "safety zone." And Page incorporates some isometric resistance—squeezing the muscles throughout the pose—to add a strength component.

For wrestling superfans, DDP Yoga offers an opportunity no other workout does, though—not just to work out *like* a wrestling star, but to work out *with* a Hall of Famer. At DDP Yoga workshops held throughout the country each year, fans can pony up $70 to join DDP for a three-hour yoga and motivational speaker event, with a 50-minute class taught by Page himself. Visit www.ddpyogaworkshops.com for dates.

TRY DDP'S CHALLENGE: THE 10-SECOND PUSH-UP

To gauge their progress with his program, Page challenges his DDP Yoga students to "10-second push-ups." These long, slow repetitions actually involve a count to 30, and put a premium on "time under tension," the length of time your muscles are under the strain of an exercise.

After a few weeks of DDP's yoga program, a friend says he improved from one 10-second push-up to 9 reps. Page himself knocked out 12 at age 64. Drop and see how many you can count out.

1. **ASSUME** the classic push-up position, with your hands directly beneath your shoulders, your body forming a straight line from head to heels. If you can, use push-up handles for this exercise to save your wrists.
2. **MAINTAINING** the rigid body line, bend your elbows to lower your chest toward the floor, taking a count of 10 to reach the bottom.
3. **HOLD** at the bottom for a count of 10.
4. **PRESS** back to start, taking a count of 10 to get back to the top. Repeat for as many reps as you can.

BUILD YOUR SHOULDERS LIKE "THE MOUNTAIN"

In the real world, the "Mountain" from *Game of Thrones* is . . . basically the same as he is on the show: The biggest, strongest, quickest knight in the seven kingdoms. Thor Bjornsson, the Icelandic actor who played Gregor "The Mountain" Clegane on the HBO mega-hit, has held the world record in the deadlift, and was crowned the World's Strongest Man in 2018. To take that crown, he had to pick up a 400-pound stone sphere, and hoist dumbbells as heavy as 220 pounds overhead.

This overhead press medley is inspired by Bjornsson's short, intense workouts that he uses to build all that strength. Use it as a finisher or as a stand-alone workout. Perform 2 repetitions of each exercise, then move to the next without resting.

EXERCISE 1: Double Dumbbell Clean and Press
Bjornsson does cleans like this with a log bar, which has handles so your palms face inward. Perform 2 reps with one dumbbell in each hand.

EXERCISE 2: Barbell Clean and Press
1. Stand holding a barbell in front of you with an overhand grip, hands slightly wider than your shoulders. Keeping your weight in your heels, bend at your hips and knees so the bar hangs in front of your knees. This is the start position.
2. From here, explode up: You'll shrug your shoulders and bring the bar up in a straight line to your shoulders and you flip your wrists so you catch the bar in front of your collarbones.
3. Dip your hips slightly, and drive through your legs to press the bar overhead. Drop it, and repeat.

EXERCISE 3: Heavy Dumbbell Hoist and Overhead Press
Grab the biggest dumbbell you can handle. From the ground, bring it to your shoulder, and press it overhead.

EXERCISE 4: Single Heavy Dumbbell Curl and Press
Bjornsson does a move like this with a metal box weighing more than 200 pounds. Your gym probably doesn't have that! Hold a heavy dumbbell by its sides, and perform a curl and press.

TAKE THE CLIMBING CLASS THAT LEBRON JAMES AND JENNIFER ANISTON SWEAR BY AND TRAIN ON AN OBSTACLE FROM *AMERICAN GLADIATORS*!

You may never get to joust with a giant foam Q-tip or dodge tennis balls while firing a Nerf bazooka, but you *can* get a workout on an obstacle from *American Gladiators*: the Versaclimber.

The aerobic mountain-climbing machine was the opening obstacle of the Eliminator for three seasons of the show, but it's not some stuck-in-the-'90s cardio machine: The Versaclimber has been shown to get users' max heart rates higher than when they're running intervals on a treadmill.

It's the centerpiece of Rise Nation studios, a chain found throughout the US that's got all the feel of a spin class—resistance knobs, neon lights, sprint intervals, and thumping music—but with the bikes replaced by Versaclimbers. Created by Jason Walsh, the trainer who turned Matt Damon into Jason Bourne, these 30-minute classes have become a conditioning favorite of Aniston, Lady Gaga, John Krasinski, and the king of the NBA, LeBron James, who has a Versaclimber in his home and visited Rise Nation classes with teammates as a Cleveland Cavalier.

This star-studded workout isn't available everywhere yet: As of now, there are Rise studios in Denver, Cleveland, Miami, Dallas, and Los Angeles. Visit www.rise-nation.com to sign up.

CAN YOU SURVIVE BEAR GRYLLS'S CORE CHALLENGE?

The next time you're waiting for your freshly caught snake to cook over the fire, or killing time waiting for your helicopter extraction from a hot zone, get in some core work with this Bear Grylls hanging leg raise challenge. It's inspired by his work with BMF—which isn't an abbreviation for something Samuel L. Jackson would say, but for "Be Military Fit," a program designed to bring British military conditioning to all the Queen's subjects.

Grylls's challenge has two levels: Level 1 is 20 strict hanging leg raises—hands shoulder-width apart on a pull-up bar, bringing straight legs up so that your toes touch the bar. If you survive 20, go wild with level 2: Hang upside down from the bar using ankle clamps, and perform 20 reps of "hands to toes." Keeping your legs straight, flex your core to do a vertical sit-up, bringing your hands up to meet your toes. Keep your body under control as you return to start. If you can do 20 of these after 20 leg raises, you're the real BMF!

TERMINATE YOURSELF WITH YOUR OWN ARNOLD-INSPIRED WORKOUT

Arnold Schwarzenegger famously said that when people told him they'd "never want to look like you," he'd quip back, "Don't worry. You never will."

You don't become an Austrian Oak by accident: Schwarzenegger's *Pumping Iron*–era workouts were insane, and considered extremely high volume by today's standards. Arnold would train every body part multiple times per week, with as many as 26 working sets for a body part in each workout. He lifted twice a day: On Monday *morning*, he would lift chest and back, then come back for 40 or more sets of legs and abs in the evening.

Keep in mind: Schwarzenegger was the greatest bodybuilder in the world, is blessed with a ridiculous work ethic, and was taking (then perfectly legal) steroids, which help athletes recover much faster.

If you'd like to experience an Arnold-level training session—or you want to try to match the GOAT when he was at his GOAT-iest with a full program—use this template to design your own.

1. Choose your body part combo to train: chest and back, arms and shoulders, or legs.
2. Choose 4 to 5 exercises per body part. For instance, for chest, you might pick barbell bench press, incline barbell bench press, dumbbell bench press, dumbbell fly, dips, and dumbbell pull-overs.
3. Perform a few warm-up sets, then do 4 or 5 sets of each exercise, increasing the weights in each progressive set. For every set, go to failure (till you can't do another repetition with correct form).
4. Rest as little as possible between sets.
5. Finish your workout with three abdominal exercises.

WORK YOUR LEGS LIKE A *CHEER* SUPERSTAR

If you watched Netflix's *Cheer*, you couldn't help but notice James Thomas. He was in the middle of almost every stunt and tumbling pass, nailing every move. There was no doubt the big-smiling, high-flying "stumbler" would be "on the mat" for the show's finale.

Also not in doubt: his athleticism. And the show, he says, drove that home for athletes in other sports: He says he's gotten "hundreds of messages" from other athletes praising his strength.

Turn your next leg day into a *Cheer* day. Try this workout that Thomas uses to help build the legs and core that make him a high-flying, mind-changing superstar.

Perform 1 set of each exercise in each pair, then move to the other exercise. Do 3 rounds of each pair.

EXERCISE **PAIR 1**

EXERCISE A: Barbell Bent-Over Row (10 reps per set)

1. Deadlift the weight off the ground so you stand holding the bar in front of you with an overhand grip, feet hip-width apart, knees slightly bent.
2. Push your hips back as if you were opening a door behind you with your butt. This starts the hip hinge.
3. Keep pushing your hips back so that your back remains flat until it is nearly parallel to the floor, with the weight hanging straight down from your shoulders.
4. Maintaining this flat back position, pull the weight toward your chest.
5. Lower the weight back to the starting position, and repeat.

EXERCISE B: High Knees onto Plyo Box (30 seconds per round)

1. Place your right foot on a plyo box or step.
2. Rapidly exchange it for your left foot. Continue.

EXERCISE **PAIR 2**

EXERCISE A: Forearm Plank (1 minute per round)

Assume a forearm plank position, with your elbows planted directly beneath your shoulders, and your body forming a straight line from head to heels. Hold for the prescribed time.

EXERCISE B: Mountain Climbers (30 reps per round)

1. Assume the classic push-up position: Your hands should be directly beneath your shoulders, your body forming a straight line from head to heels.
2. Maintaining this body line and keeping your hips parallel to the floor, lift your right foot off the ground and bend your knee so that it comes up toward your chest.
3. Return your right foot to the start position, and rapidly exchange it for your left leg. Continue alternating.

EXERCISE **PAIR 3**

EXERCISE A: Isometric Squat Hold (30 seconds per round)

In round 1, use an empty bar. Load the bar for the next 2 rounds with the most you can squat-hold for 30 seconds.

1. Stand in a normal back squat position, barbell across your shoulders, feet between shoulder- and hip-width apart, toes slightly out.
2. Push your hips back to initiate the squat.
3. Bend your knees to descend until your thighs are at least parallel to the floor, keeping your weight on your heels.
4. Hold this position for the prescribed time, then stand back up.

EXERCISE B: Jump Squats (15 reps per round)

1. Stand with your feet slightly wider than shoulder-width apart.
2. Push your hips back to squat while swinging your arms back.
3. Now drive up through your heels so forcefully that your feet leave the ground.
4. Land softly, rest, reset, and repeat.

GO VIRAL

We all know that stars aren't just on TV or the big screen anymore. From a bodybuilder doing backflips in a rubber horse mask to seven-minute ab routines to a guy who shredded his abs eating Chipotle, these viral workouts offer a taste of some of the best from the stars of cyberspace.

KEEP IT MOVING LIKE THE CORONAVIRUS "KETTLEBELL GUY"

Sometimes, push-ups won't do. In a really stressful situation, there's no substitute for slinging some iron.

But during the COVID-19 pandemic, that wasn't an option: The gyms were closed. In New York, where stress was highest of all, a hero rose to provide the weights Americans needed: Marc Miller, aka the "Kettlebell Guy."

The gym owner had to close his facilities during quarantine, so he started gathering weights from as many places as he could find to sell, then delivered them to stressed New Yorkers. Miller became a sensation, being profiled in the *Wall Street Journal*. But the Kettlebell Guy didn't just show up and drop them off: He pumped out handstand push-ups while waiting, or crammed in some kettlebell cleans.

And he still found time to slip in some intense, full-body workouts of his own. Then Miller, a "meathead at heart," mixed in a little accessory work—"I like to put the final paint on the car. A little 'curls for the girls,' " he says.

Put some paint on your own car: Try this sample upper body workout the KB guy did during the shutdowns.

PART 1: CIRCUIT

Perform 1 set of each exercise in this series, then move to the next exercise without resting. Do 4 rounds of these three exercises, resting minimally between rounds.

Circuit EXERCISE 1: Plyometric Push-Up

1. Assume a classic push-up position, with hands directly beneath your shoulders, your body forming a straight line from head to heels.
2. Maintain this rigid body line as you bend your elbows to lower your chest toward the floor.
3. Press back to start so forcefully that your hands leave the floor. Land, reset, and repeat.

Circuit EXERCISE 2: "T" Push-Up:

1. Assume a classic push-up position, with your hands directly beneath your shoulders, and your body forming a straight line from head to heels.
2. Maintain this rigid body line as you bend your elbows to lower your chest toward the floor.
3. As you press back to start, rotate your body to bring your right arm straight up over your left, forming a "T" shape with your body. In this position, your feet should be stacked, with your body forming a straight line from head to heels, but on the side.
4. Rotate back to start, and repeat, this time rotating so your left hand goes toward the ceiling.

Circuit EXERCISE 3: Dumbbell Scaption

1. Stand with your feet together, dumbbells at your sides, palms in.
2. Keeping your torso upright, lift the dumbbells out to the sides at a 45-degree angle until they're at shoulder level. The dumbbells should be positioned vertically at the top, like you're giving a double thumbs-up.
3. Control the weights as they return to your sides, and repeat.

PART 2: BARBELL BENCH PRESS

Perform 5 sets of 8 reps, resting 60 to 75 seconds between sets.

1. Lie faceup on the bench and grab the bar with an overhand grip just wider than shoulder-width apart. Unrack the bar, holding it above your sternum with straight arms.
2. Brace your core and bend your elbows to lower the bar to your chest. Your elbows should stay close to your sides, forming a 45-degree angle.
3. Pause, then press back to start.

PART 3: SUPERSETS

Perform 1 set of each exercise in the pair, then move to the next exercise without resting. Rest for 30 seconds after finishing both exercises, then continue alternating in this way for the prescribed number of rounds.

SUPERSET 1

Perform 5 rounds of Exercise A, and 4 rounds of Exercise B.

EXERCISE A: Weighted Pull-Ups

Perform overhand grip pull-ups while wearing a weighted vest or with a dumbbell between your feet. Do 6 reps per set. Miller uses a 30-pound vest.

EXERCISE B: Dumbbell Push Press

1. Hold two dumbbells at your shoulders, palms in, with your feet slightly wider than shoulder-width apart.
2. Bend your knees slightly, dip your hips, and explode up, pressing the weights overhead.
3. Return the weights to your shoulders, and repeat. Perform 8 reps per set.

SUPERSET 2

Perform 4 rounds of both moves.

EXERCISE A: Small Medicine Ball Push-Up

1. Assume a modified push-up position, with hands directly beneath your chest on a small medicine ball, and your feet slightly wider than normal. Your body should still form a straight line from head to heels.
2. Maintaining this straight body line, bend your elbows to lower your chest until it touches your hands.
3. Press back to start. Do 12 reps per set.

EXERCISE B: Cable Curl

1. Stand with your feet shoulder-width apart, holding the straight bar at arm's length in front of your thighs, palms forward.
2. Maintaining an upright torso and keeping your shoulders level, bend your elbows to lift the bar up to your shoulders. Squeeze your biceps at the top.
3. Lower your arms and repeat. Do 12 reps per set.

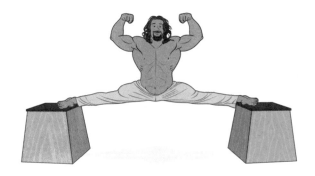

GET MOBILE LIKE THE INTERNET'S FLIPPING, SMILING STRONGMAN

E ven if you don't recognize his name, you know his videos: Jujimufu is the long-haired, hugely muscled man doing full splits on plastic chairs while holding 135 pounds overhead. He's the 235-pound man doing flips in a rubber horse mask. If those videos don't ring a bell, *stop*—put down this book and go watch his YouTube channel right now. Juji's flying, weight-flinging, and positive attitude will infect you with happiness, and leave you gasping "wow" at your screen.

How can a guy who is bodybuilder-big be so flexible? Jujimufu—whose real name is Jon Call—works at it! And fortunately for us smaller, non-flipping folks, he's happy to share that work. Here's his "Every Athlete Flexibility Routine," an 8-move sequence that takes about 45 minutes. Try it a few times a week while you're watching TV.

EXERCISE 1: Front Straight Leg Kick (8 sets of 4 reps on each leg)
1. Stand up straight with your left leg staggered just behind you.
2. Keep your supporting leg straight and your supporting heel on the ground as you kick your left leg in front of you as high as comfortably possible while keeping the leg straight.

EXERCISE 2: Rear Lift (6 sets of 6 reps on each leg)
1. Hold on to a chair or table in front of you at hip height. Bend forward slightly at the waist, and keep your back flat.
2. Keeping your leg straight, kick one leg back behind you while pointing your toes.

EXERCISE 3: Hoof Strike (2 sets of 10 reps on each leg)
1. Think of a bull getting ready to charge—that's what you're after. Stand straight and squeeze your butt.
2. Now kick your right heel back, trying to kick yourself in the butt.

WORKOUT CONTINUES >>>

EXERCISE 4: Side Bend (4 sets of 4 reps on each side)

1. Stand with your feet slightly wider than shoulder-width apart.
2. Keeping your hips square, bend down to bring your right shoulder toward your right foot.
3. Stand back up and repeat on the other side.

EXERCISE 5: Standing Torso Twist (2 sets of 10 reps on each side)

1. Stand with your feet wider than shoulder-width apart.
2. Twist your torso, maintaining control, and look the way you're twisting.

EXERCISE 6: Over-Under Band Stretch (2 sets of 10 reps)

1. Hold a resistance band or rope in front of you with your hands wide, palms down.
2. Keeping your arms straight, bring your arms up and over your head until they're behind you, with your palms now facing up.
3. Return to start, and repeat.

EXERCISE 7: Cossack Stretch (5 sets of 30 to 60 seconds each, resting 3 minutes in between)

1. Stand with your feet wide, toes facing forward.
2. Push your hips back and descend to your right by bending your right knee, keeping it tracking over your right toes. Keep your torso upright as you descend.
3. Keep descending until your body is over your right foot, coming up on your right toes while keeping your left foot flat on the ground.
4. Shift your weight to switch the position over your left foot, like a lateral squat. Shift back and forth.

EXERCISE 8: Crescent Lunging (10 minutes on each side)

1. Take a large lunge step forward with your right leg, and descend until your knees are both 90 degrees, with your rear knee grounded. Reach your arms up and overhead, and bend backward slightly, then return to upright.
2. Work in and out of the lunge—from ground to standing, and back again, twisting through your torso at the bottom and top.
3. Work through ranges of motion for ten minutes on this side, resting as needed, and then work on the other side.

HOW THE WORLD'S MOST JACKED CHEF GETS AN ARM PUMP

Move over, Steven Seagal: Andre Rush is the US military's toughest chef. He's got astounding 24-inch arms—if Rush sent you food you didn't like, you'd be afraid to send it back.

Not that you'd want to: Rush is legendary for creating gourmet meals in tiny, remote kitchens that amazed other soldiers. He's cooked for generals, ambassadors, and at the White House—where photos of him preparing a meal went viral in 2018.

But like Seagal in *Under Siege*, Rush isn't "just a cook." The retired Army master sergeant is a combat veteran, hand-to-hand combat trainer, and a master ice carver. And he finds time for 2,222 push-ups every day.

"Twenty-two vets commit suicide every day," he says. Raising awareness for that is the meaning behind all the deuces in 2,222.

In all his workouts, Rush does high reps of each exercise like this, especially on arm days: "My arm days are hell days."

Try a bit of that hell with this sample workout from Chef Rush. It's a 6-exercise circuit—a giant set—of 3 biceps exercises followed by 3 triceps exercises. You'll perform 1 set of each exercise before moving to the next exercise, with no rest in between. After finishing all 6 exercises, start again, repeating the entire sequence five times. Complete the entire sequence five or more times, and finish the workout with 50 push-ups.

EXERCISE 1: Alternating Dumbbell Bicep Curl (10 reps per round)

EXERCISE 2: Cross-Body Alternating Dumbbell Bicep Curl (10 reps per round)
Bring the dumbbell in front of your chest on each curl, keeping your palm facing up.

EXERCISE 3: Alternating Dumbbell Hammer Curl (10 reps per round)

EXERCISE 4: V-Bar Tricep Push-Down (25 reps per round)

EXERCISE 5: Straight-Bar Tricep Push-Down (25 reps per round)

EXERCISE 6: Rope Push-Down (25 reps per round)

Finisher: 50 Push-Ups

WORKOUT CONTINUES >>>

DO THE 22-PUSH-UP CHALLENGE FOR 22 DAYS

You may not be able to do 2,222 push-ups as the chef can, but you can raise awareness of suicide among military veterans. Take the 22 push-up-per-day challenge: For 22 days, do 22 push-ups—in a row, if you can—and post a video of it on social media, explaining the cause. Challenge 22 friends to join you and challenge *their* friends. And if they can, donate $22 to 22KILL, a nonprofit working to help suicidal veterans and front-line health responders.

Like Chef Rush, this challenge has gone viral before—celebrities including The Rock and Chris Evans have done it. You could make it go viral again! This could help get you started. It's a quick script for explaining the challenge in your video:

"Hi, I'm about to start the 22-day, 22 push-up challenge to raise awareness and money for 22KILL. Every day, 22 American veterans commit suicide. Today, I'm challenging [insert friends' names] to join me in this challenge, and support 22KILL with a donation of $22, or whatever you can give. You have 48 hours to answer the call: 22 push-ups per day for 22 days."

HOW ONE GUY ATE CHIPOTLE EVERY DAY—AND GOT SIX-PACK ABS

While digging into their regular bowl or burrito, every Chipotle lover has had this thought at least once: "I could eat this every day."

Devin Cunningham did—for more than a year. And he got (well, *kept*) washboard abs in the process.

"I saw some guy do it and he got featured on BuzzFeed—he ate it for 186 days straight," he says. "I was like, I could do it for a year, and I could do it with a purpose—to show people that they could eat what they want and stay fit at the same time."

So in July 2015, he started eating a bowl or burrito from Chipotle every day. And he kept eating there for 425 days—during which time he bulked up from 156 pounds at 12 percent body fat to 173 pounds at 14 percent body fat. He then cut down to 146 pounds at 8.7 percent body fat—and went viral. Cunningham was profiled in *Time*, Thrillist, and just about everywhere else online.

It wasn't just the burritos that kept Cunningham so lean. He worked out six days a week, including daily cardio sessions during the cut-down phase. Here's what he'd do on a Chipotle chest day—with cardio—while dropping those 27 pounds.

Perform each of these chest exercise for 4 sets of 8 repetitions.

EXERCISE 1: Barbell Bench Press

1. Lie faceup on the bench and grab the bar with an overhand grip just wider than shoulder-width apart. Unrack the bar, holding it above your sternum with straight arms.
2. Bend your elbows to lower the bar to your chest. Your elbows should stay close to your sides, forming a 45-degree angle.
3. Pause, then press back to start.

EXERCISE 2: Incline Bench Press

1. Lie faceup on an incline bench and grab the bar with an overhand grip just wider than shoulder-width apart. Unrack the bar, holding it above your sternum with straight arms.
2. Bend your elbows to lower the bar to your chest. Your elbows should stay close to your sides, forming a 45-degree angle.
3. Pause, then press back to start.

WORKOUT CONTINUES >>>

EXERCISE 3: Dumbbell Pull-Over

1. Lie perpendicular to a bench, with your upper back on the bench, knees bent 90 degrees. In this position, hold a dumbbell by one end over your chest with slightly bent elbows and an overhand grip.
2. Lower the weight over your head until your arms are even with your shoulders—as if they're overhead when you're standing.
3. Bring the weight back to start.

EXERCISE 4: Overhand Grip Dumbbell Fly

1. Lie faceup on a bench holding two dumbbells over your chest, palms facing as if you were holding a bench press barbell.
2. With slightly bent elbows, lower the dumbbells to the sides of your chest until your chest is stretched.
3. Bring the dumbbells back together using a wide hugging motion. Repeat.

EXERCISE 5: Single-Arm Machine Fly

Use a chest fly machine with one arm at a time. Keep your torso square.

Cardio

On the elliptical machine, sprint for 15 seconds, then go at an easy pace for 45 seconds. Repeat for 45 to 60 minutes.

Devin's "Regular" Chipotle Order

If you're a regular at the 'Potle, you've got your regular order—and Devin is no different: "A chicken bowl with extra steak, hot sauce, pico [de gallo], corn [salsa], brown rice, and cheese. That's my staple."

JAM OUT WITH THIS CHALLENGE FROM AMERICA'S MOST INSPIRING FITNESS PERSONALITY

The internet's most motivating fitness star? That's easy: Kym Perfetto, aka Kym Nonstop. As a founding instructor at SoulCycle, her client list included celebrities like Madonna and Kelly Ripa, and her upbeat inspiration is the style every other spin instructor is imitating. But—excuse the pun—she didn't stop there. Perfetto created Dryft, a mobile fitness studio at two locations in California that combines strength training and rowing. Whether you're in a class with Kym or watching her in a YouTube video, you're getting the same 10-gigawatt energy from Perfetto, and it will definitely make you want to get up and move.

Channel some Nonstop energy right now with a "song challenge" workout. Perfetto will often program one of these at the end of a fitness class—because they're fun, for starters, and because they don't require a ton of thinking by already worn-out workoutters.

For each challenge, the lyrics tell you which exercises to do. It's even easier than that sounds. Try one of these, or make a playlist for a full-body workout challenge:

"FLOWERS" BY MOBY

Using an exercise like a push-up, a squat, or a leg lift, follow along with this classic Crossfit challenge: Each time the singers say "Sally down," you descend into your exercise—bending your elbows to lower in a push-up, or squatting down. Hold that position until the singers say "Sally up," where you do the top portion of the exercise—pushing up from the ground on a push-up, for example. Continue for the full length of the song. Kym Nonstop's favorite choice? Leg lifts, "because they're really hard!"

"ROXANNE" BY THE POLICE

Every time Sting says "Roxanne," do a push-up. Every time he sings "red light," do a burpee. Sounds easy, but Sting gets pretty repetitive—and picks up the pace—later in the song!

"SWITCH" BY WILL SMITH

Do bodyweight forward lunges during the verses, and bodyweight squats during the chorus of this song. For an added challenge, do a jump squat each time Smith says "Switch" during the chorus, bringing your feet together, then back out to hip-width apart.

STILL DREAM OF DUNKING? THIS LEG WORKOUT IS FOR YOU

Dunking a basketball is the closest you'll ever come to being Michael Jordan, or, hell, Superman: You can't fly, but if you get springy enough, you can dunk—and then give yourself a lifetime of fist bumps for slamming the ball home.

You don't have to have NBA height to throw down: You just have to be like a different Air Jordan—Jordan Kilganon, the 6-foot-1 internet dunk king. More than 700,000 people follow his world tour of dunks on Instagram. And at the 2019 NBA All-Star Weekend, Kilganon blew the minds of Dwyane Wade, Reggie Miller, and others with his signature dunk, "The Scorpion" . . . while wearing jeans.

To convert his lower limbs into rocket-powered springs, Kilganon performs squats and deadlifts, of course. But he says the best workout for jumping is to practice jumping. Here's a bounce-improving workout composed of exercises he does each week.

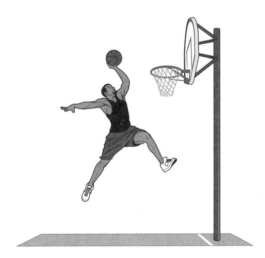

PART 1: JUMPING

Kilganon says to aim for 10 maximum-effort jumps, resting plenty between each jump. "[Dunking] is not about doing a bunch of jumps back to back," he says. You need one big jump—so practice that. When he was learning, Kilganon would practice on a shorter hoop. If that's not available, find a way to measure your jumps—touching a certain part of the net, or a spot high on a wall—and practice 10 all-out jumps.

PART 2: PLYOMETRICS

That's just a fancy word for "more jumping." You're working on maximum height, not maximum repetitions, so the sets are short. Your rest periods, as above, should be long—rest for a few minutes between each set.

EXERCISE 1: Depth Jumps (3 sets of 1 to 3 jumps, resting 2 minutes between sets)

Stand on the bottom step of a staircase. Step off with one foot, and land with both feet, jumping straight up as high as possible immediately. (The goal is to minimize the amount of time your feet are on the floor between stepping down and jumping.) Reset, and repeat. Over time, you can step from a higher platform.

EXERCISE 2: Consecutive Broad Jumps (4 to 5 sets of 5 reps each)

Stand with your feet about hip-width apart. Load your hips by pushing your hips back into a quarter-squat and raising your arms in front of you. Throw your arms forward and jump forward with two feet, landing with two feet. Immediately jump again.

EXERCISE 3: Plyometric Step-Up (3 sets of 3 reps on each leg)

Stand in front of a stable bench, box, or step. Place one foot on the box, keeping the other on the floor. Drive through your raised leg to step up so forcefully that your foot comes up off the box. Land softly with that same foot on the bench. Do all your reps on this side, then switch sides.

EXERCISE 4: Short Sprints (4 reps)

Perform 4 sprints of 20 to 40 yards each, resting fully between sprints.

THE WORKOUT THAT KEEPS THE WORLD'S MOST INSPIRING GUY ABSOLUTELY RIPPED

You've seen transformation side-by-sides, but none can match Matt Childs's: In the before, he's in a hospital bed with oxygen flowing into his nose through tubes. In the after, a year later: He's a tattooed, screaming He-Man action figure.

Childs was an alcoholic who, by his recollection, had been arrested 30 times and hospitalized 40 more. When he finally changed his life in 2015, he built a body that *Muscle & Fitness* magazine named one of its best transformations ever, and the article about him blew up.

That article, which went viral, has helped the Tennessee man reach people in recovery all over the world to offer his help. He's provided training and recovery advice to people struggling in the US and overseas, and he does it all while looking like an absolute beast—even at age 44.

To maintain that physique, Childs does a workout program built from two cycles of four days each: Day 1 is chest and back. Leg day is day 2. Shoulders, biceps, and triceps get worked on day 3. And day 4 is a calisthenics and conditioning routine that keeps him looking lean. It's his consistency that makes it work.

"Put your healthy lifestyle first, then incorporate stuff around that," he says, not the other way around. "It's discipline—that's it!"

Test your own discipline against his biweekly conditioning routine. Then see if you can stick with it to repeat the session again in five days.

EXERCISE 1: Hanging Leg Raises to Side (4 sets of 15 reps on each side)
1. Hang from a pull-up bar with an overhand grip, hands wider than shoulder-width apart.
2. Don't lean back as you pull your knees up and to the left toward your chest by bending your hips.
3. Return to start, and pull your legs up and to the right.

EXERCISE 2: Machine Crunch (4 sets of 15 reps)
Using the ab crunch machine at your gym.

EXERCISE 3: Standing Barbell Bicycle (1 set of 12 to 15 reps)
1. Stand with your feet shoulder-width apart, a barbell on your shoulders behind your head.
2. Twist your torso and bring your elbow down toward your left knee as you raise the knee up toward your elbow.
3. Return to the starting position, and do the move on the other side.

EXERCISES 4 AND 5: Battling Rope Waves and Tire Flips

1. Do these 2 exercises as a superset, performing 1 set of the first exercise, then a set of the second exercise. Repeat the pair for 4 sets.
2. For the Battling Rope Waves: Alternate your arms for big waves from a quarter-squat position. Go as fast as you can for 45 seconds per set.
3. For the Tire Flips, Childs uses a 200-pound tire. Perform a full squat to get your hands below the tire, then explode up to flip it. Perform 12 to 15 flips per set.

EXERCISE 6: Box Jumps (4 sets of 10 reps)

Stand in front of the box with feet shoulder-width apart. Dip your hips and explode up onto the box. Step down, and repeat. Perform 4 sets, progressing to higher boxes in each set.

EXERCISE 7: Lateral Box Jumps (4 sets of 5 reps on each side)

Instead of facing the box, stand with the box on your right side. Dip and explode up onto the box to your right. Hop back down, and repeat.

EXERCISE 8: Ladder Drill (12 sets)

Childs performs 12 different variations on the agility ladder (also known as a speed ladder). Do 12 rounds of your own—quick feet, in and out, and hops.

EXERCISE 9: Medicine Ball Seated Twist (4 sets of 30 seconds each)

1. Sit on the floor with your heels on the ground. Your torso should be at a 45-degree angle from the ground, and should be straight from your butt to your head. Hold a medicine ball in front of your chest with straight arms.
2. From this position, twist to the left, twisting your whole torso, not just your arms, until your hands point out to 9 o'clock.
3. Twist back to start, and then go to the right, twisting until your shoulders, chest, and hands point toward 3 o'clock. That's one repetition.

EXERCISE 10: Bleacher Sprints (42 reps)

At his local high school, Childs does 42 rounds of sprints up the bleachers, resting minimally between sets.

EXERCISE 11: 110-Yard Sprints (4 to 6 reps)

These aren't all-out sprints, Childs says, but still pretty hard runs. He performs 4 to 6 runs of this distance, then jogs for a half-mile to cool down.

PASS THIS VIRAL TEST—AND LIVE LONGER WITH LESS PAIN IN YOUR BACK

It's become a staple outside sporting events, at conferences, and in viral videos: Hang from a bar for 100 seconds, and a carnival barker–type will give you $100.

The outcome: Jacked bros and sinewy-lean fitness models fail. But hanging for a long time isn't just a party trick. Grip strength is one of the most accurate predictors of longevity.

You can improve your grip strength—and reduce shoulder pain—by practicing hangs a few times a week. Hangs may also provide some relief for cranky backs, and may lengthen your life. Most important: If you ever see one of those hang challenges, you'll walk away with a Benjamin.

Improving your time is simple: Hang from a bar. Let your whole body relax, straightening your elbows, feeling your shoulders shrug naturally toward your ears, and relaxing your spine, rib cage, and legs. Try to release any tension in your body as you hang.

Hang out and perform this workout three times a week, resting at least one day between sessions. Add these hangs at the end of your gym workout, after a cardio session, or by themselves as a break in the middle of your workday.

1. Hanging from the bar for ten seconds counts as 1 repetition. Perform 4 to 5 repetitions per set, taking a five-second break between ten-second holds.
2. Rest for three minutes between sets, and perform 3 to 5 total sets—for a total of 12 to 25 hangs of ten seconds each.
3. On the last hang of your last set, hold on as long as you can. Track your progress.

A WORKOUT TO LIVE TO 102

Most of us would be happy to still be breathing at 100 years old. At 101, George Jedenoff was still *skiing*, and working out every day to stay strong enough to do it. Over the past few years, his exploits on the slopes have become an annual video sensation, as the centenarian slashes down the slopes of Utah's Snowbird Resort.

For 45 minutes every morning, the Bay Area miner–turned–World War II officer–turned steel executive–turned-retiree gets a workout in before breakfast—a routine that most Americans half his age couldn't handle.

"You see so many people in the streets in such terrible shape. They're not going to last long," he says. And Jedenoff knows about lasting long—he told me that at the ripe age of 102. The secret: "Keep moving, keep vertical, and keep positive. Whatever comes, you've got to take a swing at it."

Now it's your turn to take a swing at a version of his always varying, but always strenuous daily workout.

MOVE YOUR JOINTS
Every day, Jedenoff spends 15 minutes bending, stretching, and "making sure all my joints work." It doesn't have to be fancy: Just spend time each day moving your joints through a full range of motion. Some of Jedenoff's favorites:

Staircase Hip Stretch
Stand at the bottom of a flight of stairs. Take a big step up with one leg to the third or fourth step, keeping your other foot flat on the ground at the bottom of the stairs. Keep your back leg straight and lean forward to stretch your hip. Move the joint around. Return to start, and do the same on the other leg.

Glute Bridge
Jedenoff does this one because he's had a stiff back for "40 to 50 years." Lie faceup on the ground with your knees bent and your feet flat on the ground. Place your arms at your sides, palms up. Keeping your feet flat on the floor, squeeze your glutes to raise your hips off the floor until your body forms a straight line from your knees to your shoulders. Pause for a second at the top of the exercise, and then slowly return to the start position. Repeat a few times.

BUILD SOME STRENGTH
To maintain muscle mass, Jedenoff does 15 minutes of strength work, using a doorjamb resistance band system and plain old floor exercises. Try some of his favorite moves:

WORKOUT CONTINUES >>>

Cable Press

1. With cables slightly behind you, hold the handles with bent elbows at your nipple line. Stand in a staggered stance.
2. Squeeze your chest and press your arms forward and together until your elbows are straight.
3. Control the cables back to the start.

Cable Fly

1. With the cables anchored high, stand between them, holding the cables out to the side with palms facing forward. Bend forward slightly into an athletic position.
2. Squeeze your chest to bring the cables down and in front of your chest, keeping your arms straight, until your fists touch.
3. Control the movement to return to start, and repeat.

Straight-Arm Pull-Down

1. Stand with the cable stack in front of you. Grab the handle with your right hand and hold it so it's just above and in front of your shoulder.
2. Keeping your core braced and your elbow straight, use your back to pull the weight down until the handle is in front of your right hip.
3. Return to start, and repeat. Do all your reps on this side, then switch sides and repeat.

Push-Up

At 102, Jedenoff does 6 to 8 push-ups on his knees—a move that many people in their 40s couldn't do as well. See if you can get 20 or more.

Sit-Up

"I'll still do maybe 6 or 8, but that's all," Jedenoff said at 102. That's almost 2,000 per year!

DO SOME CARDIO

1. To keep his ticker humming after 100-plus years, Jedenoff tackles a cardio gauntlet each morning on his exercise bike, elliptical machine, and stair climber in his Bay Area home. He uses all three each morning—only for two to three minutes each, he says, "just enough to get my legs and arms through all the motions."
2. Jedenoff finishes his 45 minutes of morning work with a jog—10 laps around his small swimming pool, a distance of a little less than a half-mile.

PART 3

WORKOUTS THAT ARE RIDICULOUSLY FUN

What fun is moving your body if moving your body isn't fun? Working out doesn't have to feel like work all the time. These workouts will help you have a blast while getting fitter.

CHAPTER 11

GRAB SOME FRIENDS

Ever had a friend who always suggests new get-togethers to get out of the rut of the same old trips to the same old watering holes? Where do they get all those ideas? For you, the answer is simple: this chapter! It's filled with plans for weekends away, adventures near home, and ways to get sweaty and stay in touch.

RUN 5 MILES, EAT 12 DONUTS

The Krispy Kreme Challenge in Raleigh, North Carolina, challenges you to do just that, taking off from the campus of NC State for a 2.5-mile run through town. At the halfway point, 3,000 or so runners dressed in donut socks, donut shirts, donut yoga pants, and more take a break to down a dozen Krispy Kreme glazed donuts. Then, they run back. The "challenge" part: Finishing the race—and all 12 glazed rings—in less than an hour.

Don't be fooled: This isn't some testosterone-fueled bro-fest. The atmosphere is fun and festive, with college-aged runners fending off hangovers amid middle-aged runners shaking off the February cold. The race includes a costume contest, so you're happily running through town surrounded by blueberries, Grateful Dead bears, and, of course, Homer Simpson.

You don't even have to finish all the donuts: Instead of the "challenger" category, you can run as a "casual," opting to finish as many donuts as you want, and running back with the rest. Some runners bring a small backpack to carry the remaining donuts back in their box; the trio I ran with in 2019 just carried our boxes back as we ran.

With all those hungover college kids, one thing can get a little intense: There's a fair amount of vomit at this race—and you'll hear warnings that you'll probably lose your breakfast, too. But if you're light on the sauce the night before, you should be fine. Just watch for puddles on the return run.

The race is run in February. Registration is available at www.krispykremechallenge.com for $45.

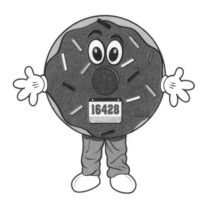

RUN A BEER MILE

The rules are simple: Chug a beer. Run a quarter-mile. Repeat three more times.

It started in Canada. In 1989, seven runners in Ontario—including a future Olympian—concocted this cockamamie race and ran its first edition at a high school track. The winning time: 7 minutes, 30 seconds.

That slap-happy evening launched what would become a worldwide phenomenon—including an annual, world championship race. And the runners have gotten serious: The record time has plummeted to 4:28, held by honest-to-goodness track athlete Corey Bellemore, also a Canadian.

For the amateurs among us, it's a little slower, but just as much fun: Your stomach will be distended and sloshing with liquid, you'll be burping—a lot—and by the time you're done, you'll have a little buzz.

Beer miles are held by breweries, running clubs, and they're just about everywhere: Just Google BEER MILE and your city or town. If you can't find one, grab some friends (so you aren't drinking alone) and organize your own. The beers need to be at least 5 percent alcohol, you've got to drink them within a 10-meter "transition zone" near the start, and you've got to keep it all down—if you throw up, you've got to run a penalty lap.

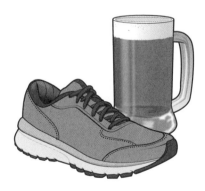

PUSH A CAR AROUND A PARKING LOT, AND FEEL LIKE SUPERMAN

Why? *Why?* Because you'll feel ridiculously powerful. I remember reading that an NFL Draft prospect was doing this around 2008, but I can't find record of it. No matter. Former NFL O-lineman Walter Jones pushed trucks around to build the power that put him in the Pro Football Hall of Fame. Studies have shown that sled pushes challenge the thighs at a similar level to squats, and tax the calves even more. A smaller study (conducted by me) has shown that it is fun, and a perfect Saturday activity with friends.

What you need:
- A car
- A friend
- A flat section of parking lot
- Some awesome music

How to do it:
1. Put the car in neutral, and shut it down. One friend stays in the car to steer, the other pushes.
2. Turn on music.
3. Push the car down to the end of your parking lot strip, then run around to the front of the car and push it back to the start.
4. Switch places with your friend, and gasp while he or she does the same.
5. Continue until you're both wiped, then go get a big lunch together.

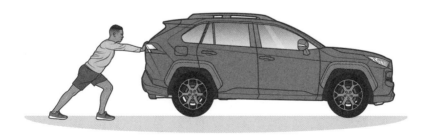

SMASH YOUR STRESS WITH A SLEDGEHAMMER

Extremely serious trainers will tell you that "Nobody needs to hit a tire with a sledgehammer."

This is true! Other things nobody needs: Cheeseburgers. High fives. *Top Gun*.

Those things are awesome, though. And so is slamming a sledgehammer into a big ol' tire. It gets your heart racing, makes your breathing heavy, and it's a stress-busting blast. It's fantastic as interval cardio, too.

It's also fantastically cheap. A new, 10-pound hammer will run you $20, and you can get the tire for free: Visit a local used tire store, and ask if they'll give you a tire that's headed for the dump—they'll happily give you their garbage! Then grab a friend, find a grassy spot (so you don't bang up your driveway), and start swinging and slamming with this simple workout.

How to do it:

You'll perform two types of swings in this workout—overhead swings and over-the-shoulder swings.

To do the overhead swing, hold the hammer behind your head with both hands. Bend your knees so you're in an athletic stance, and bring the hammer down over your head to slam the tire in front of you. Reset and repeat.

To do the over-the-shoulder swing, you'll be swinging as if you're driving a stake with the hammer. Stand facing the tire in an athletic stance. Your left hand should be at the bottom of the handle, and your right hand higher up, near the hammer head. Load your hips and bounce the hammer up from your right thigh until it's over your right shoulder. Slide your right hand down to meet your left as you slam the hammer onto the tire. Reset and repeat.

Using these two swings, do the following:

1. 20 overhead swings
2. 20 over-the-shoulder swings to the right
3. 20 over-the-shoulder swings to the left

Rest while your partner performs the same moves, and repeat. If performing the workout alone, rest one minute between sets.

Repeat this sequence until you're slammed. Then go grab a cheeseburger and watch *Top Gun*.

ELIMINATE WEAKNESS WITH NITRO'S *AMERICAN GLADIATORS* PARTNER WORKOUT

In the early '90s, the American Gladiators were superhuman stars of syndication, and the undisputed star of the show was a former Los Angeles Ram: Nitro.

Thirty years later, he's had a heart attack, two life-threatening pulmonary embolisms, and long ago hung up his spandex. But even at 56, Nitro (real name: Dan Clark) still looks like somebody who would mess you up in a game of Powerball.

His near-death experiences, which he wrote about in his book, *F Death*, made Clark reexamine his priorities: He's refocused on being with people he loves—including during his workouts. Clark loves partner workouts, and his favorites have a simple theme—"I do one. Then you do one."

Those workouts are usually 100, 200, or 300 reps of a total-body exercise or exercise pair for each participant, with the only rest being gasps while your partner finishes their round. Team up with a friend and get Gladiator strong with this challenge, one of Clark's favorites.

Perform a 3-exercise mini set, then wait while your partner does the same. Trade back and forth until you've each done 100 sets—Clark says it took him and a partner 29 minutes to complete at their last session.

EXERCISE 1: Single-Arm Dumbbell Snatch, Right Arm
1. With a dumbbell between your feet, squat down until the weight is centered between your feet. Grab it with an overhand grip.
2. Pull the weight off the floor by extending your hips and knees. As the weight passes your knees, raise your shoulders so the dumbbell comes up over your head. The weight should move in a straight line from the floor to overhead. It's kind of like trying to throw the dumbbell at the ceiling—without letting go.
3. Return the weight to your shoulder, and put it down. Do 1 rep.

EXERCISE 2: Single-Arm Dumbbell Snatch, Left Arm
Do 1 rep.

EXERCISE 3: Burpee
1. Stand with your feet shoulder-width apart.
2. Squat down until your hands are outside your feet.
3. Jump back to the top of a plank position.
4. Do a push-up.
5. Jump back to position 2.
6. Spring out of the squat and jump as high as you can. Do 1 rep.

PEDAL YOUR WAY TO PULLED PORK ON NC'S BARBECUE TRAIL

If you're a barbecue fanatic, you know there's no such thing as too much melt-in-your-mouth pulled pork or beef brisket. North Carolina knows this well: The Tar Heel State is packed with so many pits that the North Carolina Barbecue Society has designated 21 spots across the state as stops along the "Historic Barbecue Trail."

The problem? The historic barbecue joints are pretty close together: If you visit one for lunch, it's only 15 to 30 miles to the next stop—hardly enough distance by car to work up a whole new appetite. The solution: Trade four wheels for two.

Back in 2011, a friend and I parked at a Walmart in Statesville, North Carolina, and started biking: We'd ride 20 miles to one of the historic pits for lunch, fuel up, and ride another 15 to 20 miles for dinner. We'd clean up at a hotel, sleep, and repeat. After four days, we'd ridden 142 miles and eaten about 142,000 calories of pork.

You don't need to commit to half a week of riding, though, to join friends and family on a pit-stop tour of your own. And with ride-sharing apps, the whole endeavor is even easier: Park at one spot for lunch, chow down, and ride to your next pit for dinner. Take a Lyft back to your car, and your delicious day of adventure—and eating—is complete. Check the chart for biking distances between some of these historic pits, and visit http://www.ncbbqsociety.com/ for a complete list.

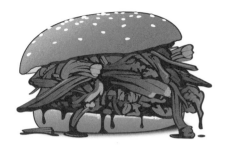

PLAN YOUR PORK-TO-PORK RIDE

A short pork stop: . . . . .Salisbury to Granite Quarry

For lunch: . . . . .Richard's B-B-Q, 522 North Main Street,
Salisbury, NC

For dinner: . . . . .M&K Barbecue and Country Cooking, 215 North
Salisbury Avenue, Granite Quarry, NC

Ride distance:. . . . . .Just 6 miles

A medium ride between meals: . . .Winston-Salem to Lexington

For lunch: . . . . .Real Q, 4885 Country Club Road,
Winston-Salem, NC

For dinner: . . . . .Smiley's BBQ, 917 Winston Road,
Lexington, NC

Ride distance:. . . . . .23.5 miles

Build up a big appetite:. . . . . .Lexington to Greensboro

For lunch: . . . . .The Barbecue Center, 900 North Main Street,
Lexington, NC

For dinner: . . . . .Stamey's Barbecue, 2206 High Point Road,
Greensboro, NC

Ride distance:. . . . . .34.9 miles

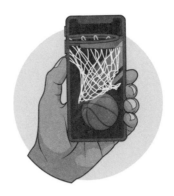

HOOP IT UP WITH FRIENDS . . . EVEN IF THEY'RE HUNDREDS OF MILES AWAY

During the 2020 coronavirus shutdowns, NBA and WNBA players played HORSE from afar, slinging videos of shots back and forth for our stay-at-home viewing pleasure. (HORSE is a game in which competitors make the identical shot of the person shooting before them. Players who miss get an "H." Players are eliminated when they've missed five times and the word "horse" is spelled.) But you don't have to be a pro to stay in touch with friends and family while getting a game in from waaaaay downtown.

Start your own game of socially distant HORSE via group text—it's like those old-timey, through-the-mail games of chess, but for the smartphone era. S.D. HORSE will help you stay in touch, get everyone outside, and give your crew the kind of ribbing, supporting, and laughing that friendly competition is perfect for. Once you've challenged a group to the game, here's how to do it:

1. Send a video (or at least a description) of your first shot to the group.
2. Everyone has 72 hours (three days) to send a video of their own attempt.
3. Those who miss (or skip the shot) get an "H," just as in a regular game of HORSE.
4. After everyone has done shot 1, shooter 2 is up.

One shot every three days isn't much of a workout, but let's be honest: Are you really going to go to a basketball court and take just *one* shot? You'll get on the court more often, shoot around, and get that heart rate pounding.

RUN 2,000 MILES WITH YOUR FRIENDS—NO MATTER HOW FAR APART YOU ARE

Fitness is all about consistency. And it doesn't get much more consistent than the "Run the Year" challenge, where runners log as many miles as the year—so in 2022, they'll run 2,022 miles.

That's 5.5 miles per day, almost 39 miles per week—an amount even seasoned marathoners don't often match. So don't do it alone: Sign up for one of these 2,000-plus-mile challenges with a group of friends to get fit—and stay in touch—together.

For Jason Tregler, being part of that kind of team helped him lose more than 150 pounds. The 47-year old Floridian has been participating in Run the Year since 2015, going from a never-runner to a multiple marathoner who has run as many as 1,800 miles in a year.

"Some people say they're 'behind schedule,' but . . . don't worry about trying to finish it too quickly. Just get out there and do something," he says. He's done the annual challenge with groups of friends, and some years just with his wife. And while you can do the challenge on your own, Tregler has participated via an online, virtual event that provides rewards for reaching milestones, tracking tools, and groups of other challengers to interact with. These other runners provide support, tips, and friendship that Tregler says helped him drop the weight and become a regular, consistent exerciser.

Organize your own Run the Year challenge with friends, or visit www.runtheyear.com to join one of their virtual challenges, which start at $25.

TURN A ROUND OF GOLF INTO A SERIOUS WORKOUT LIKE THE GOLDEN BEAR

When Jack Nicklaus needed to slim down, he sped up his game: "I would carry four or five clubs and I would go run around the course as I played," he said. The regimen helped him lose 20 pounds in the late 1960s.

Today, it's a full-fledged sport. Speedgolf combines golf with running: One stroke and one minute are scored equally—so if you shoot an 80 and finish in 58 minutes, your score is 138.

When's the last time you heard of finishing a round of golf in an *hour*? In a world where three-hour rounds won't fit our busy schedules, you can still get swings in—and enjoy time with friends and get fitter—with this growing sport.

Running may even make you better on the course by getting you out of your head: "You can't think about so many things—you look at the target, look at the hole, and don't think about your mechanics," says Scott Dawley, the founder and president of Speedgolf USA.

A former PGA tour pro, Dawley now works to grow the faster game, working with courses to increase its availability, and staging a Speedgolf pro tour.

Since it's not available at many courses yet, the tour may be your best chance to play. There are divisions for beginning runners, beginning golfers, and beginning both-ers. A nine-hole round works out to about 2.5 miles. You'll only need a handful of clubs—a wood, a long iron, a short iron, and a putter—and some friends to get started. To find a course near you or to sign up for a tournament, visit www.speedgolfusa.com.

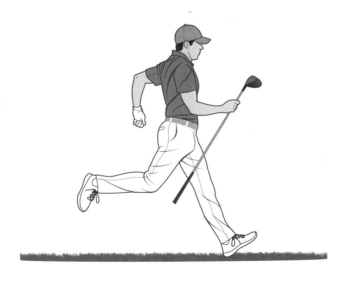

You may not be able to get Terry Crews to yell at you from across a park, but boot camping with buddies before brunch can be just as much fun as it was in *Bridesmaids*. But if you've already been to spin, danced (or tried) along with Zumba, and chanted *om* with goats at an outdoor yoga class, plan your next road trip or girls'/guys' weekend to include one of the four hardest fitness classes in America, as rated by ClassPass users. The mimosas will taste even more refreshing after this level of effort—just make sure you have a Gatorade first.

#4: Train45 at Class Studios in Dallas

"This class was 'teaching your Mom how to use Instagram' challenging," says one sweaty class-goer. For 45 minutes, you'll switch between three stations: hand weights and burpees on the mat, suspension trainer moves for strength, and the rowing machine to gas you.

#3: Megaformer Pilates at Pilates Plus in Studio City, California

Megaformer classes, which use a supercharged, multi-featured version of the Pilates Reformer machine, are the fastest-growing classes in America, according to ClassPass. There's probably an option near you, but if you're in LA, the classes at Pilates Plus are America's hardest.

#2: SCULPT Full Body Class at BODYROK in San Francisco

Another Reformer class, but with BODYROK's own custom Reformers—torture machines, basically—on which instructors urge you to lunge, plank, leg press, and jump. "It hurts to laugh, and I was hobbling home after," says one masochist. "I would totally return."

#1: Conditioning Class at Tone House in New York

Tone House's classes are like a high-intensity sports practice: You'll be divided into groups and do drills like sprints, interval sets of squats, and sled pushes—with teammates cheering you on. "I came to class already dead," says one reviewer. "Died some more and somehow came out refreshed."

PLAY TUG-OF-WAR WITH A JUMBO JET

A Boeing 757 weighs more than 220,000 pounds. But get enough friends together, and you can make that behemoth budge . . . and then lurch . . . and then roll for 12, 20, or even 30 feet.

At plane-pull events around the country, teams of 20 to 25 grab a rope and pull enormous aircraft across the tarmac—for charity, of course, often the local Special Olympics chapter.

At Cleveland's airport and at Dulles outside DC, teams of 25 pull the jets for 12 feet. At Rocky Mountain Metropolitan Airport in Colorado, teams of 10 pull a smaller jet for 20 feet. And at Newark Liberty, teams of 20 tug a 93,000-pound aircraft.

There's likely an event near you, so get a group together, and get that plane moving! Google SPECIAL OLYMPICS PLANE PULL and your nearest city to find an event.

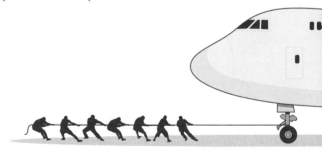

ARE YOU FITTER THAN A FIFTH GRADER?: FIND OUT: TAKE THE PRESIDENTIAL PHYSICAL FITNESS TEST AGAIN

For 1980s elementary-school students, there was only one thing in gym class scarier than the class bully with a dodgeball—the President's Challenge Fitness Test. Until 2012, when it was phased out, gym teachers would run gawky kids through this NFL Combine for pre-teens, and watch them fail to meet Herculean standards of fitness.

There were five events: pull-ups, sit-ups, the sit and reach, a shuttle run, and the mile. To win the Presidential Physical Fitness Award, you needed to score in the 85th percentile for your gender and age. To win the National Physical Fitness Award, you needed to score above the 50th percentile.

At least in my school, *nobody* could meet the higher standards, which included, for an 11-year-old boy, six pull-ups and a 7:32 mile. A 17-year-old boy would have to knock out 13 pull-ups, a standard many adults wouldn't be able to match.

Show you're finally fitter than a fifth grader—and bring your friends and your own kids along for your triumph. Use the charts below to measure your performance in these five events:

1. **SIT-UPS:** See how many you can do in a minute.
2. **SHUTTLE RUN:** Set up two cones 30 feet apart. Place two balls just beyond the second cone. Run from cone 1 to cone 2, pick up a ball, and drop it by cone 1. Repeat with the second ball, sprinting back through the starting line—when you cross the starting line, your time is recorded.
3. **SIT AND REACH:** You don't need the fancy "sit and reach" box. Sit with your back against a wall, feet straight out in front of you, and place a yardstick between your legs so it measures distance past your ankles. Lean forward with both hands stacked and reach as far as you can—the distance past your ankles is your score.
4. **MILE RUN.**
5. **PULL-UPS:** Your chin must come above the bar on each rep.

WORKOUT CONTINUES >>>

PRESIDENT'S CHALLENGE QUALIFYING STANDARDS

The Presidential Physical Fitness Award

Participants must at least reach these levels in all 5 events in order to qualify for the President's Physical Fitness Award. These levels represent the 85th percentile based on the 1985 School Population Fitness Survey.

Age	Curl-Ups (# one minute)	Partial Curl-Ups (#)	Shuttle Run (sec.)	V-Sit Reach (in.)	Sit & Reach (cm)	One-Mile Run (min:sec)	Distance Option (min:sec) ¼ mile	(min:sec) ½ mile	Pull-Ups (#)	Rt. Angle Pull-Ups (#)
6	33	22	12.1	+3.5	31	10:15	1:55		2	9
7	36	24	11.5	+3.5	30	9:22	1:48		4	14
8	40	30	11.1	+3.0	31	8:48		3:30	5	17
9	41	37	10.9	+3.0	31	8:31		3:30	5	18
10	45	35	10.3	+4.0	30	7:57			6	22
11	47	43	10.0	+4.0	31	7:32			6	27
12	50	64	9.8	+4.0	31	7:11			7	31
13	53	59	9.5	+3.5	33	6:50			7	39
14	56	62	9.1	+4.5	36	6:26			10	40
15	57	75	9.0	+5.0	37	6:20			11	42
16	56	73	8.7	+6.0	38	6:08			11	44
17	55	66	8.7	+7.0	41	6:06			13	53
6	32	22	12.4	+5.5	32	11:20	2:00		2	9
7	34	24	12.1	+5.0	32	10:36	1:55		2	14
8	38	30	11.0	+4.5	33	10:02		3:50	2	17
9	39	37	11.1	+5.5	33	9:30		3:53	2	18
10	40	33	10.8	+6.0	33	9:19			2	20
11	42	43	10.5	+6.5	34	9:02			2	19
12	45	50	10.4	+7.0	36	8:23			2	20
13	46	59	10.2	+7.0	38	8:13			2	21
14	47	48	10.1	+8.0	40	7:59			2	20
15	48	38	10.0	+8.0	43	8:08			2	21
16	45	49	10.1	+9.0	42	8:23			1	24
17	44	58	10.0	+8.0	42	8:15			1	25

The National Physical Fitness Award

Participants must at least reach these levels in all 5 events in order to qualify for the National Physical Fitness Award. These levels represent the 50th percentile based on the 1985 School Population Fitness Survey.

Age	Curl-Ups (# one minute)	Partial Curl-Ups (#)	Shuttle Run (sec.)	V-Sit Reach (in.)	Sit & Reach (cm)	One-Mile Run (min:sec)	Distance Option (min:sec) ¼ mile	(min:sec) ½ mile	Pull-Ups (#)	Rt. Angle Pull-Ups (#)
		or			or		or			or
6	22	10	13.3	+1.0	26	12:36	2:21		7	6
7	28	13	12.0	+1.0	25	11:40	2:10	4:22	8	8
8	31	17	12.2	+0.5	25	11:05		4:14	9	10
9	32	17	11.9	+1.0	25	10:30			12	10
10	35	24	11.5	+1.0	25	9:48			14	12
11	37	26	11.1	+1.0	25	9:20			15	11
12	40	32	10.6	+1.0	26	8:40			18	12
13	42	39	10.2	+0.5	26	8:06			24	14
14	45	40	9.9	+1.0	28	7:44			24	20
15	45	40	9.7	+2.0	30	7:30			30	28
16	45	37	9.4	+3.0	30	7:10			30	28
17	44	42	9.4	+3.0	34	7:04			37	30
6	23	10	13.0	+2.5	27	13:12	2:26		6	5
7	25	13	13.2	+2.0	27	12:56	2:21		8	6
8	29	17	12.9	+2.0	28	12:30		4:56	9	8
9	30	20	12.5	+2.0	28	11:52		4:50	12	8
10	30	24	12.1	+3.0	28	11:22			13	8
11	32	27	11.5	+3.0	29	11:17			11	7
12	35	30	11.3	+3.5	30	11:05			10	7
13	37	40	11.1	+3.5	31	10:23			11	8
14	37	30	11.2	+4.5	33	10:06			10	9
15	36	26	11.0	+5.0	36	9:58			15	7
16	35	26	10.9	+5.5	34	10:31			12	7
17	34	40	11.0	+4.5	35	10:22			16	7

PLAY HOCKEY AT THE BOTTOM OF A POOL

Strap on your mask and snorkel: Underwater hockey challenges players to push a puck across the floor of a pool to score. The six-on-six game is played in more than 30 countries, and by teams all over the US.

And it all happens at the bottom of the pool, with no scuba gear—so players hold their breath for as long as possible while controlling the puck. Jenny Beiner, the director of Philadelphia's team, says she's only in the action for around 15 seconds at a time—and the 28-year-old was a collegiate swimmer.

You don't need to be world-class in the water to try the game or succeed, though: Underwater hockey players wear flippers to help them swim faster, and Beiner says that if you can go to the bottom, come back up, and head back down again, you're a viable candidate for this exciting game. One founder of the Philadelphia team wasn't a swimmer at first, she says, but has become an elite player and international referee.

Beginners beware, though: Players aren't supposed to tussle at the bottom, but kicks and injuries do happen. Beiner has needed stitches above her eye before, despite players wearing mask-style goggles to protect their faces.

But if you're willing to take the risk, it's a lung-challenging thrill—and one you can try at one of the nation's many clubs. Most let new players come and try the sport for free, including providing equipment you can borrow. Visit underwater-society.org, and click on UWH to find a team near you.

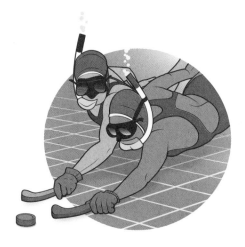

DON'T JUST TEXT: USE YOUR WORKOUT TO REALLY STAY IN TOUCH

We all need connection with those we love—and in our increasingly fast-paced, screen-based world, it can be tougher to get together. That's why meeting for a run, a race, or a workout challenge is so powerful: It improves our performance and gives us an excuse to train, but, more importantly, it helps us connect emotionally.

Even world-class athletes crave this connection. In his book *Liferider*, Laird Hamilton, the big-wave surfer, stand-up paddleboard inventor, and all-around philosopher of fitness, created a challenge that marries that physical and emotional connection in a poignant way:

"Think of someone you really like or whose company you enjoy—someone who lives within a few miles of you . . . and then do two things. First, plot a course from your home to theirs; and second, choose your mode of transport. . . . You can use a bike, a skateboard, a scooter, or your own two legs, either running or walking.

"The simple task? Undertake the journey between your home and theirs once a week for a minimum of four weeks, and challenge yourself to reduce the travel time by 10 percent on every trip."

Hamilton suggests using the travel time to think about why you're visiting this person—why you enjoy time with them, why you chose them, and why you value your relationship. Use that gratitude and those feelings to push you there—and keep you visiting someone you really cherish.

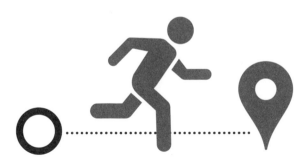

CHAPTER 12

BRING THE KIDS

These kid-friendly workouts are the best of both worlds: They're engaging enough to keep kiddos interested and challenging enough that they're a real workout for parents. Get your bond on!

DO THIS WARM-UP WITH THE KIDS BECAUSE . . . SCIENCE!

Keep everyone's legs—yours and the kids'—healthy and strong with this five-minute, scientifically proven warm-up routine: In a study of 4,000 kids, those who did this routine before soccer reduced their rate of injury by 48 percent. The best part: It's actually fun!

It's called the "11+ Kids" warm-up, and it's a five-level system that grows with kids. You can print a poster of the complete system at www.fifamedicalnetwork.com. Or start with these six activities—they're levels 2 and 3—for a ten-minute warm-up.

Activity 1: Jog and Statue
Have the kids hold a ball, standing 20 yards away. Yell "go" and have them start jogging toward you. Randomly yell "stop" and have the kids hold whatever position they're in for two seconds—on one leg, for instance. Do 5 total stops until they reach you. Repeat, with you as the ball holder, and let the kids yell "stop" for you instead.

Activity 2: Diagonal Bounds Holding a Ball
Holding a ball in two hands, perform diagonal bounds—jumping forward and diagonally from one leg to the other. Do 2 rounds of 10 total jumps (5 on each leg).

Activity 3: Plank Arm Switch
Assume the classic push-up position, but with one hand up on the ball. Keeping a rigid body line, pass the ball from under that hand to the other hand. Repeat. Do 3 rounds of 15 seconds each.

Activity 4: Single-Leg Sideways Hops
Stand on your left foot and jump to the left five times, then back to the right five times. Repeat on the other leg. Do both legs twice.

Activity 5: Crab Walk
Do a crab walk for 3 rounds of 30 to 50 feet.

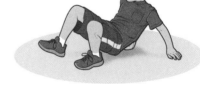

Activity 6: Somersault
Do 5 to 7 somersaults.

DO THE CHALLENGE WORKOUT OF JUMP ROPE NATIONAL CHAMPIONS

We all jumped rope as kids—but not like the Summerwind Skippers. The team of Idaho kids can hop over a rope more than 200 times in 30 seconds, and perform flips, somersaults, and other aerial tricks while still spinning the rope. The Skippers use these skills to stuff the shelves of their trophy case, including a win at the 2019 USA Jump Rope Championships in "Team Show."

The championships are like a gymnastics or swim meet, says the Skippers' coach, Kelsy Moe Porter. The jumpers perform in different disciplines—speed jumping, where team members try to jump as many times as possible in 30 seconds; and "freestyle" events, which "are similar to a gymnastics floor routine," Porter says, with flips and other tricks performed while continuing to jump. "We try to make as many difficult combinations as possible, and have to do certain elements to gain full points."

To perform these incredible feats, Porter's team practices four times a week, two hours at each practice. One drill they do at each practice is perfect to try with your own kids—it's called a "speed ladder," and takes about 10 minutes.

To do it, jump as fast as possible for 15 seconds, then rest for 15 seconds. Then go for 30 seconds, and rest for 30 seconds. Continue in this way for rounds of 45 seconds and 1 minute, then come back down the ladder, doing rounds of 1 minute, 45 seconds, 30 seconds, and 15 seconds each. See if you can keep up with your own little skipper!

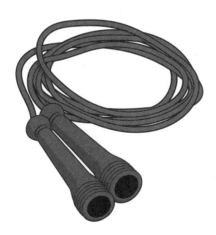

PLAY THE DODGEBALL GAME THAT TRAINS RODEO CLOWNS

First thing: They don't like to be called "clowns" anymore. The preferred word is "bull-fighters": They don't wear makeup, after all, and they're dodging one-ton steers that can kill them in a single kick.

Dane Fletcher helps keep them from getting hooked. Fletcher, a former New England Patriots linebacker and now owner of The Pitt, a gym in Bozeman, Montana, works with bullfighter Nate Jestes on workouts that will keep the cowboy in control of the bulls.

One workout Fletcher uses to help fighters make quick adjustments is an exercise ball dodgeball drill. The idea is to simulate what the bullfighter would go through—only dodging balls instead of bulls.

It also simulates something even more important for you and your kids: Fun. Here's how to play.

You will need:
- Four cones
- A stability ball

How to play:
1. Set the cones up in a big "Y" shape, with each of the points about 10 yards apart.
2. The "bull" stands between the forks of the "Y," holding the ball. The other player, the bullfighter, stands at the base of the "Y."
3. The bullfighter runs toward the fork in the "Y." As he gets close, the bull yells "left" or "right." When the fighter reaches the fork, he heads toward the cone the bull has yelled.
4. After the fighter cuts toward the fork cone, the bull throws the ball at the fighter's torso. The fighter must try to dodge the ball. Do 3 or 4 rounds of dodging, then switch positions. Keep playing until you drop!

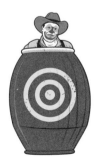

HOOP IT WITH THE KIDS TO SERIOUSLY SLIM YOUR WAIST

Spinning a Hula-Hoop around your hips and waist—or trying to—isn't just a way to have a big laugh with your kids. It can also slim your waist. In studies of "hooping," as it's now called in fitness classes, people lost almost an inch and a half off their waistline after six weeks. And they didn't spin the hoop for hours to get those results: They hooped at most for 15 minutes by the end of the study.

A weighted hoop—weighing 3 to 4 pounds—created these results, and the weight also makes it easier to keep the hoop moving around your hips and waist. Look for a hoop that's around a half pound (or 25 g), and 36 to 40 inches in diameter—they're $20 to $40 online.

Once you've got a hoop, try this 25-minute workout, adapted from the class used in the waist-slimming study.

Warm-Up
For three minutes, get your heart pumping. Do some high-knee marching, bend over to touch your toes, and perform some forward and lateral lunges.

Hoop It!
For two minutes, spin the hoop around your waist to the left. Take a breath, then spin to the right for two minutes.

Take a Break and Have Some Fun
Spin the hoop on your arms, hold it with both hands and reach overhead a few times, and march some more. Take this moving break for two minutes.

Hoop Some More
Two minutes left, two minutes right.

Movement Break
Perform 10 bodyweight squats, then hold the hoop wide and twist to the left and right 10 times. Repeat: 10 more squats, 10 more twists.

Final Hoop Session
Two minutes left, two minutes right, then 90 seconds left, 90 seconds right.

Can't get a hoop to hula? Here's a tip: Work your pelvis forward and backward instead of side to side. Sounds weird, but it works!

GET CREATIVE WHILE YOU PLAY A GAME OF SPEEDBALL

Kids don't want to exercise . . . they want to play! And, to be honest, so do adults. If I told you to run 20 all-out sprints, or join a vigorous game of soccer or basketball—you'd pick the game. But you'd still be sprinting!

"On the treadmill, I'm counting down those last five seconds. Put the same person on a basketball court—they can't get enough of it," says David Jack, founder of Activprayer, owner of a gym in Phoenix, and the most inspiring coach I know. And he loves fitness as play: "You have to *push* fitness on people. You have to *stop* play."

Jack's "Speedball" combines two-hand touch football with the wide-openness of soccer and the throwing and catching of basketball. And it rewards creativity. Even if you aren't the fastest or strongest player on the field, you can create opportunities to keep the ball by outwitting your opponents. Every kid has a chance to beat their parent—and vice versa.

1. On a large, open field, set up two equal-sized goals—it could be Hula-Hoops on the ground, garbage cans, or whatever you can create.
2. Divide into teams, and choose the number of goals you'll play to.
3. Using a small, soft ball, each team tries to move the ball down the field to score. The ball changes hands when a member of the other team scores a two-hand touch on the ball carrier.
4. Players can kick, throw, and bounce the ball to other teammates, and even to themselves—by tapping the ball in the air, players can continue moving so they're not possessing the ball when they're tagged. Getting creative about how you're moving the ball is half the fun!

PLAY 18 HOLES WITH A SOCCER BALL

You don't need fancy clubs or funny pants to enjoy the links: If you can kick a ball, you're ready for footgolf.

It's just what it sounds like—golf, but with a soccer ball. Footgolf is played on a regular golf course, next to regular golfers who are gunning for the greens. You'll just be aiming for different holes: Golf courses that offer footgolf have installed cartoonishly large holes, big enough to accommodate soccer balls. Footgolf holes are also shorter: At some courses, there are 18 footgolf holes on a 9-hole golf course—one in the middle of the fairway, and another near the green.

The game is faster, taking about two hours for a full round, and it's great for kids who are old enough to maintain a bit of on-course etiquette. But be warned: You're in for a real workout. A round of footgolf involves kicking a ball 80 times—often as hard as you can—plus 3 or so miles of walking.

Another warning to regular golfers who might join you: They might find it a bit embarrassing at first. Carrying a soccer ball around a golf course feels a bit transgressive, but after a few kicks, even stodgy duffers will be having a ball. The best part? It's offered just about everywhere: Hundreds of courses have added footgolf in the past few years, including at least one in every state. Visit www.footgolfusa.org/courses to find one.

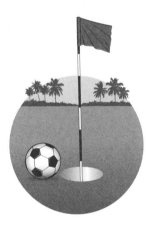

Natural waterslides are often hidden in secret, and sometimes illegal, spots that can leave you stranded in an emergency without cell service—not exactly family-friendly fun.

But the Meadow Run waterslide in Ohiopyle, Pennsylvania, isn't a secret. And it's probably the biggest natural slide you can find, stretching more than 100 feet through the park near the state's border with Maryland and West Virginia. The giant slides are so un-secret, in fact, that they're on Google Maps: Just type in MEADOW RUN NATURAL WATERSLIDES, and you'll find a parking lot for Meadow Run Trail, just steps from the slide.

That's not much of a workout, though. Work up a sweat with the kiddos and build up the sliding excitement instead: Start at nearby Cucumber Falls (also on GPS), and hike an easy 2.8 miles of the Meadow Run Trail to the slides for a big, wet reward.

Things to Know

- The water levels are high and fast in spring and fall. Visit in summer for the safest ride.
- It's a "slide," but it's still made of rocks—and not all of them smooth. Wear a shirt, sturdy shorts, and water shoes (or other shoes that you don't mind soaking).
- Details at www.ohiopyle.org.

GRAB YOUR PHONES AND GO TREASURE HUNTING

Kids are *tired* of hearing that they're on their phones too much . . . and parents are just as tired of telling them. Flip the script: Tell the kids to grab their phones—you're going geocaching.

Back when GPS was new, geocaching—a "sport" where users track down tiny treasures left by other users—was called the "sport of the future." It may not have replaced the NFL, but searching your neighborhood or a nearby hiking trail for a hidden treasure is a sneaky, fun way to get active. In 2014, scientists found that kids and parents who geocached once a week averaged 1.5 miles on each treasure hunt and hiked 10 miles per month.

Just download the free Geocaching app, and nearby caches will show up in the area around you. They could be a small bottle stashed behind a bush, or a metal lunchbox tied in a tree. Most caches contain a small logbook, so you can add your names to the list of other local adventurers.

Many caches are right near roads—these are called "Park and Grab" caches, and won't get you moving too much. Look for caches near parks, hiking trails, and other outdoor areas for a more active hunt. You can filter caches by the difficulty of finding them or the terrain nearby by upgrading to a paid version of the app—it's $6 per month. You might even start creating and placing your own—there are rules on how to do so on Geocaching.com.

CONQUER A WARPED WALL

If your kids are *American Ninja Warrior* fans, the warped wall needs no introduction: The curved tower is one of the show's signature obstacles. For the uninitiated, the wall is shaped like a banana—competitors run up the inside of the curve, attempting to get 14 feet into the air before grabbing the top and pulling themselves up to glory.

But you don't have to make it on TV to try: Warped walls have been installed at many trampoline gyms, including at many of SkyZone's 210 locations. Check their website, www.skyzone.com/locations, to see if one near you features it. The wall is also a staple of obstacle races like Tough Mudder—though those usually include a rope to grab.

Use these tips from Rose Wetzel, a two-time finalist on the show, to get to the top. She hasn't conquered the obstacle on TV yet, but has been training—and succeeding—on a wall near her home in Boulder, Colorado.

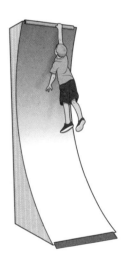

1. Think like a gymnast, instead of a runner. Many people try to sprint to get up enough speed. Wetzel has more success with "three or four powerful, bounding steps" to get moving, she says.
2. After your bounds, look up at the destination—the bar at the top of the wall you're hoping to grab.
3. Lean back a little. "If you're leaning back," Wetzel says, "you'll have more surface area for your foot" to get traction on the wall. Have a proud chest as you run, instead of putting your head down as if you were sprinting.
4. Finally: Explode. The end of a warped wall run is a jump—so think about being explosive to launch up and grab the top!

THE MOST FUN YOU CAN HAVE DOING CARDIO

The next time your kids ask go to an indoor trampoline park, join them! Bouncing can give you a workout as challenging as a treadmill: In a 1980 study, college men who jumped about three feet high on a trampoline for 5-minute bouts raised their heart rates to the same level they did running 8.5-minute miles. At those rates, a medium-weight, middle-aged man (like me) would burn 75 calories per minute! Do that for a 30-minute session, with breaks, and you've got a serious cardio workout.

Don't let it *feel* serious. It's a trampoline *park*, after all: We may not be as freewheeling as the kids, but we can still have some fun. Instead of putting on your spin-class game face, try these beginner "tricks." These help lay the foundation for the types of twists and flips your kids are probably doing—and the tricks are so much fun, the kids might just join in.

1. **SEAT DROP:** Jump high, then land on your butt. Bounce back to a standing position, and repeat without stopping. Try to get 20 to 30 seat drops in a row, rest for a few minutes, then do it again.
2. **STOMACH DROP:** Same idea, just trickier: This time, you'll land on your stomach instead of your booty. Return to start, and repeat 20 to 30 times consecutively. Rest for a few minutes, then do it again. Then try tying them together—stomach drop, seat drop, standing.
3. **HIGH JUMP:** Do two minutes of super high jumps, trying to get at least 3 feet off the trampoline. It's hard work! See if you can work up to five minutes of high jumps.

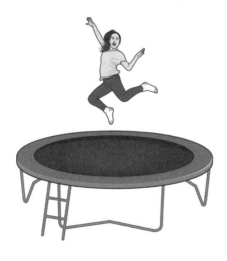

PLAY THE WORLD'S SILLIEST SPORT—AND GET A SERIOUS SPRINT WORKOUT

Like thousands of other people trying to stay in shape, John Spielman was bored with running. So he started chasing things—a baseball he'd thrown, golf balls he'd smacked. Eventually, the California dad settled on hitting a soccer ball with a baseball bat—and Cross Country Big Ball was born.

The sport's delightfully silly official site says the game is 57 percent cross-country, 29 percent baseball, 12 percent soccer, and 2 percent golf. It's 100 percent simple: Racers, each armed with their own bat and soccer ball, hit the ball in the direction of the finish line. They sprint after it, pick it up, and hit it again, continuing until they've reached the predetermined goal—across a field, around a giant circle, or whatever other course players imagine. That's one round—the game consists of as many rounds as the competitors decide to play.

It's a goofy game, but it's also eerily reminiscent of the *rarajipari* ball-chasing game of the Tarahumara tribe, described in *Born to Run*. Cross Country Big Ball is also deceptively intense fitness—because it's a race, each round is more of a series of sprints than a cross-country run. That might be normal for kids, but all that sprinting—and the smiling that comes with smacking a big ball—will make adults forget that running was ever boring.

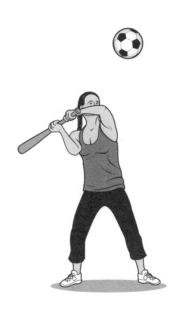

GO FOR THE GOLD WITH THIS USWNT ENDURANCE GAME

If your kids are crazy for Alex Morgan, want to pass like Christen Press, or long to raise MVP awards like Megan Rapinoe, help them hone their skills with this 8-step endurance drill. The US Women's National Team's head of performance, Ellie Maybury, uses it with our heroic soccer stars to build lungs and legs ready to take on the world—and take home the World Cup.

To do it, you'll need five cones, a soccer ball, and a goal. The USWNT does the drill for five rounds, for a 27.5-minute workout. Start with two to three rounds of 2 minutes each with your kids, and have them work their way up to World Cup levels over time. The efforts should be hard—kids (and adults!) should be pushing themselves hard throughout each 4-minute round.

Here's how to do it:
Perform the following sequence continuously for 4 minutes, running as hard as you can under control. After 4 minutes, rest for 90 seconds. Repeat three times.

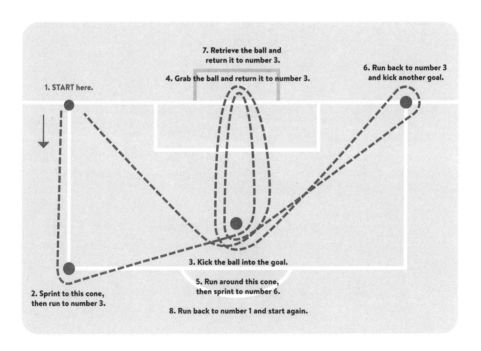

7. Retrieve the ball and return it to number 3.

4. Grab the ball and return it to number 3.

6. Run back to number 3 and kick another goal.

1. START here.

3. Kick the ball into the goal.

2. Sprint to this cone, then run to number 3.

5. Run around this cone, then sprint to number 6.

8. Run back to number 1 and start again.

BOND OVER SOME "OLDIES" AND GAME YOUR WAY TO A SERIOUS SWEAT

Dance Dance Revolution may be a game, but it *definitely* counts as a workout. In addition to anecdotes about players losing 100 pounds dancing to David Bowie, the game has been the subject of multiple scientific studies. The findings? Kids who played DDR in 10-minute chunks burned 150 to 170 calories during a 30-minute session.

More important, the game is just as infectious as it was in the early 2000s. Dust off an old dance mat, start jumping around to "Spice Up Your Life," and even the most disaffected preteen will eventually join in. Just try not to feel ancient when they call the songs "oldies."

The best part: For less than $100, you can have a setup that will help you bond together and dance to Willow Smith's "Whip My Hair." Sounds like a win.

Here's what you'll need:
- A console that can play the game: DDR was released for PlayStation 2 and 3, Xbox, Xbox360, and Wii. These machines are all on Craigslist, for $20 to $50.
- A copy of a DDR game: There are plenty to choose from for maximum song variety.
- A dance mat: These are also on eBay and Craigslist, for around $40 or less.
- A heart rate monitor (if you have one, wear it): Try to keep your heart rate over 120 beats per minute for as much of the session as you can. Or ignore the measurements, bond with the kids, and just play!

ROCK CLIMB INTO A VIDEO GAME

Since the days of the 1990s game show *Nick Arcade*, I've dreamed of climbing into a video game, interacting with a virtual world in real time, and using my body instead of buttons. VR headsets and Wii remotes create some of that experience—and they're fun—but they're still a little removed from the game experience. I'm looking for *Tron*-level immersion.

Well, the future's here, and you can give yourself—and your kids—that experience on the "Valo Climb." On this interactive climbing wall, lights pop up on hand- and footholds—touch them and the game changes. There's a Pong-like game where two players bat a virtual ball back and forth on the wall. There's a Missile Command–style game where you stop asteroids from crashing into a planet. And there are even games designed to improve your climbing skills, creating challenging routes on the wall to follow.

You can climb into these games at more than 230 locations. Visit www.valomotion.com to find one near you.

CHASE THE GOLDEN SNITCH LIKE HARRY POTTER

Get your Potter-crazy kids into a game of "muggle quidditch," a version of the snitch-chasing game played in real life by *Harry Potter* fans. Aside from not flying, it's basically the same game played at Hogwarts—and an awesome workout for parents and kids alike.

Players on each team "ride" brooms—usually PVC pipes held between their legs—while trying to score points. "Chasers" do this by throwing the quaffle—a slightly deflated volleyball—through three different hoops. Each throw through a hoop is worth 10 points. But if a chaser is hit by a dodgeball thrown by a "beater," the chaser must drop the quaffle and run back to tag their team's hoops to rejoin the game.

In the real-life game, the golden snitch—the winged golf ball chased by "seekers" like Harry Potter—is replaced by a person with a long yellow pouch on the back of their shorts. If a member of one team can grab this tail, their team scores 30 points.

Sounds pretty complicated to set up on your own: A full game requires balls, hoops, and 15 players. Luckily, there's US Quidditch, an organization that creates rules, tournaments, and youth and adult quidditch leagues around the country.

Want to try it in your own backyard? For fewer players, US Quidditch suggests a twist: Everyone's a chaser. There's only one ball (the quaffle), and all players try to score through hoops while riding their brooms. Visit www.usquidditch.com to learn the rules, get the list of clubs and teams, and find out how to build your own hoop.

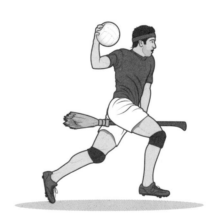

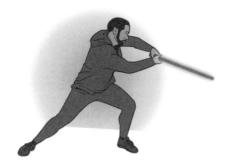

SWING A SABER LIKE A SKYWALKER

Glenn Higgins started posting videos of himself doing *Star Wars* workouts just for fun, practicing special effects to make his saber glow, and donning Comic-Con–worthy Skywalker outfits. Then, the Surrey, England–based trainer says, he started getting notes and videos from PE teachers—their students were doing his lightsaber moves to stay fit in school.

You can check out Higgins's whole library of these routines via his YouTube channel, *Glenn Higgins Fitness*. Grab your kids and some sabers—or short broomsticks—and try your hand at this Jedi workout.

Perform each exercise for 30 seconds, then rest 10 seconds before moving to the next exercise. Do 4 total rounds of the entire sequence, resting 1 minute between rounds.

EXERCISE 1: Skywalker Strikes

1. Hold your saber in your left hand, feet shoulder-width apart.
2. Raise your right knee up so you're standing on one leg, then take a lunge step to your right as you twist on the ball of your left foot and strike across your body with the saber, stabbing an imaginary opponent to your right.
3. Return to the high-knee position, and keep lunging and striking. Go for 30 seconds.

WORKOUT CONTINUES >>>

EXERCISE 2: Bridger Blocks

1. Stand holding the saber in front of you with your hands together, "blade" pointed up.
2. Push your hips back to a squat position, keeping the weight in your heels as you descend until your thighs are parallel to the floor.
3. As you press back up, twist onto the ball of your right foot and turn your torso to the left, "blocking" a strike from your left side.
4. Twist back, squat again, and twist to the right side this time. Keep alternating in this way.

EXERCISE 3: Skywalker Strikes (opposite side)

EXERCISE 4: Windu Blocks

1. Stand with your feet together, holding the saber in front of you, pointing up.
2. Put your weight on your left leg as you step slightly to the left and bend your left knee, reaching your right leg back. As you step, reach the saber up above your head with your right hand as if you were blocking a strike from above.
3. Return to start, and step to the right this time, blocking above you with your left hand.

EXERCISE 5: Alternating Lando Lunges

1. Hold the saber in both hands in front of you, pointing up.
2. Take a big lunge step forward with your right leg, descending as you step, until both knees form 90-degree angles. As you descend, twist the saber so it's facing toward the right, as if you were blocking a blaster bolt.
3. Quickly hop back up and lunge with your left leg, turning the saber to the left this time. Continue for 30 seconds.

DARE TO FAIL: LEARN TO RIDE A UNICYCLE TOGETHER

Kids are constantly learning new things, and seeing that is one of the amazing things about being a parent. But it can also get frustrating when something seems obvious to us—why can't they just *get it* already?

They're kids, that's why. Give yourself a refresher on what it's like to fail, and show them you're never too old to keep getting back up: Learn to ride a unicycle together.

One-wheelers are easy to come by: There's always a handful on Craigslist in my area, ranging from $30 to $50—I got mine for $35. Just get ready for a humbling experience. The unicycle will challenge your core, but it will really challenge your patience. Use these tips to learn to ride it together:

1. **SET YOUR SEAT:** Just as with a bicycle, when your leg is fully extended on the pedal, you want a slight crook in your knee.
2. **THE BIGGER THE WHEEL, THE BETTER:** They're easier to balance.
3. **LEARN NEXT TO A FENCE, AND PREFERABLY ON GRASS:** Hold onto the fence to get on the cycle, and use it for your first few sessions of learning to maintain your balance. Grass will add balance and a soft landing if you fall.
4. **DON'T PEDAL RIGHT AWAY:** First, get your balance. Your first time on the unicycle, just try to feel your center of gravity. Move the pedals back and forth a little, moving forward and backward slightly along the fence.
5. **DON'T HAVE ANYONE IN FRONT OF OR BEHIND YOU:** While learning against the fence, you're not very likely to fall sideways. More likely, you'll lose your balance forward or backward—and the unicycle will come shooting out from underneath you. Make sure the kids are clear from both areas!
6. **DON'T EXPECT TO RIDE YOUR FIRST TIME OUT:** Plan for a few sessions with the kids over the course of a few days—10 to 15 minutes at a time will be enough to test your patience. Within a few sessions, you'll all be rolling around.

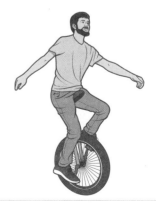

CHAPTER 13

DO IT FOR
THE 'GRAM

Sometimes, you just want a picture that makes you look awesome. Time to fill your life with likes: This guide will help you get the photos and have fun getting there, whether it's hiking to an incredible view or participating in a class that's unbelievably fun. Get ready to make people jealous.

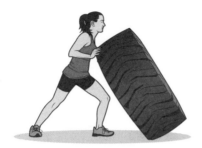

FLIP YOUR OWN GIANT TIRE

You are powerful. You can move mountains. Well, maybe not *mountains*. But you *can* flip one of those giant, 600-pound tractor tires. And you'll *feel* like you can move mountains.

Sure, you could just lift a barbell. But it's not the same. And giant tires have a bonus: They're cheap . . . or even free! You don't have to go to an expensive gym to get your mitts on one of these gargantuan rings of rubber: Google local FARM TIRE or TRACTOR TIRE supply places, and call to see if they've got any scrap tires. They're expensive for these businesses to get rid of, so they'll be happy to give you one for free. You may even find these big boys on Craigslist with a quick search for TRACTOR TIRES.

Start with a tire in the 300-pound range, which is used by many athletes in training. Feeling stronger? Strongman athletes use tires that are 650 pounds or more. When you're perusing the junk wares you're being offered, just Google the name and model from the side of the tire to find its weight. Then roll it up a ramp, truck it home, and get ready to Hulk out. Here are two workouts to get you started.

WORKOUT CONTINUES >>>

WORKOUT 1: FLIP FOR TIME

Flip the tire as many times as you can in 2 minutes. Rest for 2 minutes, and repeat. Go for 3 or 4 rounds. Over time, try to improve the number of flips in each round. Too hard? Start with a minute. Too easy? Go for 30 extra seconds each round.

To flip the tire, stand in front of it with your feet about hip-width apart, your toes almost touching the tire. Push your hips back to squat deeply, and place your hands under the tire, either inside or outside of your feet. Keeping your chest upright, explode out of the squat so the tire rises up with you with enough momentum that you can flip your grip so your palms now face the sky. In this position, the tire will be around chest level. Push with your legs and arms to get it over. Keep flipping in that direction, or run around to the other side and flip it back.

WORKOUT 2: TIRE FLIP TRIPLE CHALLENGE

Three exercises, done three times each for three minutes . . . repeated a total of three times. Perform each of these exercises for 3 reps, then move to the next exercise without resting. Continue the cycle for three minutes. Rest for three minutes. Do 3 total rounds of three minutes each.

EXERCISE 1: Tire Flip

Same as above.

EXERCISE 2: Squat Jump

Squat down next to the tire, then explode up so forcefully that you jump up onto the side of your tire. Jump back down, and repeat.

EXERCISE 3: Decline Push-Up

Place your feet on the side of the tire, your hands on the ground. Maintain a rigid body position as you bend your elbows to lower your chest toward the ground. Press back up, and repeat.

DO DOWN DOG IN TIMES SQUARE

On the summer solstice, Times Square is packed—just like any other day. But the first day of summer is different: The lights are still flashing, but the gathered thousands are hushed. They're doing yoga.

"It's a surreal experience, hearing that intersection be so quiet," says Amanda Jedeikin, who used to help organize the event while an editor at *Shape*. "The atmosphere is transformed. Usually it's so chaotic, but instead you have thousands of people engaged in a collective, quiet activity."

The activity isn't *that* quiet, though: Your fellow yogis will be taking selfies, have their phones on their mats, and, as with any huge yoga event, it can be tough to hear the instructor. "It's not a really good workout—it's probably the worst yoga class you can take," Jedeikin says with a laugh.

That doesn't mean it's not worth doing! Outside of a zombie apocalypse, it's probably your only chance to experience such a calm Times Square. Keep track of the next class by clicking SEASONAL EVENTS at www.timessquarenyc.org.

"MIND THE GAP" AS YOU RUN A MARATHON AROUND LONDON—AND UNDER IT, TOO

Explore central London—and 42 of its Underground stations—in one long run. The "UnderRound" challenge is an "anytime" marathon challenge that has runners loop around Zone 1 of the UK capital while dipping into—and out of—each of 42 different Tube stations without boarding a single train.

It's the brainchild of Rory Coleman, a Welsh coach and speaker who has run more than 1,000 marathons—including 2 rounds of his own street-and-subway challenge.

The toughest part: navigating the stairs. Covent Garden station, number 19 on the route, has 193 stairs from platform level back up to the street. And Coleman's first UnderRound, undertaken a week before Christmas, added another obstacle to those steps: throngs of holiday shoppers.

If you finish, there's no ribbon, medal, or T-shirt. There's just a place on Coleman's leaderboard, which doesn't even exist online—it lives only on Coleman's home computer in Cardiff. If you want to join their ranks, email Coleman at rory@colemancoaching.co.uk, and he'll send you a complete set of maps, instructions, and directions for £10—about $15. A small price to pay for an adventure you'll never forget.

BIKE THROUGH A TWISTING TUNNEL OF NEON STRAIGHT OUT OF *TRON*

If you're near Des Moines, this is a side trip you've got to take: Thirty miles out of town, stretching across the Des Moines River, are the spiraling, bright-blue LEDs of the High Trestle Trail Bridge. It looks like a graphic from the opening of 1986's *Transformers: The Movie* or a set piece from *Big Trouble in Little China*. Basically, it's the 1980s, but a bridge. And you can ride (or run!) right through this landmark.

The artwork is called *From Here to There*, and it's meant to simulate looking down a mine shaft. A series of metal squares, lined with blue LEDs, give off a spiraling effect that makes it look as if the half-mile bridge could suck you into an alternate universe. What definitely won't suck: the photos! Taken during the day or when the bridge is lit from dusk until midnight, this is a marvel you'll want to remember in your camera roll forever.

You can easily do an out-and-back ride to the bridge from the Whistlin' Donkey bar in nearby Woodward, Iowa—the bar is just half a block from the trailhead, and less than a 3-mile ride to the bridge. For an all-day affair, park one car at the Whistlin' Donkey, and drive another 20 miles to Ankeny (with your bikes). Park at the city's sports complex, use the restroom, and grab a pre-ride pint at Firetrucker Brewing. Then mount up for a 20-mile ride. Snap a bunch of photos, and finish with a celebratory beer—and plate of tater tots—at the Whistlin' Donkey.

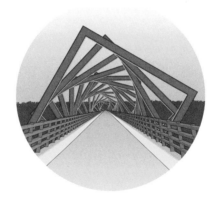

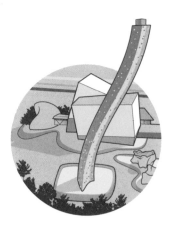

CLIMB THE DIZZYING, SPINNING DUTCH CLIMBING WALL OF YOUR DREAMS

It's not the world's tallest climbing wall (that one's in Georgia—see chapter 2), but Excalibur might be the most famous. Rising out of the ground like King Arthur's sword from the stone, this 120-foot, twisting wall above Groningen in the Netherlands has inspired countless breathless Instagram posts and wow-check-this-out drone videos. And it's easy to see why: Excalibur looks like it's physically impossible—like a Leaning Tower of Pisa with handholds.

You can grab those handholds for a mere 12 euros: That's the cost of a day pass at Bjoeks Climbing Park, home to this yellow giant. But you'll need some climbing experience: Excalibur is only open to "independent climbers" who can belay for themselves. You can take a course to become qualified for 100 euros, and you can climb the convex side of the wall with top-roping experience only—no anchoring along the way is necessary.

Things to Know

- Groningen is two hours from Amsterdam by car, or three hours by bus. Bus rides are $10 to $20 per person each way.
- If you don't have your own gear, Bjoeks will lend you harness and belay equipment for free. Climbing shoes rent for 3 euros per day, and an 80-meter rope can be rented for 4 euros per day.
- If you don't have a friend coming along, you can find another solitary climber to partner with you for the day via WhatsApp. There are details on the Bjoeks website.
- You'll need to arrange a time to go and to climb—visit www.bjoeks.nl to register.

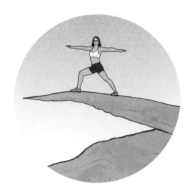

HOVER OVER A CALIFORNIA VALLEY AT POTATO CHIP ROCK

At the peak of Mount Woodson, about 30 miles northeast of San Diego, you can perch on a wafer-thin slice of rock that's hanging over oblivion, with a panoramic view of a verdant valley below. Photos of hikers on "Potato Chip Rock" look Photoshopped—but they're real, and so is the hike you'll do to earn this 'grammable moment.

From the Mount Woodson trailhead in Pomay, California, to the peak, it's a 7-mile round-trip hike that gains 2,000-plus feet in elevation. It's not all about the summit, though: You'll enjoy plenty of scenery as you climb stone steps, navigate through giant boulders, and walk above the waters of Lake Poway below. The ascent will probably take around 2.5 hours. But you'll get plenty of rest at the top: Waits can be up to an hour to get your potato chip photo at the top. But this is one of San Diego County's most popular photo spots for a reason. The wait is worth it!

Set your GPS to MOUNT WOODSON TRAILHEAD, POWAY, CA. The parking lot opens at 6 a.m. Parking is $5. The trail is well marked and easy to navigate: Just follow the signs for MT. WOODSON SUMMIT.

Things to Know

- Don't worry about the rock snapping off and sending you tumbling—it's an optical illusion! The sliver of rock is only suspended about a story and a half above some rocks below.

SWING ON THE TRAVELING RINGS IN SANTA MONICA

It doesn't get much more iconic California than the original Muscle Beach, where gymnasts and strongmen have gathered since the 1930s to perform feats on the Santa Monica sands. And it doesn't get much more "Muscle Beach" than the steel rings hanging from upside-down U-shaped frames along the beach.

You don't have to be a stuntperson to fly along the rings, though: You just have to get in line. Anyone can swing—for the shortest wait, go during weekday work hours. The apparatus gets going after work, starting around 4 p.m., and is crowded on weekends.

Rings like these were touted as fitness aids as far back as the 1880s. And the physics of getting going hasn't changed: Grab the first ring, then sprint for the next one so you're holding two rings. Once you've grabbed ring 2, pull on the first ring by bending your elbow to create momentum. Release your hand from ring 1 and swing to ring 3. Continue in this way, trying to get them all—and don't forget to get a picture!

Things to Know

- To find the rings via GPS, put in the Spokes 'n' Stuff bike-rental shop, and look across the street.
- You'll want some chalk on your hands. You might find some near the rings, or you can buy a block at the bike-rental store.
- These aren't the only traveling rings in the US. There are sets in Virginia Beach, San Antonio, and more. A rings enthusiast keeps a tally of all of them at www.travelingrings.org.

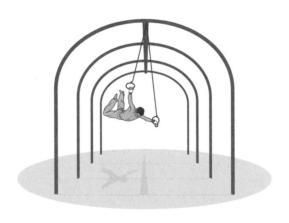

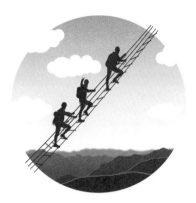

FLOAT ABOVE THE ALPS ON AUSTRIA'S "STAIRWAY TO HEAVEN"

H awaii's "Stairway to Heaven" is a classic spot for a travel pic that will leave viewers breathless—but it can also put you behind bars. The hike is illegal, and those who skirt those rules put themselves at risk and leave trash along the otherwise unspoiled Oahu mountain.

For a legal—and even more breathtaking—"Stairway to Heaven" photo, Austria's "Sky Ladder" needs to be on your list. The alpine nation's Gosaukamm Mountains are filled with *via ferrata* routes, where steel rungs, ladders, and cables have been hammered into mountains to make them more accessible—creating something that's harder than hiking, but easier than climbing. The crown jewel of these reinforced routes is the Sky Ladder, a 130-foot-long steel cable ladder that hangs high above a gorge, leaving hikers suspended in the air for a white-knuckle adventure . . . and an unbelievable photograph where they're flying above the Alps.

The ladder is on the Donnerkogel *via ferrata* route, rated a "Class D"—there's lots of exposure and overhanging, so while the rungs make the route *easier* than climbing, it's still not *easy*. You'll need a *via ferrata* gear set, including ropes, helmet, and harness. All of this—plus guiding for the area's various *via ferrata* hiking—can be found in the town of Gosau, where you'll start your adventure. Visit www.lasereralpin.at.

(For *via ferrata* routes closer to home, see the "Iron Rung Routes" of Maine's Acadia National Park on page 12.)

PRACTICE ASANAS IN THE WORLD'S MOST BEAUTIFUL AMPHITHEATER: JOIN 2,000 OTHER YOGIS AT SUNRISE FOR OHM-MY-GOD VIEWS

The Red Rocks Amphitheater outside Denver is the world's only naturally occurring, "acoustically perfect" concert space: Two sandstone rocks, each 300 feet tall, frame the space for perfect sound amplification and gorgeous views. For more than a century, it's been used for unique concert experiences. And for the past few years, it's been home to a different kind of gathering: sunrise yoga sessions.

Held at 7 a.m. weekly throughout the summer, these "Yoga on the Rocks" sessions draw 2,000 practitioners to the space to learn from local and internationally known teachers, bending and posing at 6,450 feet above sea level.

Fair warning: Like any gigantic yoga class, this will probably not be the best or hardest yoga class you'll ever take. Your classmates will likely be snapping photos and chatting. But soaking up the sunrise and staring down the bleachers at thousands of others is worth the subpar vinyasa experience. If you still want a workout afterward, you can hike the acres of trails surrounding the amphitheater, or wait until it clears out: The concert venue's stairs are a popular running challenge, with 145 high-altitude stairs from the stage to the top.

Yoga on the Rocks sessions are $16, and you've got to book them online: Visit www.redrocksonline.com, and book early—they sell out!

'GRAM, FORREST, 'GRAM!

When Forrest Gump "felt like running," he headed out for a journey that lasted three years, crisscrossing the US for a seven-minute montage of unbelievable beauty shots. Here's how to re-create some of those shots yourself—and get a good run in, too.

Shot 1: "I Just Felt like Running"
As Forrest crosses the Mississippi, he's interviewed by reporters on a white steel bridge.

How to Find It

The bridge is the Woods Memorial Bridge in Beaufort, South Carolina, a town also featured in *The Big Chill*.

Make It a Run

Any great workout should end with a great post-workout snack: Start at Harry C. Chambers Waterfront Park, head across the bridge, and run 1.5 miles to Dairy Queen on the other side.

Shot 2: Running Up Mountain Switchbacks
Gump pounds around curves in—as it turns out—North Carolina.

How to Find It

For many of the shots in this montage, film fans have done the work for you: They've added GPS markers for Forrest's runs. These switchbacks are near Linville, North Carolina, overlooking Grandfather Mountain. Just search FORREST GUMP CURVE, and your GPS will take you there, where a posted sign says FORREST GUMP RAN HERE.

Make It a Run

Park at the entrance to Grandfather Mountain, on US-221, and head uphill—it's about 1.5 miles to the Curve, and another half-mile to the top.

Shot 3: Turning around at a Lighthouse

While describing his run, Gump says he came to one ocean, turned around, and went back. While saying this, he approaches a white lighthouse along a wooden deck, then turns around.

How to Find It

It's the Marshall Point Lighthouse in Port Clyde, Maine, north of Portland on the scenic drive up US-1.

Make It a Run

Don't make things too complicated: Get some lobster. Park at the Drift Inn Canteen in Port Clyde. Then run an out-and-back 5K to the lighthouse before chowing down.

Shot 4: Forrest's Finish Line:

In the montage's concluding shot, Gump finally stops running on a hill in a picturesque desert with towering mountains behind him.

How to Find It

This location is in Utah's Monument Valley, at mile 13 on Route 163 near the Arizona-Utah border. It's been marked on GPS as Forrest Gump Hill, and there's even a parking lot selling souvenirs.

Make It a Run

The area is flat, arid, and hot, and the road is very, very straight. For safety's sake, you're probably best just doing a quick mile along the road. But for a longer jaunt, try to make it early in the day and run to—or from—the Canyonlands Hotel in nearby Mexican Hat, an 8-mile journey each way.

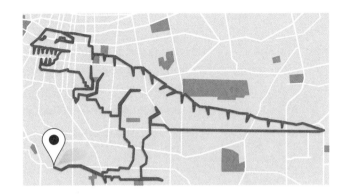

TURN YOUR RUN INTO A WORK OF ART

Y ou could pound out a 5K training run, or draw a giant corgi across your town.
"When you map a shape . . . you're giggling while you go. You slowly forget about any kind of pain you have," says Claire Wyckoff. The LA-based comedy writer would know: Her GPS drawings—mostly not safe for work, and shared via her Instagram, @og_dick_run_claire—have been seen by thousands. CNN, Perez Hilton, *Outside*, *Cosmo*, and other outlets have all written about her drawings of T-Rexes, poop emojis, and lots and lots of genitalia.

Making dirty drawings with her runs has helped Claire go farther and harder than she ever would have if not to finish a masterpiece: "In San Francisco, I mapped half of one run up this massive hill. I never would have run up that hill otherwise," she says.

Here are some tips from Wyckoff on creating your own GPS masterpiece.

Grab a Map
Wyckoff starts her drawings in one of two ways—either she has a shape in mind she'd like to run, or she looks at the map for obvious shapes. "Something might pop out at you, like a smiley face. Or you might think, 'Oh, that looks like a tree,' " she says.

Using www.mapmyrun.com, she then meticulously pre-creates the drawing so she'll have a guide when she hits the road. "You don't want to mess up. With this kind of art, you can't just grab a new canvas," she says. If you make a mistake at mile 6, you'll have to start over. So map your plan first.

Use Parks and Pauses to Bring Your Vision to Life

To create round shapes, Wyckoff will make part of her drawings include parks—that way, she can run the exact section of a shape she'll want through an open field. Her tip for diagonal lines: If you pause the app on one street corner, run to the next point, and resume your run in the app, the GPS will simply draw a diagonal line between those points—so you can create diagonals that cross city blocks.

Check the Satellite

While mapping your shape, turn on the "satellite" function of the map. You may find that the field you planned to run through is actually a restricted area with a fence, or there's a private driveway in the middle of your shape. Wyckoff once had this problem with the White House lawn: She'd drawn a shape across DC, forgetting that you can't just cut through the East Wing!

Bring a Friend

Wyckoff takes a screenshot of her running plan map, and texts it to herself with directions. Then her husband comes along for the run—he keeps track of the run they've planned on the screenshot, while Claire looks at a live view on the GPS.

Bringing a drawing buddy will also add to the fun . . . and that's the point. "GPS drawing is a running endeavor, but it's also a 'having fun with life' endeavor," she says. And it'll be even easier to laugh—and run farther—with a friend.

SWIM THROUGH SWARMS OF JELLYFISH

Don't worry, they don't sting! It's one of the world's most unusual experiences: Gliding through clouds of jellies in "Jellyfish Lake" in the Pacific nation of Palau. Two non-stinging species of jellyfish, Moon and Golden, are adapted to the conditions of the lake, which is separated from the ocean by limestone. So the jellies—and the tourists who come to swim with them—are basically all you'll find in these green waters.

The lake is found on Eli Malk Island, one of roughly 340 that make up Palau; it's a 45-minute boat ride from Koror, the nation's main hub. That's a long way to go from the US just for the jellyfish, but there's more to do there: Palau has world-class scuba diving on its nearby reefs and a bevy of World War II shipwrecks.

Things to Know

- Visitors to the lake must buy a pass. It's $100 for 10 days of access—this provides access not just to Jellyfish Lake, but to diving and other activities on the surrounding Rock Islands.
- Tours are available from various operators in Koror.
- There's another jellyfish lake in Indonesia. Look up LAKE KAKABAN for details.

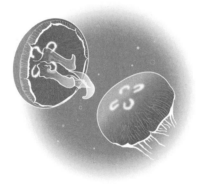

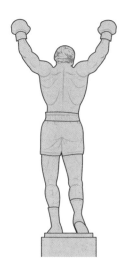

STAR IN YOUR OWN *ROCKY* TRAINING MONTAGE

I f you want to get in shape to shock the heavyweight champion, avenge your slain trainer, and end the Cold War, you're gonna need a montage.

In just a few minutes of quick cuts, Rocky Balboa sprints up stairs, punches meat, and chases chickens to become a stallion fit to take down giants. Star in a sweatsuit-soaking montage of your own: Crank up "Eye of the Tiger" and do this workout, drawing from four decades of *Rocky*.

GET FIRED UP: JUMP ROPE

Five minutes should do the trick: Try jumping for 20–30 seconds at a time, then rest for 20 seconds. To make your jumping more Balboa-esque, do 1 round of high-knee jump roping, bringing your knees up toward your chest. Then do a round of alternate feet jumping. Continue alternating in this way until you're warmed up and breathing heavily.

GET STRONG LIKE A STALLION

If you want to "eat lightning and crap thunder," you've got to move fast. Perform these exercises as quickly as possible while maintaining good form.

EXERCISE 1: Medicine Ball Push-Ups

Rocky does a lot of one-armed push-ups—in the gym, in front of sunsets, jumping back and forth. Med ball push-ups are a little easier, and he uses them to train for his fight in *Rocky Balboa*. Assume a classic push-up position, but with a medicine ball under one hand. Maintaining a rigid body line, bend your elbows to lower your chest toward the floor. Press back up to start. Do 8 reps, then switch arms, and repeat. Perform 4 sets on each arm.

WORKOUT CONTINUES >>>

EXERCISE 2: Bent-Over Lateral Raise

In *Rocky 2*, Balboa does 50 of these. Start a little slower: Stand holding dumbbells in your hands with feet hip-width apart, knees slightly bent. Push your hips back to bend forward with a flat back, hanging the dumbbells in front of you. Maintaining this flat-back position, pull the dumbbells apart to the sides so that your upper body forms a "T" shape. Return to start, and repeat. Perform 8 reps per set for 4 sets, working up to 5 sets of 10 over time.

EXERCISE 3: Barbell Jump Squats

Rocky does these with a log over his shoulders in a junkyard. You can just use a light barbell—or even a broomstick. Stand with your feet slightly wider than shoulder-width apart and the barbell or broomstick over your shoulders. Push your hips back to squat. Now drive up through your heels so forcefully that your feet leave the ground. Land softly, reset, and repeat. Do 4 sets of 8 squat jumps.

EXERCISE 4: Land-Mine Press

When Rocky does this move in his Siberian training cabin in *Rocky IV*, he presses a huge horse cart filled with his friends overhead. No horse cart? Use a barbell!

Place one, unweighted end of a barbell into a land-mine anchor. Hold the weighted end of the barbell in front of your chest with both hands. Bend your knees slightly to assume an athletic stance. Press the barbell forward and up with both arms, then slowly lower it down. Perform 4 sets of 8 reps.

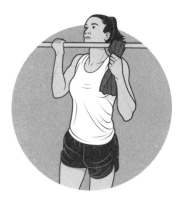

EXERCISE 5: One-Arm Chin-Ups

If you can knock out 5 sets of 5 one-armed chin-ups, go for it. But to work up to Rocky's level, grab a towel. Drape it over the bar where one hand would normally go, and hold this with one hand with your other hand in a normal chin-up position, palm facing your body. Concentrate on using the hand that's on the bar as you perform a chin-up, using the towel hand as a stabilizer. Go for 5 sets of 5 on each arm.

EXERCISE 6: Dragon Flag

This move is too tough for pretty much everyone. But if you're in a snow-covered Russian cabin in front of a fire, you might as well try it. Lie faceup on a bench and grab the bench next to your ears so that your elbows are bent and your upper arms are next to your head. Your hands are there simply for support—don't pull with them or you'll wrench your neck. Use your core to roll up onto your shoulders until your body is straight and perpendicular to the ground—basically, you're stacked on top of your shoulders. From here, slowly lower your body under control using your core, maintaining a straight body line. Work toward bringing your body down until it's hovering just above the bench. Then bring it back up to the start, and lower slowly again.

GONNA FLY NOW: CARDIO TIME

You've got to have the conditioning to go the distance. You can get most of your road work in on the streets of Philly—see page 16 for a route through the most scenic sections of Rocky's runs. But if you can't make it to the city of Brotherly Love, get some cardio in with other montage moves.

EXERCISE 1: Shadowboxing

Boxing is in three-minute rounds, so do the same: Throw three punches—left, right, left—then shuffle left three steps. Repeat, this time shuffling right. Continue for a three-minute round. Rest for a minute, then try to do 4 three-minute rounds.

EXERCISE 2: Stair Running

You don't need to run up the Philadelphia Museum of Art stairs to give you a heart-pumping, Rocky-worthy workout. Find a long set of stairs and run up them as quickly as you can. Jog back down at half that pace, and repeat. Go for 6 rounds to start, and work your way up to 20 over time.

In *Rocky IV*, almost 10 percent of the movie's total running time is training montages.

When you do, you'll get a visceral understanding of political injustice—not many workouts can do that.

A quick recap: "Gerrymandering" creates political boundaries that give one party a political advantage that disenfranchises the voters of the region. That's not my opinion: Federal judges ruled in 2016 that two of North Carolina's congressional districts created voting blocs that artificially disenfranchised minority voters.

The League of Women Voters in Asheville, North Carolina, on the border of the state's 10th and 11th congressional districts, organized a "Gerrymander 5K" to make these convoluted borders real for runners. The 3-mile route turns 13 different times, sometimes including one section of a suburban planned community, but not another.

The NC event has spawned similar events across the country, and a Facebook group, "Make My Own Gerrymander 5K," where folks from other squiggly jurisdictions can organize their own runs. Find one near you at facebook.com/groups/gerrymander5k. Or visit one of these spots to have a physical experience of congressional lines on your own.

Cuyahoga Falls: Near Akron, Ohio

Seven "highly irregular" districts in Ohio came under fire, as Republicans won 75 percent of state House seats with 51–59 percent of the vote. One—Congressman Tim Ryan's 13th district—looks like a jigsaw puzzle piece where it meets the neighboring 14th district.

You can jog a quick, suburban 2 miles that cross the lines between the two districts five times—including a street where most of the houses are in Ryan's district, but the cul-de-sac has a different representative!

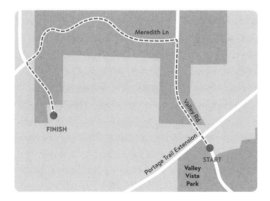

1. Begin at Valley Vista Park in Cuyahoga Falls, at Valley Road and Maitland Avenue.
2. Run northwest to Meredith Lane. During this stretch, you've crossed into the 14th district, and back into the 13th. Turn left.

3. Run to the four-way intersection at Pine Brook Trail—you crossed back into the 14th. Turn left onto Pine Brook Trail.

4. About 0.2 miles into this run down Pine Brook, you've crossed back into the 13th. So these neighbors have a different congressional representative than those at the four-way. Keep going.

5. In another 0.5 miles on this same street, you'll cross back into the 13th district. You'll then come to a "Y" intersection. The cul-de-sac on the left of the "Y" is in the 13th district. The cul-de-sac on the right is in the 14th district. Total distance: 2 miles.

Christophers Crossing: Near Frederick, Maryland

Though most cases of partisan gerrymandering that have gone to the courts in recent years were the results of Republican redistricting, Maryland Democrats redrew the 6th congressional district to create another blue stronghold in the Old Line State. This 3.2-mile run makes ten turns in the same neighborhood.

1. Begin at Christophers Crossing and Poole Jones Road. As you look at Poole Jones, the house in front of you and the farm field behind it have different representatives. Wild! Face right.

2. Run 0.43 miles to Greenvale Drive. Turn right. As you run down this street—the houses on either side are in different districts!

3. After 0.2 miles, you'll come to a "T" intersection. Turn left on Glendale Drive.

4. After a quarter-mile, you'll come to Falstone Drive. Turn right, go one block, turn left on Overlook, and then left again on Clearfield . . . to return to Glendale. Look back at where you turned off, one block back—that's a different district!

5. Stick with Clearfield, and at your run's 1.4-mile mark, turn right on Glendale again.

6. After 0.2 miles, turn left on Meadowview Drive, then right on Sunnybrook. Run toward the "T" intersection, noting that the houses on either side of this street have different representatives on the gerrymandered map.

7. Turn left on Stone Ridge at the "T," then make a right on Yellow Springs Road.

8. At Christophers Crossing, turn right to head back to the start.

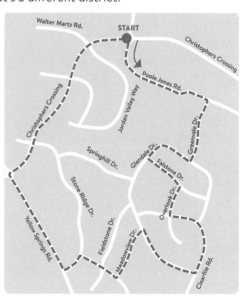

WORKOUT CONTINUES >>>

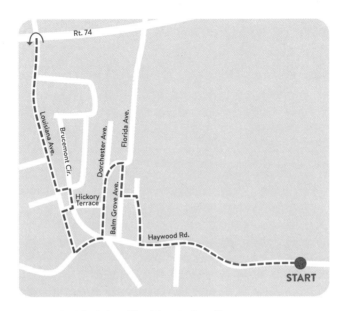

The Route That Started It All: Asheville, North Carolina

Get ready for ten turns in the first 1.2 miles!

1. Begin at The Admiral restaurant, 400 Haywood Road. Go west.

2. After 0.38 miles, turn right on Martin Avenue to go north.

3. You'll quickly turn left on Balm Grove Place, then right again on Balm Grove Avenue.

4. You've only gone 0.64 miles: Turn left on Florida Avenue, heading southwest, then bear left on Dorchester Avenue to go back to . . . Haywood Road, where you started.

5. Turn right on Haywood at the 0.88-mile mark. After 0.08 miles, turn right again on Louisiana Avenue.

6. At the 1.08-mile mark, make a right on Crown, a left on Majestic, and another left on Brucemont Circle to come back to Louisiana Avenue. This cuts a single block out of the district. That's 1.22 miles.

7. Head 0.4 miles up Louisiana Avenue—no turns, I promise!—to Patton Avenue. Turn around and retrace your steps.

CHAPTER 14

ANYTIME, ANYWHERE FITNESS ADVENTURES

You don't need a big budget, a two-week vacation, or even transportation to turn moving your body into an adventure machine. You've got all you need at home or at your local gym to have a mind-expanding, heavy-breathing experience. Here's your guide.

PUT SOME PLAY IN YOUR WORKOUT

When you were playing tag in kindergarten, you weren't thinking, "I'm really getting in some high-intensity sprinting!" You were exercising, but you weren't exercising: You were playing!

The playground can still give you a workout. It's a convenient option to exercise when you're busy—while your kids have soccer practice, slide over to the playground to knock out a quick strength session. And it doesn't get stale: Even after years of these workouts, it's still fun for playground workout aficionado Al Kavadlo, because the unique layouts let him get creative.

"You're improvising, using your surroundings—[the playground] allows you to do that," says Kavadlo, the internet's foremost calisthenics acolyte and author of books including *Zen Mind, Strong Body*. He suggests building your playground workout around four key movements: pushing, pulling, squatting, and trunk flexion. Here are some suggestions for each category. Try doing four sets of each exercise you choose in each category.

Pushing Options
1. Push-ups.
2. Push-ups with hands elevated on a bar or step (easier).
3. Push-ups with feet elevated (harder).
4. Shoulder press push-up.

Pulling Options
1. Chin-ups.
2. Inverted row.
3. Monkey bars.

Squat Options
1. Step-up.
2. Swing split squat: Put one foot in the seat of a swing, and the other farther in front. Push your hips back to squat down so your planted knee bends 90 degrees. Press back to start.
3. Jump and touch: Find something high to jump and touch. Squat down, then jump!

Trunk Flexion Options
1. Hanging leg raise.
2. Lying leg raise.

GO PLOGGING

Sounds like something you'd need to look up in the Urban Dictionary, but plogging isn't gross—not in that way, anyway. It's a Swedish workout of jogging while picking up trash—in Swedish slang, to "plocka up."

Groups have sprung up around Europe to join in, but you don't need a group to make your run into an Earth-cleaning experience. Just grab a pair of gloves and bring along a trash bag. And don't worry about losing your intensity: On my first plog, I ran 2.5 miles in 26 minutes—not fast, but enough for a great cardio session while removing a giant bag of trash from my neighborhood.

ROW LIKE A GOLD MEDALIST

There's one piece of heart-pumping equipment in your gym that Navy SEALS, ultramarathoners, and Crossfitters all agree on: the rowing machine. But if you want the best rowing workout possible, who do you talk to? A rower!

Lauren Schmetterling is among the best in the world on an erg—and one of the best rowing outside, too. The Team USA rower won gold in the Women's Eight at the 2016 Olympics, and has earned three gold medals at World Championships, too. But she's also lightning fast on a rowing machine: Schmetterling finished fourth at the World Indoor Rowing Championships in 2019, where rowers compete on the stationary machine for individual glory.

To prepare for Olympic-level races—and to compete inside—Schmetterling uses the same types of rowers you'll find in your gym. Try to keep up with her typical training day with this workout—or use the toned-down version for a more manageable rowing-machine challenge.

LAUREN SCHMETTERLING'S WORKOUT
After a warm-up, row for 5,000 meters (Schmetterling completes this in around 20 minutes). Rest for 2 minutes. Repeat 4 more times, for a total of 5 rounds.

To make this a little more manageable, Schmetterling suggests 3 rounds of 2,000 meters each, resting 5 minutes between rounds. In each round, she says, you should be aiming for 22 to 24 strokes per minute, trying to make each 2,000-meter effort faster than the last.

C hances are, your gym has equipment you're not using. Some isn't worth your time—looking at you, 130-pound dumbbells. But some other stuff might just be intimidating—it looks fun or useful, but you don't want to waste your time or look like a fool. You're paying for it, though! Here's how to make all those pieces of equipment work for you.

PUNCH AWAY THE STRESS

Hitting a heavy bag is one of the most fun, stress-busting activities any health club has to offer. And it'll get your heart pumping faster than you think: "If you're not used to doing it," says Arturo Reyes, "you'll start to lose your breath in the first 30 seconds."

Reyes should know: Once the WKA's number two kickboxer at 124 pounds, he now coaches at Urban Boxing DC in the nation's capital. But while the bag is fun and efficient, it can also be intimidating—you don't want to look like a goof when you strap on the gloves, and you don't want to get hurt.

Don't worry, Reyes says. With just two simple punches (see sidebar), you can create combinations to get your heart pumping and your lungs heaving. Try this three-round workout to start—try for 3 minutes per round, resting 30 seconds in between. If that's too hard, try for one-minute rounds to start.

HOW TO DO IT
In each round, you'll perform three different punch combinations for one minute. After you've done all three combos, rest for 30 seconds, and repeat. Try to do 3 rounds to start.

Combination 1: Jab, Jab, Cross
Stay light on your feet, but stay in one spot while you do this combo: Jab, jab, then cross. After one minute, move to combination 2 without resting.

Combination 2: Jab, Cross, Step, Step
Bounce a little for this minute. Do a jab, a cross, then move left two steps. Repeat, but this time, step right two steps. After one minute, move to combination 3 without resting.

Combination 3: Double Jab
Perform two jabs, take a beat, then repeat. Go for 1 minute. After you've done all three combos, rest for 30 seconds, then start again with combo 1.

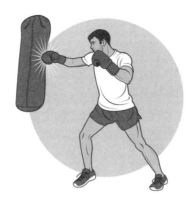

TWO PUNCHES, ONE MILLION WORKOUTS

With just these two basic punches, Reyes says, you can create unlimited workouts.

1. **The Jab:** Boxing's most basic punch creates openings for fighters, and will also tell you how far to stand from the bag—your lead hand should just hit the bag when your arm is fully extended.

    Stand in a ready position, with your dominant hand farther from the bag: hands up, elbows in, back foot at a 45-degree angle from the bag, front foot slightly angled. Move only your lead arm—extend it from this position until it hits the bag, with a slight bend in your elbow. Snap it back to start.

2. **The Cross:** From the same ready position, keep your lead arm up, guarding your face as you twist your hips, back foot, and upper torso to bring your rear arm forward to punch the bag. Keep a slight bend in your elbow as it hits the bag. Return to start.

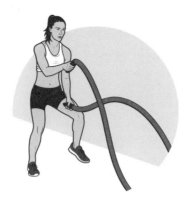

TORCH FAT AND HAVE FUN WITH THE BATTLING ROPES

In dramatic sports drink commercials, super-hot athletes wave these big, braided ropes to enhance their super-hotness (and their need for electrolytes). Those ropes are in your gym! You can look just as badass!

Some killjoy may tell you that they are not badass, just bad—that the ropes won't give you a good cardio workout.

That's not exactly right: Training with the ropes only got trainees in one study to 68 percent of their maximum possible effort, compared to going all-out on a treadmill. But you're unlikely to go all-out on the treadmill, anyway—and there's a 100 percent chance that doing so is not as much fun as the ropes.

So mix them in! Start by getting into a quarter-squat and doing some easy alternating waves on the rope to warm up. Then perform each of these moves as fast as you can for 15 seconds, then rest for 45 seconds before doing the next move. Try for 3 total rounds of all three moves. Try to increase the amount of time you work for each interval, working toward 30 seconds on, 60 seconds off.

EXERCISE 1: Alternating Big Waves
Bring your hands from above your head down to your thighs on each swing.

EXERCISE 2: Two-Hand "X" Waves
Bring both hands up and together above your head to the right, then whip them down to your left knee. Then come up to the left of your head, and down to your right knee. You'll make an "X" in the air.

EXERCISE 3: Double-Arm Slams
Big waves, big slams. Bring your hands together straight in front of your head, and slam the ropes down between your legs. Keep going, slamming big, loud, and fast.

THEN SLAM!

Sure, you can reduce stress with deep breathing. Or you can grab a medicine ball and slam it into the floor. So don't just use those balls for ab work.

Throwing a medicine ball helps build power—and it will make you *feel* powerful, too. You'll be working your arms, legs, back, and abs simultaneously—oh, and those smile muscles, too. Grab a ball (for maximum safety, choose a soft-sided ball), and try this 3-move workout.

In each set, do the slam or throw, then get the ball and reset. You don't want these to be cardio workouts—each rep should be powerful, so make sure you're reset before each throw. Rest one minute between sets and exercises.

EXERCISE 1: Medicine Ball Slam
Stand with your knees slightly bent, holding a medicine ball at your chest with both hands. Raise your arms up over your head, and then forcefully slam the ball down in front of your feet. Perform 3 sets of 5 reps.

EXERCISE 2: Rotational Slam
Stand in the same position as Exercise 1, but place the ball outside your right foot. Bend down and pick it up, rotating your arms like a rainbow over your head as you stand up. Once the ball is over your head, slam it down next to your left foot (but don't hit your foot!). Pick it up and rainbow over to the other side, slamming it on the right. Perform 3 sets of 3 slams in each direction.

EXERCISE 3: Two-Armed Side Throw
Stand with a wall on your right side about 4 feet away, and the ball on your left hip, held with both hands. With knees slightly bent, twist through your torso to swing the ball around toward your right hip, releasing it so it flies against the wall around chest height. If it bounces back, catch the ball and rotate back to start. If not, pick it up and reset. Do 2 sets of 5 throws on each side.

DOUBLE YOUR WALKING CALORIE BURN WITH THIS MILITARY SECRET

For centuries, the US Army has used a secret tool to help soldiers get into World War–winning shape: a backpack.

Loading up a pack turns a simple march or jog into a combination strength and cardio workout—in training camps, soldiers do weighted marches of 20-plus miles, carrying packs weighing 50 to 100 pounds.

Even if you don't walk that far or load that heavy, "rucking"—named for the military "rucksack"—can pump up your heart rate throughout your walk, turning a normal stroll around the block into a calorie-crushing workout. Carrying a 40-pound pack increases my average heart rate by more than 15 percent on a 30-minute walk. According to the *Compendium of Physical Activities*, a 200-pound man will burn 378 calories when rucking for 30 minutes, compared to burning just 141 without the pack.

Rucking can do more than separate you from your gut, though. It can bring you together with other like-minded fitness folks: Rucking clubs across the country carry flags to honor soldiers, and go for long marches and engage in conversations while wearing packs. There are also rucking challenges—races without the race part—happening all over, all the time. Find clubs and events at www.goruck.com.

But you don't need others to get rucking: Instead of 100 pounds, start with around 10 percent of your bodyweight—load a dumbbell (wrapped in a towel to stabilize it), some bricks, or heavy books into a backpack, and head out for a walk. You'll burn nearly triple the calories with the same stroll.

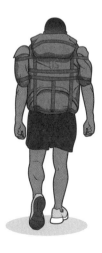

MAKE FUNNY FACES, LOOK YOUNGER: IT'S REAL! SCIENCE BACKS UP THE RESULTS

You don't see people showing up in droves to chains like "Planet Faceness," even though the muscles on our mugs can sag just as much as those on our arms and thighs.

Maybe that's because, even though facial exercises have been touted for a century, there's been little proof that they work. But scientists at Northwestern studied Gary Sikorski's "Happy Face Yoga" system, finding that when women did a 30-minute session of his exercises three to four times a week for 20 weeks, they looked two years younger.

Sikorski's 18-exercise system increases blood circulation to the face, but also incorporates outside resistance—just like lifting weights. But instead of strapping barbells to your nose, all you need is your hands. Try this three-pack of Sikorski's exercises for six weeks, and see if you look younger. You can find his full, scientifically backed program at www.happyfaceyoga.com.

EXERCISE 1: The Lion
Smile! Inhale deeply, then exhale forcefully. As you exhale, open your mouth wide, stick out your tongue, roll your eyes up, and tighten all the muscles in your neck, chest, abdominal area, and butt. Repeat three times. Now do it again, but this time, press your middle and index fingers across the top of your forehead. Create a tight band on your forehead and flex your eyebrows up as you exhale. Do this second part three times.

EXERCISE 2: Scooping
This exercise will help tighten the area on, around, and under the jaw, Sikorski says. Open your mouth and say "ahh." Fold your lower lip over your lower teeth and hold tightly, jutting your lower jaw forward. Using only your lower jaw, scoop up very slowly as you close your mouth. Repeat, pulling your chin up a little higher each time you scoop, tilting your head backward over 10 repetitions. On the final repetition, your chin will be pointing at the ceiling. Hold this position—chin toward the ceiling—for 20 seconds. Repeat three times.

EXERCISE 3: Lower Eyelid Firmer
As we age, Sikorski says, our eyes narrow. By working the large muscle around the eye, this makes our eyes look bigger, brighter, and younger. Place your middle fingers near the inner sides of your eyes at the top of your nose. Place your index fingers outside the eyes. Using these fingers, you're holding that big muscle, the obicularis occuli, in place throughout the move.

Squint your lower eyelids—imagine you're looking up at bright sun. Squint up, then release 10 times, keeping your upper lids as wide as possible throughout. On the 10th squint, hold for 20 seconds. Repeat the 10 squints one more time, finishing with another hold.

*B*aby Shark has been viewed more than 7 billion times on YouTube. And if you've had a kid in your life since 2015, you probably feel like a million of those views can be chalked up to you.

But the shark family can exercise more than just your patience: It can also work your core. The "Baby Shark Ab Challenge" is nearly as big a hit as the song itself, reaching more than 8 million viewers in different videos. Even the Washington Nationals, who used "Baby Shark" as a theme song, have tried it!

For each line of the song—Baby Shark, Mommy Shark, etc.—you'll do a different ab move, mostly from a V-Up Hold position, while trying to move to the song's undeniably catchy beat. See if you're up to the challenge, and then try your own Shark Week: Try to go faster over time, getting more repetitions of each movement each day.

Here are the exercises to do for each "verse" of the song:

Baby Shark: V-Up Hold with Foot Clap

1. Begin by assuming a V-Up Hold position: Lie on your back with your arms and legs extended. Brace your core and pull your upper body up into a half-sit-up, with your back straight and your arms straight in front of your shoulders, while lifting your legs up off the floor, knees straight and legs slightly separated. In this position, your body will form an open "V" shape. This is the starting position, the "V-Up Hold" position.
2. Maintain this position and bring your feet together to "clap" them on each beat, returning your legs to the original position. Continue through the "Baby Shark" portion of the song.

Mommy Shark: V-Up Hold with Alternating Straight-Leg Raise

1. Continue to hold the V-Up Hold position. On each beat, lift your right leg up toward your face while keeping your left leg in the original V-Up Hold the position. Keep your knees straight.
2. Return your right leg to the V-Up Hold position, and lift your left leg up in the same way.
3. Keep scissoring your straight legs in this way through "Mommy Shark."

Daddy Shark: V-Up Toe Touch

1. Continue to hold the V-Up Hold position. On each beat, crunch your abs so your legs and arms both come up, touching at the top.
2. Return to the V position, and repeat on each beat through "Daddy Shark."

Grandma Shark: V-Up Hold Bicycle

1. Continue to hold the V-Up Hold position. On the beat, bend your right knee and bring it toward your face while keeping your left leg in the V-Up Hold position.
2. Return the right leg to start and bring your left knee toward your face. Continue bicycling your knees in this way through "Grandma Shark."

Grandpa Shark: V-Up Hold Double Knee

1. Continue to hold the V-Up Hold position. Perform this as with "Grandma Shark," but bring both knees toward your chest together, instead of one at a time.
2. Continue in this way through "Grandpa Shark."

Let's Go Hunt: V-Up Hold Flutter Kick

1. Continue to hold the V-Up Hold position. Flutter kick your legs, moving them up and down slightly, in a scissor motion, while keeping your knees straight.
2. Continue in this way through "Let's Go Hunt."

Run Away: Mountain Climber

1. Flip over and assume the classic push-up position: Your hands should be directly beneath your shoulders, your body forming a straight line from head to heels.
2. Maintaining this body line and keeping your hips parallel to the floor, lift your right foot off the ground and bend your knee so that it comes up toward your chest.
3. Return your right foot to the start position, and repeat with the left leg, switching rapidly through "Run Away."

"Safe at Last" and "It's the End"

Perform a static V-Up Hold through these two verses.

TRX suspension trainers are in every gym in the world today, with everyone from pro athletes to senior citizens using the straps to perform hundreds of exercises. But 15 years ago, there was just one TRX—in an undisclosed location in Malaysia.

If you don't know the story of the TRX's invention—the brand name is an acronym for "Total Body Resistance Exercise"—here's the short version: Randy Hetrick, a Navy SEAL, was waiting for days with his team for a mission to start. There wasn't much to do, so the SEALS trained. Without equipment, though, they couldn't work on pulling strength—something Hetrick wanted to target. So he took a jiujitsu belt, knotted it, and threw it over a door. "Close the rotation, reach up to the top of the door with the other hand—that's the first move I ever created," he says.

Within a few hours, he and his teammates had 20 moves for his nascent invention. A few years later, while working to launch his on-base apparatus as the "TravelFit," Hetrick did this 45-minute workout on Veterans' Day. The mission: Celebrate sweat, strength, and gratitude. Grab your gym's TRX straps and try this workout, which its inventor created in 2007.

This workout is in three strength sections of 12 to 13 minutes each. In each block, the exercises are performed for 60 seconds each. After each block, rest 1 minute, then move to the next block.

BLOCK 1: LOWER BODY

EXERCISE 1: TRX Lunge

1. Stand with one foot behind you in the strap, so your knee is bent 90 degrees and the strap is angled slightly forward. Your other foot should be flat on the floor.
2. Bend your front knee and sink your hips backward so that your suspended leg goes backward until you're in a lunge position, with both legs bent 90 degrees. The strap will now be vertical.
3. Stand back up, and repeat. Do 30 seconds on this leg, then switch feet and repeat.

EXERCISE 2: TRX Lateral Lunge

1. Stand holding the straps at chest level, with your feet together, toes pointed forward.
2. Take a big step to the right, pushing your hips back and descending as you step by bending your right knee, keeping it tracking over your right toes. Keep your torso upright as you descend, using the straps for balance as needed.
3. Press back to start, and perform the move to the left. Continue for 60 seconds.

EXERCISE 3: Crossing Balance Lunge

1. Stand underneath the straps, holding one in each hand at your sides. Lift your right foot off the ground slightly so you're standing on your left leg.
2. Send your right leg back as if you were going into a reverse lunge, but keep your right knee and foot hovering over the ground—use the straps for balance.
3. Stand back up. Repeat for 30 seconds, then switch legs.

EXERCISE 4: Knee Strike

1. No straps: Stand with your arms in a boxing position.
2. Strike your right knee up and across your body.
3. Reset and repeat for 30 seconds, then do the same with your left knee. After this move, rest 1 minute, then move to Block 2.

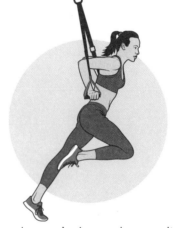

BLOCK 2: UPPER BODY

EXERCISE 1: TRX Chest Press

1. With your hands in the straps, lean forward so you're in a push-up position at a 45-degree angle.
2. Maintain a rigid body line as you bend your elbows to the bottom of the push-up position.
3. Press back to start. Repeat.

EXERCISE 2: TRX Power Pull

1. Hold the straps in your right hand and lean away at a 45-degree angle with your feet about shoulder-width apart. Your left arm should be behind you, so your torso makes a "T."
2. Maintaining a straight body line, pull with your right arm to row yourself up. At the same time, twist your core so you're facing forward, and reach up past your right hand with your left, as if you were going to climb a ladder.
3. Twist back to the start, and repeat. Do 30 seconds on this arm, then switch and do 30 more.

WORKOUT CONTINUES >>>

EXERCISE 3: TRX Fly

1. Start as you did for the chest press, but with your arms wide in a "V" shape.
2. With a slight bend in your elbows, hug your arms toward your chest—the angle of your body will get shallower as you fly.
3. Control your body to return to start. Repeat for 60 seconds.

EXERCISE 4: TRX Curl

1. Face the handles and hold them at the top of the curl position. Lean back slightly with your feet shoulder-width apart.
2. Slowly uncurl your arms, maintaining a rigid body line so your body falls backward slightly.
3. Curl back up. Repeat for 60 seconds.

EXERCISE 5: TRX Tricep Extension

1. Assume the position you had for the chest press. Bring your hands closer together, almost touching.
2. Keep your hands together and elbows close to your sides as you lower your body toward your hands.
3. Press back up. Repeat for 60 seconds.

EXERCISE 6: Speed Squat

Perform bodyweight squats as fast as you can for 60 seconds. After this move, rest one minute, then move to Block 3.

BLOCK 3: CORE

EXERCISE 1: TRX Overhead Squat

1. Stand with your feet slightly wider than shoulder-width, holding the handles taut with your arms in a big "Y" shape.
2. Keep your arms up as you push your hips back to squat, descending until your thighs are at least parallel to the floor.
3. Press through your heels back to the starting position.

EXERCISE 2: Side Plank

Get in a side plank position, but with your feet elevated in the TRX straps near the ground. Hold for 30 seconds on each side.

EXERCISE 3: Pike

1. Get in a classic push-up position, with your arms directly beneath your shoulders, but your feet in the TRX handles just off the ground.
2. Use your core to lift your hips and bring your feet toward your face into a pike position, keeping your back and legs straight.
3. Return to start, and repeat.

EXERCISE 4: Hamstring Curl

1. Lie faceup with your heels in the handles of the TRX straps, so your feet are just off the floor with legs straight.
2. Squeeze your butt to lift your hips up, and form a straight line from head to heels.
3. Pull your knees toward your chest until your thighs are perpendicular to your torso.
4. Extend your legs back out, and repeat for 60 seconds.

EXERCISE 5: Rolling Side Plank

1. Assume a side plank position on your left side: Prop yourself up on your left elbow and stack your feet in the TRX handles close to the ground. Your body should form a straight line from head to heels. Point your right arm perpendicular to your torso so it's pointed toward the ceiling.
2. Maintaining your plank, bring your right arm down and under, threading the needle under your left arm.
3. Return back to start. Do this for 30 seconds on this side, then switch sides and do 30 more.

EXERCISE 6: Crunch

1. Just a regular old crunch. Go for 60 seconds.

"HASH" WITH YOUR LOCAL DRINKING CLUB WITH A RUNNING PROBLEM

When the original Hash House Harriers drew up their running club's constitution in 1950, the group had four goals: To promote physical fitness, run off their weekly hangovers, persuade older members they're not as old as they feel, and "acquire a good thirst and to satisfy it in beer."

That's the kind of club I can get behind—and I'm not alone. Since its initial founding by British officers prior to World War II, Hash House Harrier clubs have formed all over the world, and in every state of the US. In weekly or monthly runs, they follow similar objectives as the original: The club runs (or sometimes walks) along a path of sawdust, flour, or chalk laid by one member, called a "hare." At the end of the run, they drink—usually beer.

Each run is called a "hash," and while some clubs are more serious about the running portion (with others focused on the refreshments), they're all undeniably fun. They're also incredibly welcoming: Many hashes present multiple trails of different lengths—a 3-mile trail that's all on the roads, a 6-miler that includes some trail running, and a 10-miler for the hard-core hashers, for instance—and groups usually include runners of various speeds, so you won't be left in the dust.

Bottom line: Hashing is one of the most fun ways you can do cardio, and the clubs are *everywhere*. Search HASH HOUSE HARRIERS and your town, or check the map at www.half-mind.com/regionalwebsite/index.php.

THREE EXERCISES THAT WILL HELP BANISH BACK PAIN FOR LIFE

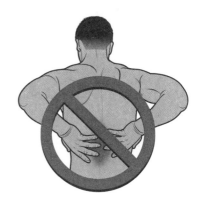

NFL PLAYERS AND UFC FIGHTERS SWEAR BY THIS TRIO, AND YOU SHOULD, TOO

It may not be as sexy as climbing a mountain, but keeping a lid on low back pain will help keep you ready to tackle all those bucket-list adventures. And chances are, back pain's coming for you: Half of all Americans suffer some back pain symptoms every year.

But your pain is as individual as you are: "There is no such thing as non-specific back pain," says Stuart McGill, professor emeritus of spine biomechanics at Ontario's University of Waterloo, and one of the world's foremost experts on pain-free spines. In his book *Back Mechanic*, McGill gives readers a system to determine what's causing their pain, and to create a customized plan to alleviate it. Ninety-five percent of patients who were told they needed back surgery were able to become pain-free without surgery using these techniques. So if your back *really* hurts, check it out.

Just about everyone, though, can benefit from McGill's "Big Three" exercises. This simple trio improves "proximal stiffness," a fancy way of saying that you're strong in the center—providing a stable springboard for all the movements your body needs to do, like twisting, jumping, pressing and pulling. The "Big Three" also helps build muscular endurance so you can maintain that stiffness for longer without pain.

Add ten minutes of the Big Three to your daily routine, and you'll be ready for bigger adventures with less back pain. If a single stretch of ten minutes is too much, break it up throughout the day.

No matter how long your session, one repetition is equal to a 10-second hold for each move. Keep that time consistent, even as you get stronger. Instead, add reps to the workout. For now, do 3 sets, resting 20 seconds between sets. In set 1, do 6 reps. In set 2, do 4 reps. In set 3, do just 2 reps.

WORKOUT CONTINUES >>>

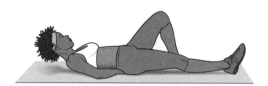

EXERCISE 1: McGill Curl-Up

1. Lie faceup with your hands under your lumbar spine, palms facing down. Your elbows will be just off the floor. Brace your core, and raise your head, neck, and shoulders off the ground—just a little bit!
2. Hold for 10 seconds for 1 rep, then return to the ground and repeat.

EXERCISE 2: Side Plank

1. Start with a bent-knee side plank. Stack your knees and prop yourself up on your left elbow. Your elbow should be directly beneath your shoulders, and your body should form a straight line from head to knees. To get into this position, Dr. McGill recommends not raising the hips laterally off the floor, but from a hinged hip—press your hips forward as you come up and establish the rigid body line.
2. Hold the side plank for ten seconds for each rep, repeating on the other side.

If you have shoulder pain or a rotator cuff injury, perform a wall plank instead. Lean against a wall with your elbow with your outside foot in front of your inside foot. Maintain a rigid body line for ten seconds.

EXERCISE 3: Bird Dog

1. Get on all fours with your hands directly beneath your shoulders and your knees directly beneath your hips. Brace your core and raise your right hand and left leg off the floor, sweeping them out toward the front and back as you raise them. Only raise the hand and leg until they are parallel with your torso—not higher.
2. Hold this position for ten seconds, then return to start. Do all your reps on this side, then switch arms and legs, and repeat.

If this is too hard, start by raising only your leg, keeping both arms on the floor.

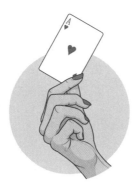

SHUFFLE THE DECK TO GET SWEATY ANYWHERE

Sometimes, when you can't get to the gym or don't have access to equipment, you can get stuck—searching online for the right workout or trying to design one yourself. Solve this paralysis by analysis with a simple tool: a deck of cards. Those 52 can give you a different HIIT workout every time you deal.

HOW IT WORKS

Each suit represents an exercise, and the value tells you how many repetitions to do. Draw four cards at a time, do the moves, then rest 25 seconds and repeat.

The Moves
Hearts: Push-Ups
Spades: Squats
Clubs: Lunges
Diamonds: V-Ups

The Reps
For numbered cards, do the number: For example, the eight of spades is 8 squats.

For face cards: Jacks are 12. Queens are 13. Kings are 14. Aces are 15.

Example: If you draw the two of clubs, the six of diamonds, the four of hearts, and the eight of clubs, you'll do 2 lunges, 6 V-ups, 4 push-ups, and 8 more lunges. Rest 25 seconds, then draw four more.

The Challenge
Make it through the whole deck. Too hard? Get as far as you can. Too easy? Reduce the rest periods on your next shuffle, or double the repetitions, making the deck twice as hard.

TURN GAME TIME INTO *GAINS* TIME LIKE AN MLB SLUGGER

Most of us are just going to watch the game, not play it. But you can do that like a champ, too: When Juan Soto was sidelined due to a positive COVID-19 test, the Washington Nationals slugger known for his "shuffle" between pitches predictably couldn't stop moving. While he waited for medical clearance to return to the team, Soto watched his teammates . . . and worked out.

"I've been riding my bike when my team is on defense, on the offense I try to do shoulder, core, whatever . . . some leg stuff," he said before returning to the team. "I've been trying to keep my body in shape."

And it worked: In his first 11 games back with the team, Soto smashed six homers. So take a page from his playbook: Get off the couch for a few innings, grab a resistance band, and do this workout inspired by Soto's routine. Perform this workout for around three innings of the game—longer if you're feeling ambitious.

IN THE TOP OF THE INNING
Ride an exercise bike or perform high-knee marches throughout the half-inning.

IN THE BOTTOM OF THE INNING
Grab a resistance band and do this 6-exercise circuit. Perform 9 repetitions of each exercise, then move to the next exercise. Repeat all 5 moves three times. If the home team is still at the plate, rest for two minutes, and do some more.

EXERCISE 1: Squat
1. Stand with your feet around hip-width apart, toes slightly pointed out. If you're using a resistance band, stand on the band with the handles in your hands at shoulder height.
2. Push your hips back to initiate the squat.
3. Keeping your weight in your heels, bend your knees and lower until your thighs are at least parallel to the floor, maintaining a flat back.
4. Press through your heels to stand back up.

EXERCISE 2: Overhead Press
1. Stand with the band under your feet, holding the handles at your shoulders, palms facing in. Change the width of your feet to adjust the tension on the band.
2. Keeping a proud chest, press the bands directly overhead until your arms are straight.
3. Return to start, and repeat.

EXERCISE 3: Push-Up

1. Assume a classic push-up position, with hands directly beneath your shoulders, your body forming a straight line from head to heels.
2. Maintain this rigid body line as you bend your elbows to lower your chest toward the floor.
3. Press back to start.

EXERCISE 4: Resistance Band Curl

1. Stand with the band under your feet, holding the handles at the sides of your thighs.
2. Maintaining an upright torso, bend your elbows to lift your hands up to your shoulders. Squeeze your biceps at the top.
3. Lower your arms and repeat.

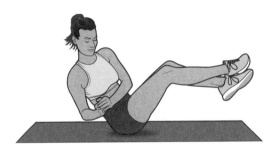

EXERCISE 5: Seated Russian Twist

1. Sit on the floor with your heels on the ground. Your torso should be at a 45-degree angle from the ground, and should be straight from your butt to your head. Place your arms in front of you as a guide.
2. From this position, twist to the left, twisting your whole torso, not just your arms, until your hands point out to 9 o'clock. To use your hands as a guide, your shoulders and chest should remain in the same position relative to your hands as you twist.
3. Twist back to start, and then go to the right, twisting until your shoulders, chest, and hands point toward 3 o'clock. That's 1 repetition.

GRAB A BROOMSTICK AND STAY LIMBER FOR MORE ADVENTURES

You don't need a double-blind study to tell you that as you get older, you're less mobile. Here's one anyway: In a study of 6,000 people, scores on a flexibility test went down 0.6 percent for each year of age. For every two years you live, your joint flexibility is reduced by 1 percent.

By the time you're 35, you're feeling it—no longer bounding over every fence you see or effortlessly bending over to pick up a dropped set of keys. But you're not stuck with the mobility you've got . . . if you've got a stick.

Stick Mobility is the brainchild of two trainers, Neal Valera and Dennis Dunphy, who wanted to help their clients get stronger and move better simultaneously, using a long, flexible stick. Like a yoga block, the stick lets you access stretches that your current flexibility levels might not allow.

The system has grown into a full-blown series of classes, where athletes, golfers, kids, and mobility-seeking adults swing and stretch on their signature bright orange sticks. But you can try their stretches right in your living room and get inspired to find a class near you. Grab a sturdy broomstick or a long PVC pipe, and try the first three stages of the "Ninja Flow Lunge," the move Valera and Dunphy recommend for first-timers.

For stage 1 of the ninja flow, assume a wide stance, with your feet about double your hip-width apart, feet facing forward and a slight bend in your knees. Hold the stick in your right hand at eye level, with the base inside your right big toe. Tuck your hips under by squeezing your butt, and squeeze your core. Keeping your shoulders and hips square, pull the top of the stick backward, stretching your chest and the front of your shoulder. Hold for ten seconds. Repeat on the other side.

To step this up to stage 2, return to the start position. With your right hand still high on the stick, hinge forward at the hips, maintaining a flat back as you lean forward. Your elevated arm will make you feel a big stretch in your chest and shoulder. If this is too much, return to the first position. If it's OK, reach down with your other, non-stick-holding arm, increasing the stretch. Hold for 10 to 15 seconds. If you need support during the stretch, reach across with your left hand, grabbing lower on the stick. Repeat on the other side.

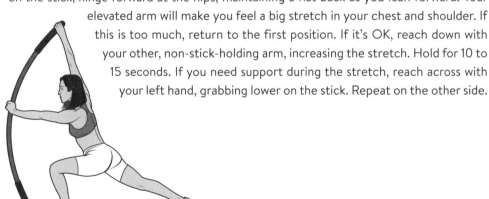

DESIGN YOUR OWN FITNESS ADVENTURE—IN YOUR OWN BACKYARD: USE THESE TIPS FROM A GLOBE-TROTTING, OCEAN KAYAKING EXPLORER

By now, you know you don't have to go to the ends of the Earth to find active adventure. Now it's time to create your own signature "bucket list" workout right in your area. And there's no one better to help than filmmaker Beau Miles. While the Aussie cut his teeth on expeditions like a 2,000-kilometer kayak trip around the Horn of Africa, Miles has spent the past few years focusing on adventures closer to home—climbing (and sleeping in) a centuries-old tree, and cramming activity in between mile-long laps for a 24-hour marathon.

"[On 'bigger' adventures], one day out of ten was exceptional. The rest was just bloody hard work," he says. "What's the point of having one magnificent moment, when you can have 100 moments that are just shy of that?"

Here are some ways Miles finds those near-perfect moments—and you can, too.

1. **Indulge Your Curiosity, and Add a Physical Challenge**

   When Miles filmed *Run the Line*, about a defunct rail line near his home, he was already interested in the train's history. Instead of just learning more from books, he tacked on a physical challenge—running the line, even as it cut through properties and farms that didn't exist half a century ago. He wound up meeting farmers, exploring new places, and experiencing the history firsthand. Take something you're already curious about, and add a challenge for your body.

2. **Combine Something You're Good at with Something You're Bad at**

   "I want to use a skill set that I have—like rowing or running—and I overlay something I'm not particularly good at," he says. In *Mile an Hour*, Miles combined running with a lack of sleep—which none of us are good at—and other tasks like mending a button or fixing a chair. But the "not good at" activity can be even simpler: "It might be talking to people. I'm not very good at talking to people."

   Layer the known with the unknown, and you're an explorer.

3. **Document It**

   "We're all storytelling animals and we're reflective by default," Miles says. The process of editing films lets him experience his adventures again, and experience the emotions he felt during them. We can't all be filmmakers, but we can all document our exploration—whether it's in a note to a friend, a personal journal, or on social media. Documenting your emotions before you start, during planning, and in the hours and days after your adventure can help you relive it—and accurately remember what you liked and didn't—so you can plan an even better-for-you adventure the next time.

PART 4

WORKOUTS THAT WILL CHALLENGE YOU

Time to test your limits: See how you fare against the standards set by mega-athletes, multiple marathon finishers, world record holders . . . and even yourself.

CHAPTER 15

TEST YOURSELF

It's not just half-marathons and triathlons that can test you. These 29 challenges will push you to your edge and tell you how strong you are—and how far you've come—in all aspects of fitness.

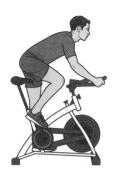

THE "REAL" TABATA WORKOUT IS INSANELY HARD

The "Tabata protocol" has spawned a thousand imitators, but there's only one *real* Tabata workout—proven to give you 60 minutes of cardio work in 4 minutes. It's the same one that Izumi Tabata (so *that's* where that name came from!) used in the study that started it all.

In the study, Tabata compared two groups on bikes for six weeks: One group rode for an hour, 5 times per week, at 70 percent of their maximum capacity. The other group rode for just four minutes, 4 times per week, riding at 170 percent of their VO$_2$Max for 20 seconds, then resting for 10 seconds before repeating.

Here's the thing: 170 percent of your VO$_2$Max is *insanely* hard. VO$_2$Max indicates how much oxygen your body is using when you're breathing or exerting your hardest. So if you're at 170 percent of that, you're going so fast and so hard that you don't have oxygen flowing to your muscles to keep you going. This is called "anaerobic" training, and it's key to getting the benefits.

If you want to really try a "Tabata" workout, get on a bike—preferably one with arm action, since you can work your whole body to exert yourself even harder. After a warm-up, try going all-out for 20 seconds—really hard, so that you can pedal and pump no harder! Ten seconds of rest won't feel like enough. See if you can do it for 4 minutes, and then laugh in the face of any other workout with the gall to call itself "Tabata."

BE LIKE MIKE (JORDAN, OF COURSE): DO THIS RUNNING TEST

The test is simple:

1. Go to a local track.
2. Run as many laps as you can in 12 minutes.
3. Stop, pant, and figure out how far you've gone.

That's it. It's called the "Cooper Test," named for Kenneth Cooper—the inventor of aerobics. The test has been used for 50 years to measure VO_2Max, which indicates how much oxygen your body is using when you're breathing or exerting your hardest. The American Heart Association uses VO_2Max as an indicator of overall fitness.

VO_2Max is often talked about and measured when discussing endurance athletes—Greg LeMond famously had a world-beating max, and the record for the highest intake ever recorded was by a cross-country skier. But short-burst athletes have been tested in this way, too: Michael Jordan when he was at the University of North Carolina at Chapel Hill, soccer great Pele when he was starring for Brazil, and—formerly—the referees of FIFA.

A VO_2Max above 51 is excellent. Between 43 and 51 is "good." If you score 34 to 42, you're fair or average. And anything under is, well, not good. Use the chart below with your age and distance run to see which of these ranges your VO_2Max falls into.

Age		Very Good	Good	Average	Bad	Very Bad
13–14	M	2700+ m	2400–2700 m	2200–2399 m	2100–2199 m	2100- m
	F	2000+ m	1900–2000 m	1600–1899 m	1500–1599 m	1500- m
15–16	M	2800+ m	2500–2800 m	2300–2499 m	2200–2299 m	2200- m
	F	2100+ m	2000–2100 m	1700–1999 m	1600–1699 m	1600- m
17–20	M	3000+ m	2700–3000 m	2500–2699 m	2300–2499 m	2300- m
	F	2300+ m	2100–2300 m	1800–2099 m	1700–1799 m	1700- m
20–29	M	2800+ m	2400–2800 m	2200–2399 m	1600–2199 m	1600- m
	F	2700+ m	2200–2700 m	1800–2199 m	1500–1799 m	1500- m
30–39	M	2700+ m	2300–2700 m	1900–2299 m	1500–1899 m	1500- m
	F	2500+ m	2000–2500 m	1700–1999 m	1400–1699 m	1400- m
40–49	M	2500+ m	2100–2500 m	1700–2099 m	1400–1699 m	1400- m
	F	2300+ m	1900–2300 m	1500–1899 m	1200–1499 m	1200- m
50+	M	2400+ m	2000–2400 m	1600–1999 m	1300–1599 m	1300- m
	F	2200+ m	1700–2200 m	1400–1699 m	1100–1399 m	1100- m

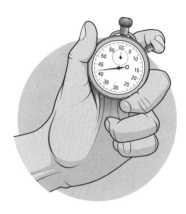

THE ONE-HOUR WORKOUT THAT WILL PREDICT YOUR MARATHON TIME

If you're training for your first marathon—or trying for a new personal record—this workout is like a crystal ball: In about an hour, you'll know (roughly) how fast your race time will be. It's trusted by legends, developed by a champion, and you don't need a *Beautiful Mind* to do the math. It's called "Yasso 800s," and all you need is a track.

Developed by Bart Yasso—a marathon winner, former *Runner's World* "Chief Running Officer," and just generally a really nice guy—the workout couldn't be simpler.

1. Convert the hours from your goal time into minutes, and the minutes into seconds. So if your marathon goal is 3 hours and 30 minutes, the important time for your Yasso 800s is 3 minutes and 30 seconds.
2. Head to a track, or find a spot where you can measure out 800 meters easily (at a track, that's two laps). After warming up, try to run 800 meters in your minutes/seconds time from step 1.
3. After you finish, jog for the same amount of time it took you to finish the 800. Repeat.

Use this workout starting a few months before your goal race, beginning with just 4 repeats of 800 meters, adding 1 round each week. As you get within a few weeks of race day, run this workout as a test. If you can run 10 repeats of the 800-meter effort at the goal time from step 1, chances are you can finish the marathon in your goal time. It's that simple!

ADD 40 POUNDS TO YOUR SQUAT IN ONE MONTH

All you need is a barbell: Load it with the amount of weight you think you can lift 10 times. Then lift it 20 times.

Don't say you can't. You can! You just need time: Instead of pumping through the set like a piston, breathe as many times as necessary between reps, taking as long for the single set as you need. Later in the week, do it again—but with 5 more pounds on the bar.

For more than half a century, lifters hoping to add strength and size have been doing this 1-set workout, inspired by lifting guru John McCallum, the book *Super Squats*, and throwback-loving strength coaches. McCallum, in his 1960s magazine columns, claimed to have put on 100 pounds (of mostly muscle) over time by doing little more than tons of squats in this way.

And it really works! Try it for a month and see how strong you can get. After thoroughly warming up, here's all you do.

EXERCISE 1: Overhead Press
Do 3 sets of 12 reps.

EXERCISE 2: Squats
Perform 1 set of 20 reps.

EXERCISE 3: Dumbbell Pull-Over
Do 2 sets of 20 reps with a 20-pound dumbbell.

Perform this workout twice a week, adding 5 pounds to the squat bar at each workout.

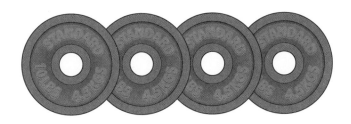

THE WORLD RECORD BURPEE CHALLENGE

f you think 30 seconds of burpees at the end of your workout is torture, try doing them for 12 hours straight.

Bryan Abell did, burpee-ing 4,689 times to set a Guinness World Record in 2019. Then a student at Michigan State University, Abell trained for just 30 days before setting the record. The 23-year-old did the feat as a fundraiser for his charity, the Stronger Warrior Foundation, which provides care packages to active-duty military members and supports veterans charities.

"I had probably done fewer than 500 burpees in my whole life [when I started training for the record]," he says. In the 30 days of training, he practiced the six-position move 30,000 times.

Abell didn't do all those burpees in a row: He used an "every minute on the minute," or "EMOM" workout. To do this kind of workout, you perform the exercise you're working on at the start of every minute, and rest with any time left in that minute. When the second hand strikes :00 once again, you repeat.

For his EMOM burpees, Abell would do 7 or 8 reps at the start of each minute, then rest the remainder of that minute. In his training, he'd repeat that for 90 minutes most training days—and on the day of the record attempt, for 12 hours straight. Just get a taste: Try it for 10 *minutes* to start.

BURN 346 CALORIES IN 13 MINUTES

When scientists tested this workout, participants burned as many calories as you'd get from an Oreo McFlurry in just 13 minutes—almost as much time as it would take to eat it!

The workout looks easy, but it's deceptive: Even though you're only lifting half of your max on each exercise, 30 seconds is a long set. And with the short rest, you may find your reps falling from 18 per set down to 11 by the third go-round. But there's good news: Keeping the blood flowing into the muscle like that will give you a wicked pump—making this the perfect workout to do before your next trip to the beach.

For each exercise, choose a weight that is 50 percent of your 1-rep max—that's a weight you could only do once. Perform the exercise for 30 seconds, then rest 15 seconds. Repeat twice more, then move to the next exercise.

EXERCISE 1: Barbell Bench Press (3 sets of 30 seconds, resting 15 seconds between sets)

1. Lie faceup on the bench and grab the bar with an overhand grip just wider than shoulder-width apart. Unrack the bar, holding it above your sternum with straight arms.
2. Bend your elbows to lower the bar to your chest. Your elbows should stay close to your sides, forming a 45-degree angle.
3. Pause, then press back to start.

EXERCISE 2: Barbell Bent-Over Row (3 sets of 30 seconds, resting 15 seconds between sets)

1. Deadlift the weight off the ground so you stand holding the bar in front of you with an overhand grip, feet hip-width apart, knees slightly bent.
2. Push your hips back like you're opening a door behind you with your butt. This starts the hip hinge.
3. Keep pushing your hips back so that your back remains flat until it is nearly parallel to the floor with the weight hanging straight down from your shoulders.
4. Maintaining this flat back position, pull the weight toward your chest.
5. Lower the weight back to the starting position, and repeat.

WORKOUT CONTINUES >>>

EXERCISE 3: Barbell Bicep Curl (3 sets of 30 seconds, resting 15 seconds between sets)
1. Stand holding a barbell (or EZ-curl bar) in front of your thighs.
2. Curl the weight up to your shoulders without swinging your body.
3. Return to start, and repeat.

EXERCISE 4: Skullcrusher (3 sets of 30 seconds, resting 15 seconds between sets)
1. Lie faceup on a bench holding a short barbell or EZ-curl bar with an overhand grip, your arms straight out from your shoulders.
2. Bend your elbows—without flaring them to the sides—as you bring the bar down toward your head. Stop when your elbows are bent 90 degrees.
3. Press the weight back to the start position. Repeat.

EXERCISE 5: Leg Extension (3 sets of 30 seconds, resting 15 seconds between sets)
1. Use the leg extension machine.

EXERCISE 6: Lying Leg Curl (3 sets of 30 seconds, resting 15 seconds between sets)
Use the lying leg curl machine.

Tip! Figure out all your weights first and, if you can, gather them. Getting from station to station this quickly is tough!

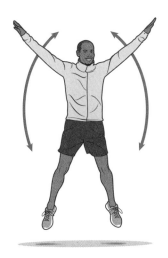

THE 7-MINUTE WORKOUT

In 2014, the "7-minute workout" went viral when the *New York Times* said it "essentially combines a long run and a visit to the weight room into about seven minutes of steady discomfort."

Well, kind of. In innumerable studies, hypertrophy and strength gains come from total volume lifted: So if you do 10 sets of 10 with 10 pounds, or 2 sets of 10 with 50 pounds, you'll get the same strength and muscle size benefits. Seven minutes of bodyweight-only maneuvers aren't going to get you the volume of a heavy lifting session.

But what you can improve in that seven minutes is VO$_2$Max, your body's ability to use oxygen at maximum effort. And that maximum effort is key: As you perform these exercises, go all-out.

This is the 7-minute workout that launched an app, an "advanced" 7-minute workout, and 50 billion copycats. Perform each exercise for 30 seconds at as fast a pace as you can while maintaining your form, resting 10 seconds between exercises. That protocol will take 7 minutes. The authors of the original study suggest performing the circuit two to three times, pushing the workout to 14 or 21 minutes.

EXERCISE 1: Jumping Jacks
Perform traditional jumping jacks.

EXERCISE 2: Wall Sit
1. With your back against a wall, slide down the wall and bend your knees until they're at a 90-degree angle.
2. Hold this position for the prescribed time.

WORKOUT CONTINUES >>>

EXERCISE 3: Push-Up

1. Assume a classic push-up position, with hands directly beneath your shoulders, your body forming a straight line from head to heels.
2. Maintain this rigid body line as you bend your elbows to lower your chest toward the floor.
3. Press back to start, maintaining the straight body line.

EXERCISE 4: Abdominal Crunch

Perform classic crunches, with knees bent and feet flat on the floor.

EXERCISE 5: Alternating Step-Up onto a Chair

1. Stand in front of a sturdy chair.
2. Keep your torso upright as you place your right foot on the chair and press through your heel to bring your left foot up so you're standing on the chair.
3. Return to the ground, and repeat with the other leg.

EXERCISE 6: Squat

1. Stand with your feet hip-width apart, toes pointed slightly out from parallel.
2. Push your hips back to initiate the squat. Bend your knees to descend until your thighs are at least parallel to the floor, keeping your chest up and your weight on your heels.
3. Keep the weight of your body in your heels and press back to standing.

EXERCISE 7: Triceps Dip on a Chair

1. Sit in front of a sturdy chair (preferably pushed against a wall).
2. Place your hands on the chair behind you, your fingers pointed forward (toward your butt). Bend your knees 90 degrees with your feet flat on the floor. Move your butt just in front of the seat.
3. Bend your elbows to 90 degrees, lowering your body. Then press back up. Repeat.

EXERCISE 8: Forearm Plank

1. Assume a modified push-up position on your forearms, with elbows directly beneath your shoulders, your body forming a straight line from head to heels.
2. Squeeze your glutes, legs, and core, and maintain this rigid body line for the pre-scribed time.

EXERCISE 9: High-Knee Run in Place

Lift your knees high, and run in place.

EXERCISE 10: Alternating Forward Lunge

1. Stand with your feet shoulder-width apart.
2. Take a large lunge step forward with your right leg, descending as you step until your knees both form 90-degree angles.
3. Press through your right foot to stand back up. Repeat on the other side. Keep alternating.

EXERCISE 11: "T" Push-Up

1. Assume a classic push-up position, with your hands directly beneath your shoulders, and your body forming a straight line from head to heels.
2. Maintain this rigid body line as you bend your elbows to lower your chest toward the floor.
3. As you press back to start, rotate your body to bring your right arm straight up over your left, forming a "T" shape with your body. In this position, your feet should be stacked, and your body forming a straight line from head to heels, but on the side.
4. Rotate back to start, and repeat, this time rotating so your left hand goes toward the ceiling.

EXERCISE 12: Side Plank (Left)

1. Lie on your side with your left forearm on the floor directly under your shoulder, and your feet stacked.
2. Prop yourself up on your elbow and form a straight line from ear to ankles. Hold this position for the prescribed time, then repeat on the other side.

EXERCISE 13: Side Plank (Right)

1. Lie on your side with your right forearm on the floor directly under your shoulder, and your feet stacked.
2. Prop yourself up on your elbow and form a straight line from ear to ankles. Hold this position for the prescribed time, then repeat on the other side.

Sunday	Monday	Tuesday	Wednesday	Thursday	Friday	Saturday
	X		X		X	

GET STRONG IN JUST 40 MINUTES PER WEEK

If you want to be strong, but don't want to get "bulky," this 13-minute workout is for you. When scientists had participants perform this 7-exercise session three times per week, men who did just one set of each exercise during each workout increased their strength over eight weeks just as much as others who did the same moves for 5 sets in each session. But the 1-set workouts were much shorter: Just 39 minutes per week, compared to more than three hours per week for the 5-setters.

Ready to get strong, fast? Here's how to do it.

For each exercise, do a set of 8 to 12 repetitions until you reach "momentary concentric failure"—when you can't do another repetition with correct form. Perform each rep for one second on the way up, and two seconds on the way down. Give yourself up to 2 minutes to change to the next exercise, and you should be done in 13 minutes.

EXERCISE 1: Barbell Bench Press

1. Lie faceup on the bench and grab the bar with an overhand grip just wider than shoulder-width apart.
2. Unrack the bar, holding it above your sternum with straight arms.
3. Bend your elbows to lower the bar to your chest. Your elbows should stay close to your sides, forming a 45-degree angle.
4. Pause, then press back to start.

EXERCISE 2: Seated Barbell Overhead Press

1. Unrack a barbell with an overhand grip at or slightly narrower than your shoulders.
2. Keeping your torso upright, press the barbell overhead until your arms are straight.
3. Pause, then slowly lower back to the starting position.

EXERCISE 3: Wide-Grip Lat Pull-Down

1. Grab the bar of a lat pull-down station with a wide, overhand grip. Pull your shoulder blades back and down.
2. Keeping your core braced, pull the bar down to the top of your sternum.
3. Return to start. Repeat.

EXERCISE 4: Seated Cable Row

1. Sit at a horizontal cable row station, using a V-bar. Grab the handles and pull your shoulder blades back and down.
2. Keep your torso upright and a proud chest as you row the weight until the V-bar reaches your chest.
3. Control the weight back to start. Repeat.

EXERCISE 5: Barbell Back Squat

1. Stand in a normal back squat position, barbell across your shoulders, feet between shoulder- and hip-width apart, toes slightly out.
2. Push your hips back to initiate the squat.
3. Bend your knees to descend until your thighs are at least parallel to the floor, keeping your chest up and your weight on your heels.
4. Keep the weight of your body in your heels and press back to standing.

EXERCISE 6: Leg Press

Use the leg press machine.

EXERCISE 7: Single-Leg Machine Leg Extension

1. Perform this workout three times a week, resting at least one day between workouts.
2. Use the leg extension machine, but only use one leg at a time.

GET FIVE HOURS OF FOCUS: WORK OUT LIKE A CHESS MASTER

How fit do you really need to be to sit still and move pawns around?

Very fit. The stress of a chess tournament can have pretty startling effects on the body: Grandmasters like Cristian Chirilă can lose as much as 15 pounds during the course of a ten-day tournament—from forgetting to eat, but also just from intense concentration. In one tournament, it was found that a Russian grandmaster had burned 560 calories in two hours of chess—more than most people burn running 5 miles.

"You have to keep focus for five hours at a time," says Chirilă, who lives in St. Louis. "If you lose that focus at any moment, you can blunder something and the game is over."

To build that mental endurance, Chirilă and his fellow competitors need lots of physical endurance—so they train long and hard. In 2017 and 2018, while acting as a chess and workout training partner of Fabiano Caruana, the world's second-ranked player, Chirilă says, "I was waking up, and doing this [three-exercise circuit] every morning." It prepared his body—and mind—for an intense day of concentration.

HOW TO DO IT

Perform each exercise for 50 repetitions, then move to the next exercise. Repeat all three exercises four times, for a total of 200 repetitions of each. Rest as little as possible, trying to reduce the total time needed to complete the workout. Chirilă's time: 20 minutes.

EXERCISE 1: Push-Ups
EXERCISE 2: Sit-Ups
EXERCISE 3: Bodyweight Squats

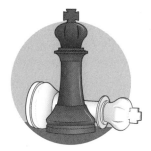

USE THE A-B-Cs TO SHRED YOUR A-B-S

Take your planks to 26 new levels with this stability-ball challenge—writing the alphabet with your arms.

Prop yourself on the ball in plank position—elbows on the ball, feet on the floor, your body forming a straight line from head to feet. Clasp your hands together and imagine you're holding a giant pencil pointed at the ground. Maintain your rigid body line and move your elbows beneath your shoulders to write a letter "A" with the pencil. Then continue, writing all the letters of the alphabet. If you can make it to "Z," take a breath, then do it again—this time in lowercase.

DO YOUR FIRST MUSCLE-UP

It doesn't matter whether you "need" to do it or not: When you get yourself up over the bar for the first time, you won't just wow the people around you—you'll wow yourself, too.

A muscle-up starts out like a pull-up. But the muscle-upper flings their body up until the bar is at their waist, and the entire upper body is above the bar. Then they press their arms straight—so they started with the bar above them, and finish with it below.

If you can do 10 pull-ups, you're probably strong enough to do it—but you still might not get it right away.

"There's timing and technique to it as well," says Al Kavadlo, author of calisthenics books, including *Raising the Bar: The Definitive Guide to Pull-Up Bar Calisthenics.* Here's how to practice the technique.

1. **Feel the Technique**

   A muscle-up is a pull-up *plus*: Kavadlo suggests you practice two moves, explosive pull-ups and negative muscle-ups, to get the *plus* part.

   To do an explosive pull-up, make sure the area beneath your pull-up bar is safe—put down a pad or mat, and try not to do it over concrete. Pull up with enough speed and force to leave the bar, then re-grab it before coming back down. Practice a few of these during each pull-up session.

   For the negative muscle-up, place a bench next to where you'd like to do your muscle-ups. Use the bench to get your body up over the bar, in the final position of a muscle-up. From here, slowly reverse the move: Bend your elbows to the bottom of the dip position. Then flip your grip so your body is near the top of the pull-up, and descend to the bottom. Use the bench to get back to the start, and repeat.

2. **Grip It and Rip It: Do Your First Muscle-Up!**

   You've got the technique. It's time to do it! To make your first muscle-up easier, Kavadlo has three tips:
   - **Narrow your grip.** When you transition from the pull-up to the top of the bar, this will let your elbows stay closer to your body, so you can drive the elbows back to transition up.
   - **Pull the bar down.** It's a mental switch that could make the difference. Think of pulling and driving the bar down past your chest and abdomen.
   - **Don't give up!** Remember, the muscle-up is a skill. So practice it. Even if you don't get it on your first attempt, you've got the strength to do it. Keep at it!

EMBRACE DISCOMFORT FOR TWO MINUTES TO BUILD ENDURANCE AND POWER

Over 2.5 million years of evolution, finding comfort in an uncomfortable world kept us alive, safe, and able to spread our DNA.

But avoiding discomfort in our modern circumstances has made us "the fattest, least fit, most disease-ridden, and unhappy population in the history of man," says Michael Easter. In his book *The Comfort Crisis*, Easter argues that our drive for comfort is killing us.

The solution? Embrace discomfort. "Hunger, different forms of physical effort, outdoor exposure . . . even being bored is something we no longer face," he says. "But it's linked to improvements in creativity, mental restoration, and happiness."

It works for workouts, too—when you go beyond your comfort zone, you can reach new heights. This workout from Easter, an interval weight-training routine he learned at Gym Jones, one of the world's most uncomfortable gyms, is "arguably the single most effective way to build world-class endurance, strength, and power in the shortest time possible."

SECTION 1

Alternate between these 2 moves three times, then rest for 2 minutes. Repeat that— 3 rounds, 2 minutes' rest—two more times. Rest for 5 minutes, then do Section 2.

Strength Move 1: Goblet Squat
1. Stand with your feet hip-width apart, toes pointed slightly out from parallel. Cup one end of a dumbbell in both hands in front of your chest with your elbows pointing down—in this position, the dumbbell and your arms will look like a goblet.
2. Push your hips back to initiate the squat. Bend your knees to descend until your thighs are at least parallel to the floor, keeping your chest up and your weight on your heels.
3. Keep the weight of your body in your heels and press back to standing.

Perform 10 reps. Goal weight: 70 pounds.

Cardio Challenge 1: Rowing Machine
Row for 2 minutes. Goal distance: 575 meters.

SECTION 2

Alternate between these 2 moves three times, then rest for 2 minutes. Repeat that—3 rounds, 2 minutes' rest—two more times.

Strength Move 2: Dumbbell Push Press

1. Hold two dumbbells at your shoulders, palms in, with your feet slightly wider than shoulder-width apart.
2. Bend your knees slightly, dip your hips, and explode up, pressing the weights overhead.
3. Return the weights to your shoulders, and repeat. Perform 8 reps per set.

Perform 10 reps. Goal weight: 35-pound dumbbells.

Cardio Challenge 2: Run

On a treadmill, run as far as possible in two minutes. Goal distance: 0.37 miles.

DO 10,000 KETTLEBELL SWINGS IN 10 DAYS . . . LIKE A MADMAN

When people do a four-week, 10,000-swing kettlebell challenge, they come out leaner. Their abs are more visible. Their squats and deadlifts improve.

For a truly mind-bending challenge, though, James Heathers compressed all those swings into a mere 10 days. Heathers, a sometimes profane, always frank, and funny scientist, is a gym rat and amateur strongman. And he wanted harder abs, sure. But he also wanted to see what he was made of.

"[It] started as an exercise in pure masochism," he says. If you did 60 swings per workout, three times a week, it would take a little more than a year to do 10,000. Heathers spent 10 days slipping in sets of 10 to 50 swings whenever he could to reach that big, hairy number.

You may or may not lose fat—three of the five people who joined Heathers's challenge lost 3 to 5 percent of their body fat over 10 days. You'll build a ton of work capacity—the ability to do more work in your workouts, allowing you to have more gains, more quickly.

But doing this kind of challenge in 10 days isn't about any of that. Abs are temporary. Knowing you have guts is forever.

So if you want to test the limits—of your patience, your tolerance, your ability to manage work and life and exercise—follow Heathers's lead. For 10 days, swing.

Note: An improper swing can wrench your back. If you don't already know how to do a kettlebell swing proficiently, skip this workout or replace the move with squats.

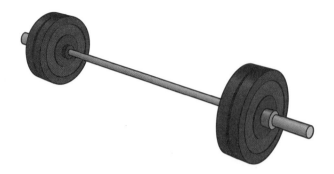

BENCH TWO PLATES WITH THE PLAN FROM A WORLD-RECORD LIFTER

Robert Herbst has set more than 38 world records in powerlifting—and, in his 60s, is still chasing new ones. You may not want a world record, but are probably gunning for records in your own world—personal bests. For many benchers, that goal is 225 pounds—two 45-pound plates on each side of a bar.

Try this Herbst-style benching program for six weeks, aiming to increase your maximum weight by 2.5 pounds per week. Then take two easier weeks before attempting your goal weight.

WORKOUTS FOR WEEKS 1–6

Training Day 1: Speed Day

The Goal: Move weights explosively—as fast as possible while maintaining control.

1.   Choose a weight you can press six to eight times.
2.   Perform 9 sets of 3 repetitions with a shoulder-width (or slightly narrower) grip—this puts the focus on your triceps. Perform each repetition explosively, pressing the bar up as quickly as possible while maintaining control. Rest one minute between sets.
3.   Finish the workout with 3 sets each of close-grip incline bench press, barbell floor press, overhead press, and barbell curls.

Training Day 2: Heavy Day

Start by subtracting 15 from your goal weight to determine your "Heavy Day Base Number," or HDBN. We'll use it below to set your weights in this workout, and you'll try to increase it by 2.5 pounds each week.

But if some weeks you can't hit the calculated weight, don't give up, Herbst says: "Your strength can vary 3 to 4 percent, based on the amount you slept, what you ate," and other factors. "Just keep plugging."

Rest three to five minutes between all sets in this workout.

1.   Perform 2 warm-up sets of 10 reps each.
2.   Perform 5 reps using 85 percent of your HDBN for this week.
3.   Perform 2 sets of 3 reps each using 95 percent of your HDBN.
4.   Perform 1 or 2 sets of 2 reps each using 97 percent of your HDBN.
5.   Finish by loading the bar with a weight that's heavier than your overall goal weight. Ask a spotter to help you unrack the bar, and hold it at the top of your bench press position for 5 to 10 seconds. Then rerack the bar.

WORKOUTS FOR WEEKS 7–8

Taper and Crush Your Goal

In week 7, perform the speed workout, and perform a lighter version of the heavy day—working up to your 5-rep weight instead of the 2-rep weight.

In week 8, don't do the heavy day at all. Rest up and crush your goal!

I sometric exercises, where a position is held at maximum tension for a short period of time, can build strength fast: In the 1950s, scientists found that 1 max contraction per day could increase strength by 5 percent per week.

But scientists at the Soviet Union's amazingly named "department of maximology," which conducted studies on the nation's elite athletes, felt isometrics had limitations: They could strain tendons, and only made practitioners stronger in one part of a movement. So they developed "dynamic isometrics," where short holds are performed at various stages of an exercise.

They're perfect if you only have access to light weights, don't want to work out for long, or are looking for a maximology-approved challenge. You can build strength—and wear your legs out—in just 90 seconds with a 3-repetition set of dynamic isometric squats. Load up a bar with less than you'd normally squat, and try it.

Stand in a normal back squat position, barbell across your shoulders, feet hip-width apart, toes slightly out. Push your hips back to squat and slowly bend your knees, lowering your body until your knees are bent at about 160 degrees—barely bent at all. Hold this position for three to four seconds, then continue bending until your knees are at about a 145-degree angle. Hold three to four seconds. Then lower to 115 degrees, do a three- to four-second hold, and finish at 90 degrees with a three- to four-second hold. Stand back up at a moderate speed, and repeat for 3 total repetitions. For an added challenge, push up out of each squat so explosively that you jump off the ground.

DO 500 SQUATS

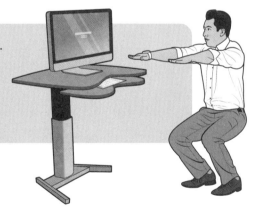

For the days when you don't want to think at all. Stand. Squat. Repeat. Maybe cry. See God. Time yourself.

(Workout from Jeremy Frisch, owner of Achieve Performance, Clinton, Massachusetts.)

PUT YOURSELF THROUGH A HALF-MILE OF HELL

Sometimes, you just need to see what you're made of. Martin Rooney creates challenges that do just that: His legendary "Hurricane" workouts, composed of 3 all-out rounds of five minutes each, have helped MLB, NBA, NFL, and combat sport athletes—and regular folks—hone their bodies and minds. And the author of *Warrior Cardio* brings his unique brand of mind/body training to thousands with Training for Warriors, his fitness system practiced at more than 100 locations around the world.

Try one of Rooney's most intense challenges: The Half-Mile of Hell. You'll need four kettlebells, 40 yards of walking space, and some *grit*. Your mission: Complete the following regimen in less than 15 minutes.

1. Pick up a pair of 32-kg kettlebells and walk 40 yards, down and back.
2. Put down the 32s and pick up a single 28-kg kettlebell in your right hand. Hold your left arm up and out—pointing to the side—and walk 40 yards, keeping your shoulders level. Switch hands and walk back, now with your right arm pointing to the side.
3. Drop the 28-kg bell and pick up a 24-kg kettlebell in your right hand. Press the kettlebell overhead, keeping your shoulders level. Walk 40 yards. Switch so the weight is in your left hand, press it overhead, and walk back to start.
4. Repeat this sequence for 4 total rounds. Goal time: 15 minutes.

Too heavy? Use lighter weights to start! Work your way up to this challenge, trying it out every week or two.

MAKE YOUR OWN NFL COMBINE

Saying NFL players are "strong, fast, and athletic" is like saying a Ferrari is a car. Technically true, but understating things *just* a bit. Give yourself a feel for just *how* superhuman these gridiron stars are by staging your own "underwear Olympics," trying out the same drills that prospects do at the annual NFL Combine.

Event 1: 40-Yard Dash

Run 40 yards as fast as you can. Everyone gets two tries—count your fastest time.

How do you measure up?

At the 2019 NFL Combine, the fastest 40 was run by defensive back Zedrick Woods in 4 minutes, 29 seconds. The slowest time was 5 minutes, 41 seconds, by Nate Herbig, an offensive lineman.

That's still pretty fast. For an easier standard, NFL Network analyst Rich Eisen runs the distance each year in a suit and tie. His best-ever time: 5.97 seconds.

Event 2: Bench Press

Athletes lift 225 pounds for as many repetitions as possible.

How do you measure up?

In 2019, offensive lineman Iosua Opeta set the standard with 39 presses. The lowest score was 6.

Too heavy for your group? For the 301-pound Opeta, 225 is just about 75 percent of his body weight. Go for as many reps as you can at that percentage of your own weight.

Event 3: Vertical Jump

Have each participant in your Combine stand next to a wall with their arm raised straight overhead against the wall. Mark the top of their fingers with chalk or tape. This serves as the basis for their jump.

When it's your turn to jump, stand next to the wall by your marking, holding another piece of tape. Jump straight up and place the tape as high as you can on the wall. The height difference between the tape marks is your vertical.

How do you measure up?

In 2019, safety Juan Thornhill jumped 44 inches. Ross Pierschbacher, an offensive lineman, set the low bar at 22.5 inches.

Event 4: Broad Jump

From a standing position behind a line, jump with two feet as far forward as possible.

How do you measure up?

The best broad jump in 2019: 141 inches by wide receiver Emanuel Hall. The shortest: 89 inches.

Event 5: Three-Cone Drill

Set up three cones as shown to form a 90-degree angle, with 5 yards between cones 1 and 2, and 5 yards between cones 2 and 3.

When the timer starts, run from cone 1 to cone 2, then back to cone 1. Next, run around cone 2 to the left (so the cone is on your right), then around cone 3 so it's on your left. Then run back around cone 2 to cone 1. The timer stops when you pass cone 1 on this final sprint.

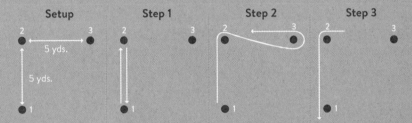

How do you measure up?

In 2019, cornerback David Long finished this drill in 6.45 seconds. The slowest time: 8.34 seconds.

Event 6: 20-Yard Shuttle Run

Set up three cones in a straight line, each 5 yards apart. Start by standing at the center cone, facing perpendicular to the line of cones.

From this position, sprint out to your right, touching cone 2 on your right with your right hand. Then sprint to cone 3, touching it with your left hand. Sprint past cone 1 to finish. When you pass cone 1, the timer stops.

How do you measure up?

At the 2019 Combine, David Long finished in 3.97 seconds. The slowest time: 5.28 seconds.

DO THE ONE-HOUR WORKOUT OF THE 1,000-MARATHON MAN

Rory Coleman started 1994 like thousands of others: He wanted to lose weight, quit smoking, and live a healthier life. He never set out to run a marathon at all.

"I set out to go and run because I liked it," the Cardiff, Wales coach and speaker says of his then-31-year-old self. When you run, he says, "all your problems are put to the side, and you enjoy that 'me time.' All you're thinking about is the next step."

He liked it so much that he wanted a *lot* of next steps. He started running shorter races, which turned into marathons, and "I started clocking them up. It became what I did."

Coleman ran marathons on road courses, ultras on trails, and events through canyons and deserts—including the Marathon des Sables, "the world's toughest footrace." Coleman has run the 156-mile event 15 times—more than anyone else from the UK. Even being paralyzed couldn't stop him: After a running of the Marathon des Sables in 2016, Coleman was stricken with Guillain-Barré syndrome, which left him paralyzed from the neck down for a month. Less than three months later, he ran a marathon—and has run more than 75 since. He's finished more than 1,000 overall.

Coleman coaches thousands of runners to their first marathon through his company, Coleman Coaching. And one of his signature workouts is the Power Hour, a 60-minute treadmill interval session.

It's simple: Run four minutes at your marathon pace, then one minute at your 10K pace—the difference between these two paces should be about 1.5 mph on the treadmill, Coleman says. So if you're hoping to run nine-minute miles as your "marathon pace," set the treadmill to 6.6 for four minutes, then 9.1 for one minute. Repeat this for an hour.

"It's not the minute going quick that's hard. It's the minute right after," Coleman says, when you're trying to recover. Over time, though, you'll get more efficient at recovering from the faster bouts—meaning you're getting stronger. Try this workout once a month or once a week, and track your progression.

DROP AND GIVE ME 50

I f you could only do one exercise for the rest of your life, your best bet might be the push-up: It works not just your arms and chest, but your core and even your legs. And if you can knock off 50 in a row, you've got roughly double the muscular endurance of the average person, according to the Canadian Society for Exercise Physiology.

If you can already do 10 in a row, use this four-week program to build up to 50—or at least get close. (Can't do 10? Cut all the repetition numbers in half, and work up to 25 to start.)

You'll do push-ups two days in a row, rest for one day, then repeat, doing at least four sessions per week. The first three days each week are the same. The fourth session finishes with a burnout set, testing how many push-ups you can do. Read this sample plan for week 1, then use the chart to change the number of repetitions done in each session for weeks 2, 3, and 4.

WEEK 1, DAY 1: TWO ROUNDS OF 5X5

On days 1 through 3, you'll do 2 rounds of 5 sets. Rest completely between rounds—maybe do some leg exercises to break it up, or do 1 round in the morning, and another round in the evening.

In each round, perform 5 sets of 5 reps of push-ups, resting 15 seconds between sets. On the last rep of your last set, hold your body at the bottom of the push-up position—with chest hovering above the floor, elbows bent—for as long as possible.

Week 1, Day 2
Repeat day 1.

Week 1, Day 3
Rest.

Week 1, Day 4
Repeat day 1, but do 6 reps in each set.

Week 1, Day 5
On your fifth day of each week, do 1 round the same way you've done it on the previous three days. But for your final round, do 1 set: Do as many push-ups as you can in a row. Mark down your number so you can beat it next week!

	Reps/Set on Days 1 and 2	Reps/Set on Days 4 and 5
Week 2	7	8
Week 3	9	10
Week 4	11	12

THE CHALLENGE WORKOUT THAT HELPED A 35-YEAR OLD REALTOR RUN AN OLYMPIC-STANDARD 5K

Keira D'Amato has no sponsors. She has to balance her training with her job as a Realtor and her life as a mother of two. But at age 35, the Richmond, Virginia runner is flying: In 2020, she ran a 5K in 15 minutes, 4 seconds, faster than the Olympic standard—and faster than her fastest 5K as an All-American 15 years before.

"My biggest rebuttal to 'You slow down as you age' is . . . who says?" D'Amato notes. But D'Amato says she's not competing with her college self of younger times, and thinks that's key for any "aging" amateur athlete. "I'm comparing myself to last week and last month, trying to get a little bit better."

To keep getting a bit better, D'Amato logs 70- to 100-mile running weeks and twice-weekly strength workouts, as well as this challenge workout early in every season—40 rounds of 200 meters each.

"[Each effort is] intense and short, but the real battle is purely mental," she says. "A lot of wild things happen in your head: 'How many do I have left? Thirty-five? Oh my God!' It's a mental struggle to stay focused, to stay relaxed, and to keep your eyes on the prize. By the end, you feel really proud. You stayed focused. You stayed with it."

To do this workout, head to a local track. Get warmed up, and get ready to count!
1. Run 200 meters, half a lap of the track, at your best mile pace. (Two hundred meters is about one-eighth of a mile, so if you're an eight-minute miler, aim to finish each 200 in one minute.)
2. Jog 100 meters to recover—a quarter lap.
3. Repeat 40 times.

CLIMB EVEREST WITHOUT LEAVING YOUR HOMETOWN

The challenge of "Everesting" is simple: Jump on your bike and climb up a hill. Ride back down. Repeat until you've climbed 29,028 feet—the height of Mt. Everest.

Finish the climb in a single ride—with breaks as needed, and tracked on Strava or virtually on Zwift—and your name can join 10,000 other cyclists' in the Everesting Hall of Fame at www.everesting.cc.

The challenge has its roots in the first *real* Everest ascent: In 1994, George Mallory, a grandson of one of the climbers on the original Everest expeditions in the 1920s, completed the first "Everesting" ride. He pedaled 8 laps up and down Mount Donna Buang, a 3,507-foot hill in Australia's Victorian Alps.

You don't have to head to a mountain range to follow in Mallory's pedal strokes: You could Everest up the highest hill in your town, a rise in your neighborhood, or even your driveway—though that might take a *lot* of laps. There's a calculator at www.everesting.cc to help plan your Everesting "expedition," as well as rules and instructions on how to submit your ride (or run) for the Hall of Fame.

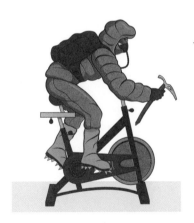

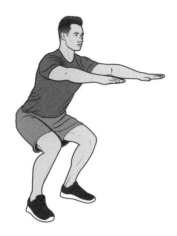

THE 1,000-REP LEG DAY CHALLENGE

D on't skip leg day: Embrace it with this 1,000-repetition challenge from Dana Linn Bailey, one of the biggest badasses in the fitness world. Since winning the Olympia in 2013, Bailey has appeared on *America Ninja Warrior*, competed in powerlifting at the Arnold Classic, and posts daily tips and workouts in her DLB Daily series—including this grueling leg session.

You'll perform 100 reps of a weighted exercise, then 100 reps of bodyweight "air" squats. Repeat until you've done all 5 main exercises and 5 rounds of air squats for 1,000 total reps.

Break up the 100 reps into as many sets as you like—Bailey did 5 sets of 20 reps each when she completed the challenge. Choose a weight that's about half the amount you would normally use for that exercise. Rest as needed between sets—just finish!

EXERCISE 1: Barbell Squat (100 reps)

1. Stand in a normal back squat position, barbell across your shoulders, feet between shoulder- and hip-width apart, toes slightly out.
2. Push your hips back to initiate the squat.
3. Bend your knees to descend until your thighs are at least parallel to the floor, keeping your chest up and your weight on your heels.
4. Keep the weight of your body in your heels and press back to standing.

EXERCISE 2: Bodyweight "Air" Squat (100 reps)
Perform this squat as you did with Exercise 1, just without the barbell.

EXERCISE 3: Leg Press (100 reps)
Use the leg press machine.

EXERCISE 4: Bodyweight "Air" Squat (100 reps)

EXERCISE 5: Leg Extension (100 reps)
Use the leg extension machine.

EXERCISE 6: Bodyweight "Air" Squat (100 reps)

EXERCISE 7: Lying Leg Curl (100 reps)
Use the lying leg curl machine.

EXERCISE 8: Bodyweight "Air" Squat (100 reps)

EXERCISE 9: Dumbbell (or Barbell) Lunge (100 reps on each leg)

1. Stand with your feet shoulder-width apart, dumbbells at your sides or barbell on your shoulders.
2. Take a large lunge step forward with your right leg, descending as you step until your knees both form 90-degree angles.
3. Press through your right foot to stand back up.
4. Repeat on the other side.

EXERCISE 10: Bodyweight "Air" Squat (100 reps)

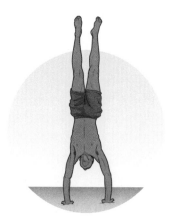

DO A HANDSTAND:
YOGA'S QUEEN OF UPSIDE-DOWN TEACHES YOU HOW

Near the end of most yoga classes, it's inversion time—getting your legs up above your head via legs up the wall, or popping up into a headstand. But for Heidi Kristoffer, one of New York's most popular yoga teachers—and a self-proclaimed "inversion addict"—headstand's a no-no.

"Headstand should be considered one of the most advanced poses in yoga," she says. It requires more core strength and body control than most yogis imagine in order not to damage the cervical spine. Kristoffer has her students start with what seems like a more advanced pose: handstands.

You really can do one! Here are some strengthening starter poses from Kristoffer to help you get there.

GROUP 1: BUILD ENDURANCE

You'll need core strength and shoulder endurance to hold a handstand. Build both with these three moves, practicing them every day. Once you're feeling confident in the "L" handstand, start practicing group 2.

EXERCISE 1: Straight-Arm Plank

Do lots of planks—30 seconds each. Do them throughout your workout and throughout your day. You'll strengthen your wrists and your core.

EXERCISE 2: Wall Shoulder Stretch

1. Stand facing a wall at arm's distance. Plant your palms on the wall at face height, shoulder-width apart.
2. Slowly drop your torso, keeping palms connected; relax your head between your arms and relax your shoulders. Perform this exercise for 30 seconds a few times throughout the day.

EXERCISE 3: "L" Handstand

1. Facing away from the wall, bend down and plant your hands on the ground close to the wall. Then put your feet on the wall behind you, and walk your feet onto the wall to waist height.
2. Walk your hands out until your body forms an "L"—straight torso, straight legs, 90-degree angle.
3. Hold for 5 rounds of 30 seconds each.

GROUP 2: BALANCE PRACTICE

Once you're feeling strong in the "L" handstand, add these to your routine every day, or every other day, if you want to give your wrists a rest. Once you're feeling brave enough to do wall handstands without the wall, you're ready to handstand for real!

EXERCISE 1: Crow Pose

1. Squat down with your feet close together and your knees far apart. Plant your hands on the ground around shoulder-distance apart, 6 to 8 inches in front of your feet.
2. Shift forward and come on your toes, straightening your arms a little as you come forward toward your arms.
3. Your knees should be planted above your elbows and stay bent as your feet lift off the floor.
4. Do 5 holds of 5 seconds each here.

EXERCISE 2: Wall Handstands

1. Facing the wall, plant your hands about shoulder-width apart on the ground in front of it.
2. Kick one foot, then the other, up the wall into a handstand position, using your heels and legs against the wall for support.
3. Practice this position to strengthen your muscles and develop a sense of balance. Over time, move a little farther from the wall. Do 5 rounds of 5 seconds each, with your holds getting longer each day.

CHAPTER 16

GO COMPETE

Get out there! Run, bike, swim, and climb against the best with these unique and must-do races and events. You may not win, but you'll see what you can really do.

SET YOUR 5K PR, THEN WATCH THE WORLD'S BEST RUNNERS FLY BY

The Carlsbad 5000 is the "World's Fastest 5K": Sixteen world records have been set on the course, a scenic, relatively flat loop by the Pacific Coast. And it's got a great way to get your finishing kick for a personal record: The last quarter-mile is downhill!

But running your fastest 3 miles isn't the only reason this April race is worth the trip to the West Coast. Unlike most road races, where "regular" runners toe the line after the elite global runners have started flying down the course, the Carlsbad 5000 does the opposite: Race day starts with five groups of "regular" runners, spaced out to keep the course from getting too crowded. Once they're finished, the elites take off—meaning you could set your own personal record, then watch champions take a crack at a world-beating time.

The race is each April. Registration is $49 at www.carlsbad5000.com.

Things to Know

- If 5K isn't enough, you can also do the "All-Day 20K." Instead of running with just one of the "regular" groups, you run in all four age group races—four consecutive 5Ks, taking a break between each 3.1-miler to hear the "Star-Spangled Banner" again.

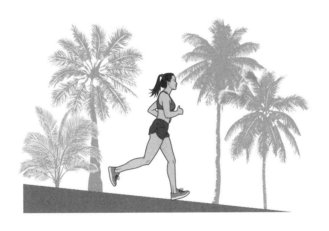

The question isn't *why* run Boston . . . it's *how*. The world's oldest annual marathon is also one of America's most popular—so popular that it's one of very few marathons in the country that requires a swift finish in a previous race. Yes, you can get in by raising $5,000 or more for charity, but, for many runners, running a Boston qualifying time—"BQ-ing"—is the ultimate fitness goal.

That time is no joke! To qualify for the 2021 race, men would need a time around 3 hours (depending on age group), and women would need a finish around 3 hours 30 minutes. And sometimes, there are too many qualifiers, so the time gets reduced even more.

Dreaming of Hopkinton and Heartbreak Hill? Get your training on, and sign up for one of these three races—ridiculously high percentages of their runners qualify for Boston.

Last Chance BQ.2 Marathons

When: June and September • Where: Geneva, Illinois (in June and September) and Grand Rapids, Michigan (September) • Runners Who BQ: 49–58 percent in 2019
The BQ.2 marathons are designed to help runners BQ. They're small races, run on super-flat courses in the Midwest—Geneva is a suburb of Chicago—with pacers focused on helping runners qualify. The catch: You have to qualify for these qualifying runs. Check the race group's website, www.bq2races.com.

REVEL Mount Hood

When: June • Where: Portland, Oregon • Runners Who BQ: 34 percent in 2019
The REVEL race series specializes in fast times—each of the entries in the six-race series is slightly downhill, which the company says "provides a unique opportunity for runners to qualify for exclusive events." Other REVEL races also have high BQ rates, but Mount Hood stands on top. Beware: Running downhill for 26 miles can be tough on your knees, so research training methods to keep your legs from blowing up.

Light at the End of the Tunnel Marathon

When: June • Where: North Bend, Washington • Runners Who BQ: 36.9 percent in 2019
North Bend, about 30 miles east of Seattle, has three marathons with high BQ times—all with BQ rates above 30 percent. But it's not just about qualifying for Boston. These steadily downhill, gravel-track marathons have a unique quirk—a 2-mile run through a tunnel. That, plus the gorgeous mountains around Seattle, make this a marathon worth running even if you don't BQ.

ARE YOU MORE POWERFUL THAN A LOCOMOTIVE?

You don't have to be Superman to test yourself against a train—you just have to go to Colorado.

Each May at the Iron Horse Classic bike race, hundreds descend on Durango, Colorado, to do just that. An antique steam engine whistles to start a 50-mile dash to Silverton—and cyclists try to beat the train through groves of aspens and pines. The locomotive takes 4.5 hours to arrive at the finish, but beating it there is no small feat: The route climbs two consecutive 10,000-foot peaks along the way.

It's grueling, the air is thin, and there are precious few downhill stretches before the climbs are done—but the views are spectacular, cowbell-ringing locals line the course, and the town of Silverton is so sweet with charm it'll rot your teeth. Oh, and one more thing: You get to race a train!

Registration for the race is $126, plus $40 for transit on a bus back from Silverton. Registration begins in late February or early March for the May event. Visit http://ironhorsebicycleclassic.com for details.

Things to Know

- If you're not a geography buff, Durango is *far* from Denver. You can fly to Durango directly, or drive from Denver (six hours) or Albuquerque, New Mexico (four hours).
- There are plenty of road bikes to rent in Durango, though prices go up for this annual event.

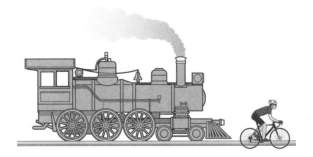

CLIMB 17 STORIES IN ONE MINUTE

Potrero Hill in San Francisco climbs more than 200 vertical feet in less than a third of a mile, topping out at a 21 percent grade. And at the annual Red Bull Bay Climb, the fastest cyclists conquer that hill in around a minute. That's faster than the average hotel elevator can climb, and many riders do it on a fixed-gear bicycle—no gears!

If you've got the thighs for it, you can join in. The climb is held each September—details and signups are at www.redbull.com. Can't make it then? You can try it on your own, but fair warning: You'll have to deal with cars. The race route goes on DeHaro Street from 18th Street to the hill's peak at Southern Heights Avenue.

RUN UP THE SEARS—ER, *WILLIS*—TOWER

Elevator? Pfft. You don't need no stinking elevator. The only thing that stands between you and panoramic views of the Windy City are 2,109 stairs.

Each November, SkyRise Chicago pits 3,000 runners against the 103 floors of the Willis Tower. Because the race admits more entrants than other iconic stair climbs (like the Empire State Building Run-Up), SkyRise is relatively easy to get into: Registration is $70, and you've got to raise $150 for the race's charitable partner.

Once you're in, things get tough, says five-time SkyRise racer Mark Ewell. The Colorado real estate broker is America's sixth-best stair-climb racer, according to Tower Running USA. And he says Willis's stairs are tougher than most.

"The average building has steps that are 7 inches, up to 7.5 inches. The Sears Tower is 7.7 inches," the 46-year-old says. Doesn't seem like much, but "You feel that [difference] after 2,100 of them."

So you'll be huffing and puffing, but not for long: Elite runners like Ewell finish the race in about 15 minutes, while the average participant takes closer to 40. The reward is worth the steep ascent, though: SkyRise finishes on the 103rd story's glass-enclosed sky deck level, where you can catch your breath, take in the views, and snap some epic post-race photos.

SkyRise is held the first weekend of November, with registration opening in summer. Follow the race's Facebook page for updates.

Sound like your jam? If you're intrigued by stair-climb racing, check out one of these other tower runs, recommended by Ewell.

EMPIRE STATE BUILDING RUN-UP (NEW YORK)

This race is the Boston Marathon of stair runs—the granddaddy of 'em all. Unlike many other stair races, where the stairwell looks, well, like a gray, concrete stairwell, the Empire State's stairs have architectural touches all the way up its 86 floors. And when you finish, what a view: Runners emerge onto the Empire State's outdoor observation deck, doing a half lap to the finish as NYC stretches around them in every direction.

The trouble with this race is its size—it's a huge building, but, for safety reasons, a tiny field of runners. The event takes ten of America's elite step-climbers, like Ewell, and then has a lottery for the rest of the spots—about 50 slots. Registration for the lottery opens in late January, with the race taking place each May. Keep your eye on www.nycruns.com for details.

SPACE NEEDLE CLIMB (SEATTLE)

The Base 2 Space race takes just a few minutes, but the uniqueness of the 832-step race makes it stand out, Ewell says. That's because the Space Needle's stairs are outside—winds whip past as you vault up to the roof of Seattle, taking in the sights all the way to the top.

The race is held in late September, with sign-ups—including early-bird discount rates—beginning in early summer. Follow the Space Needle's Facebook page, facebook.com/spaceneedle.

BIKE IN THE WORLD'S WINDIEST RACE

The Dutch Headwind Cycling Championships pit humans against nature: Held on a dam in southern Holland, the annual race sees Olympians and everyday cyclists with their faces peeled back against hurricane-force winds.

Riders in pajamas, suits, and other costumes strain to reach the speed of a brisk walk. And while it may look silly, the challenge is very real. The 5.2-mile course is pancake-flat and ramrod straight, but wind gusts up to 75 mph slam into the faces of riders, pitting riders against forces of drag 64 times greater than a normal, stiff breeze. And they're not doing this on carbon-fiber bikes with ultralight everything: All riders use the same, commuter-style bikes with no gears. All this adds up to humbling times and major struggles—recent editions of the race have added a vomiting station near the finish.

Hard as it is to complete, it's even harder to enter: The race is not scheduled for a specific date, but is whipped together based on storm conditions. Three days before the race is held, organizers put out a call via social media: A storm is coming, and it's time to sign up. There are only 300 spots for individuals, and 11,000 people signed up for them in 2020, filling the race in less than four hours. Some additional spots for four-person teams remained open a bit longer, but if you want to ride against this wind, you've got to be ready to act fast: Follow the race on Twitter (@NKTegenwind) and Facebook (https://www.facebook.com/NKtegenwindfietsen), and set an alert to go off when they post.

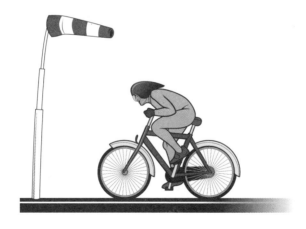

RUN ON THE GRASS AT YOUR FAVORITE STADIUM—WITHOUT GETTING ARRESTED

You don't have to go streaking to get on the field of your favorite team. Spartan Race's "Stadion" series lets you run—and climb walls, flip tires, and do lots of burpees—on that expertly cut turf without the risk of getting flattened by security.

Stadion races are run at legendary stadiums, including Wrigley Field, Fenway Park, and Lambeau Field (where you can also run a marathon; see page 39), as well as newer parks like Philadelphia's Citizens Bank Park and Busch Stadium in St. Louis. Veteran Spartan racers say they're some of the most fun races on the annual circuit—"kind of like a party, but you're redlining the whole time," says one participant.

These stadium races are missing one obstacle-course staple: mud. The groundskeepers wouldn't take too kindly to turning center field into a pigsty, so the dirt, grime, puddles, and slips of normal Spartan races are replaced by obstacles that make the Stadions feel more like a group workout: Rope climbs, wall jumps, lots of burpees, and *tons* of stairs—you'll be running through the stands in addition to on the field for around 3 miles of fun.

For a sports fan, trading in the mud for some inside access is more than worth it: You'll get to see the inner workings of your favorite stadium, run through the tunnels, and be paraded through parts of the park that normal fans never see. Oh, and you'll get the screaming fans, too—spectators can cheer you on from the seats as you work your way to the finish.

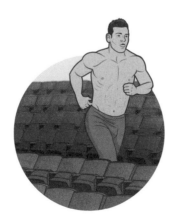

"If you raced with men on foot, and they have worn you out, how can you compete with horses?"

This question is asked in the Bible's book of Jeremiah, and since 1983, ultramarathoners in Arizona have answered it: People fare pretty well. In the annual "Man Against Horse" race, runners and riders climb Mingus Mountain near Prescott, about 100 miles north of Phoenix. And man triumphs over horse regularly: From 1999 until 2014, the runners beat the riders every year.

The reason is distance: Horses can't cool down by sweating while running, so riders have to stop to let their mounts recover. And the terrain offers an edge for humanity, too: While the horses smoke people on the flats, the Man Against Horse climbs 5,000 feet, including a 3-mile hike that includes 1,500 feet of elevation gain—taller than climbing the Sears (aka Willis) Tower, and it's only part of the race. And unlike the tower, you're not climbing stairs: Mingus Mountain is rocky, slippery, steep, and narrow—meaning both horse and human need to be nimble.

Similar races are held each year in Wales, Scotland, and New Zealand. The Prescott edition is run each October, with 12-, 25-, and 50-mile distances. It pays to go long: Finishers of the 50-miler get a belt buckle. Registration is $110. Check out www.managainsthorse.net.

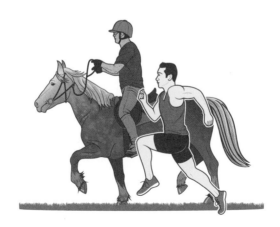

RACE YOUR BIKE AROUND A VIRTUAL WORLD

If you've been leaving your bike in the garage all winter, dust it off! Use it inside to bike through London, the Alps, and in virtual races against real people from around the world—all on your laptop or tablet.

Since the days of the Nintendo Power Pad, video games have tried to incorporate fitness. Zwift has mastered it: By connecting your bike to a "smart turbo trainer," which can sense your power output and speed—and adjust resistance based on it—you can enter 10 different virtual races per day. Instead of staring at the wall while you work out, you can interact with more than a half-million other riders to take on a section of the Giro d'Italia, virtually climb the Tour de France's legendary Alp d'Huez, or ride through a fantasy forest teeming with dinosaurs. Zwift doesn't skimp on the "video game" part of gaming, either: There are power-ups, virtual bikes with different speeds, and customizable outfits. If they add a blue, leader-seeking turtle shell, it'll be perfect.

Things to Know

- You'll need a bike, of course, and a smart turbo trainer that straps onto—or replaces—your back wheel. The "smart" part indicates that the trainer will connect to a mobile device—and Zwift's app—via Bluetooth. Find options on Zwift's website and other enthusiast sites.
- Zwift's app is free for 7 days; then it costs a monthly fee.
- Don't worry: You don't have to be a budding pro to race. Zwift includes a 20-minute test to determine your level, so you can choose races where you'll be competitive.

RACE UP A SKI JUMP

It's even crazier than you imagine: You climb the equivalent of 40 stories in a quarter-mile. Still not impressed? Try this: The hill is so steep that the race has a rule—if you kick a rock loose, everyone has to yell "Rock!" to keep runners below from getting a faceful of boulder.

It's all part of the completely bonkers Red Bull 400 series, a tour of ski-jump races around the world—in Russia, Slovakia, and in US states, including Utah, Colorado, and Michigan. The races start with a sprint up grass and dirt that's so steep there's a cargo net to help runners hold on, and finishes with the ski-jump climb—at an average 37 percent grade, steeper than any street in the US. It's called a "run," but everyone finishes the race using hands and knees.

The good news: It's over quickly. Unlike slogging through a multi-hour marathon or even a 30ish-minute 5K, the Red Bull 400 races are finished in around 10 minutes, with the course records under 5. Those 10 minutes are tougher than anything you've ever done, though—which is why there's oxygen available at the top.

Keep track of the year's races and sign up at www.redbull.com/int-en/events/red-bull-400-int.

None close to where you live? Try a "Vertical K" race—these other super-steep races climb 1,000 meters in 5K or less.

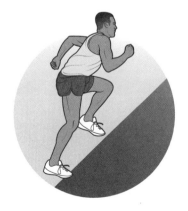

The Trans Tahoe Relay is how: Each July or August, teams race across the lake for an 11.5-mile swim that crosses state lines.

Sounds hard enough, but that's before you factor in the elevation—ringed by mountains, Lake Tahoe is at an oxygen-poor height of 6,200 feet, 1,000 feet higher than Denver. And it's brisk, with water temperatures ranging from 55°F to 60°F. Oh, and there's one more challenge: swimming in a straight line. The Trans Tahoe doesn't have bright, inflatable buoys like many other open-water races, so staying on course in the choppy water is tough.

But if you're a strong swimmer, and can find five friends who are, too, participants say it's a blast. Teams of six board boats on a beach in Nevada to start. Each team member swims for 30 minutes, then swaps out for another. After everyone has done their half-hour, team members take 10-minute swims until reaching another beach on the lake's California shore. While each team member swims, the others follow along, cheering, on the boat beside them.

Trans Tahoe teams don't take the race too seriously, as their names suggest—groups like the "White Claw Warriors" and "Shivering Timbers" have braved the frigid waters in years past. For upcoming editions, visit www.transtahoerelay.com. You'll need to fill out an application, including getting a membership in USA Masters Swimming. Registration is $800 for each team of six.

RACE THROUGH SAN FRANCISCO WITH PINK GORILLAS, NAKED RUNNERS, AND 50,000 MORE FRIENDS

Bay to Breakers is one of the world's biggest races, drawing between 50,000 and 100,000 participants each May. It's one of the world's oldest races, having been run continually since 1912 (with the exception of 2020, when it was canceled due to COVID-19). It's one of the world's most beautiful races, traveling 7.46 miles west from downtown San Francisco to the crashing breakers of the Pacific.

Most important: It may be the most fun race on Earth. Racers toss tortillas back and forth to pass the time before the start, many wearing costumes—thousands of pink gorillas, Elvises, and furry creatures toe the line, often having tipped back a few drinks prior to the race. Groups of 13 or more run tethered together by bungee cords in the "centipede" division. And many runners wear nothing but a smile: Hordes of naked racers take to the streets to cut through the fog, baring it all.

Unless you can get into one of the elite corrals in the front, don't expect to set a personal record at Bay to Breakers: The race is crowded, pumped up by participants who didn't bother registering. And with all that liquid courage consumed prior to the start, there's plenty of walking—especially when runners reach the Hayes Street Hill, an 11 percent grade at the 2-mile mark. It's a moving party—and not always a quick one. But it's a run you'll never forget.

The race is held the third Sunday of May each year. Registration is $65 at www.capstoneraces.com/bay-to-breakers.

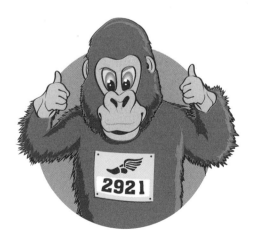

BEFORE YOUR RACE: CALM YOUR MIND LIKE A SOVIET OLYMPIAN

The night before a big event, it could be your mind that's racing—going over your preparation, worrying about bathroom breaks, thinking about how to pose for the race photographers. Those pre-race jitters can affect your precious pre-race sleep.

Mother Russia has a plan for you: As part of their psychological training, USSR Olympians were taught mental techniques to pump extra adrenaline into their bodies in competition, and calm down the night before. Try this Soviet sports psychology bedtime routine before your next race (or big meeting):

Part 1: All-Over Relaxation
Breathe in a relaxed way. Now, beginning at your feet, concentrate on each muscle group in your body—feet, ankles, legs, abdomen, spine, chest, arms, shoulders, and face. Tense each one for a moment, then release completely. Continue until you've worked all the way from feet to head.

Part 2: Auto-Suggestion
Now that you're relaxed, you're ready to instill confidence-building ideas in your mind. Start by simply thinking the phrase, "I quiet myself." Think "I" as you inhale, and "quiet myself" as you exhale. Continue a few times. When you're relaxed, think these phrases—"I" as you inhale, and the rest of the phrase as you exhale:

- I feel myself quiet and assured.
- I am prepared to struggle for victory.
- I am thoroughly ready to compete.
- I am full of strength and energy.
- I feel light and free.

Continue thinking these phrases as you breathe until you feel calm and ready for sleep. Hit the hay: You've got a race to crush tomorrow!

CHAPTER 17

THE WORLD'S TOUGHEST WORKOUTS

There's tough stuff throughout this list, but these final workouts are for the real masochists: nine races and challenges only the fearless would try.

TRY TO PASS SIMONE BILES'S WARM-UP TESTS

The women of USA Gymnastics are perhaps the greatest athletes on Earth. Not only can they flip and twist and land perfectly, but they do all of it better than anyone else. Team USA has won team gold on the regular of late, and the team's star, Simone Biles, not only has a growing pile of World and Olympic medals, but four acrobatic moves named after her.

Five times each year, the team comes together from their individual training homes to a camp in Texas, like a balance beam Justice League. There, they bond while high-performance team coordinator Tom Forster helps hone their skills. But before they get started, Forster makes sure they're up to team standards with a series of warm-up tests called "verifications," short benchmarks of fitness and gymnastic skills designed to make sure the athletes are staying on course for their next international victory.

Aside from the gymnastics tests, which are a little out of reach for the average gym-goer—things like splits and front flips—the verifications make up one of the toughest workouts you'll ever try. See if you can stack up to this world-beating warm-up.

EXERCISE 1: Hanging Leg Lifts
Hanging at arm's length, lift your legs from a straight body line up until they touch your hands at the top, maintaining straight knees and pointed toes throughout. Perform 20 repetitions as quickly as possible. (The fastest time, Forster says, is 24 seconds.)

EXERCISE 2: Standing Vertical Jump
See if your jump increases in height each time you test it: One easy way to do this is to jump with a piece of tape in your hand. Jump up and place it on the wall. Snap a photo of where you put it. Next time, try to put a new piece even higher.

EXERCISE 3: L-Shape Rope Climb
Holding the body at a 90-degree angle in an "L" shape—with legs pointed straight out in front, toes pointed—climb up (and then back down) a 16-foot rope using only your hands.

EXERCISE 4: Handstand Hold
Hold a handstand for one minute.

EXERCISE 5: Press Handstand
Sit on the floor in a straddle position. Press your hands into the floor between your legs, raising your body up into a handstand. Return to the starting position, and repeat 10 times.

RUN THE WORLD'S MOST NOTORIOUS RACE—IF YOU CAN GET IN

It takes a certain type of person to even *want* to run the Barkley Marathons.

"They're people who hear, 'You don't want to try this chili pepper,' and think, 'OK, I'll take a bite!'" says Nickademus de la Rosa, who was 13th runner to complete the event—only 15 runners have ever finished the race. For the then 23-year-old, the need to finish the race was, he says, a foreshadowing of mental illness for which he sought treatment in the ensuing years.

The brainchild of Gary "Lazarus Lake" Cantrell, the Barkley gives racers 60 hours to finish five loops of an unmarked 25-mile course through the forests of Tennessee's Frozen Head State Park, climbing more than 50,000 cumulative feet. Oh, and the five loops aren't in the same direction—racers do three loops in one direction, and two in the other. Still not sadistic enough for you? Two or three loops are run at night.

Even if all of that sounds good to you—as it did to de la Rosa before his first attempt in 2011—it's almost impossible to get into. It's limited to 40 runners, but even where to sign up to be one of those 40 is a mysterious course to be navigated.

"You have to send an email to the right person at the right time of the [right] day," de la Rosa says. The email address and the timing, de la Rosa says, must come from a previous participant. But those previous participants aren't supposed to reveal those details, like Fight Club.

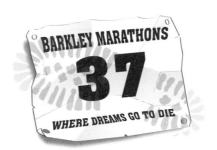

RUN A RACE THAT NEVER ENDS

The last runner standing wins. That's the idea behind a "backyard ultra": Runners toe the line for a 4.1-mile run each hour, starting on the hour. Any extra time is rest. So if a racer finishes the lap in 48 minutes, they've got 12 minutes for eating, drinking, micro-naps, and convincing themselves to do another lap.

And the people who do these races convince themselves to do a *lot* of laps: Then 39-year-old Maggie Guterl won the 2019 Big Dog's Backyard Ultra—the original and most famous race of its kind—by running for 60 hours, covering 250 miles.

If you're stubborn enough to try, more than 50 of these races are held annually. Find one near you at www.backyardultra.com.

SWIM TO ESCAPE THE WORLD'S THIRD-LARGEST WHIRLPOOL

In the Gulf of Corryvreckan, there's a maelstrom like few others in the world. In this narrow strait, separating two of Scotland's 790 offshore islands, a whirlpool grows with such force that its roaring can be heard 10 miles away. When a life jacket–wearing mannequin was tossed into its swirling waters, the dummy was pulled 860 feet down to be dragged along the sea bottom.

So, naturally, people swim across it. At slack tide, the whirling eases slightly, giving people about 40 minutes to cover what can be between three-quarters of a mile and nearly 2 miles (or 1.2 and 3 km), depending on how much the tide pulls at their wet suits.

This is not a swim for the weak of stroke or the faint of heart—nor is it one you'd probably want to undertake without an experienced guide. If you're crazy enough to try it, Highland Open Water Swim organizes a crossing each year that benefits Children with Cancer UK. You'll need to pass an acclimation swim and prove that you've done other open-water swims to get on board with one of their ten-swimmer groups. Visit www.highlandopenwaterswim.com to sign up.

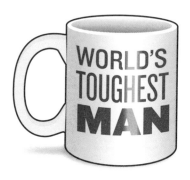

TWO DAYS OF HELL FROM THE WORLD'S TOUGHEST MAN: CHALLENGE YOURSELF LIKE AN ULTRAMARATHON-RUNNING NAVY SEAL

David Goggins willed himself to become the toughest man on Earth: He went from a 300-pound man with a dead-end job to America's 36th African-American Navy SEAL—finishing "Hell Week" training *twice* to earn the honor. In the years afterward, he became an elite ultramarathoner and broke the world record for pull-ups in 24 hours—completing 4,030 reps in 17 hours.

Goggins tells his unbelievably motivating story in his book, *Can't Hurt Me*, where he outlines how he overcame obstacles to accomplish all that and more, and peppers in lines that will make you want to get up and get moving: "Victory," he writes, "often comes down to bringing your very best when you feel your worst."

One way to test that out: The 4-by-4-by-48, a two-day challenge that Goggins does annually: He runs 4 miles every 4 hours for 48 hours straight.

"If you can't run 4 miles, walk. If you can't walk, ride your bike. If you can't ride your bike, do calisthenics," he says. The effort should take 30 minutes to 1 hour at the start of every 4-hour block. "If you take this 48 hours, you can put it in your cookie jar. Your cookie jar is a reminder of how badass you are when times get hard in your life."

You'll have to "smile at pain," as Goggins says, to do it: Running 4 miles every 4 hours is 48 miles in two days. But if you finish, it's two days that could change your life—or at least give you an unforgettable challenge and story.

THE "300 WORKOUT"

To get the eye-popping abs of Spartan warriors, Gerard Butler and his *300* castmates worked with Mark Twight, founder of Gym Jones in Salt Lake City, and author of such enviable celeb physiques as Henry Cavill's hulking take on Superman in *Man of Steel*.

One workout Butler did became legendary: The "300 Workout" is a notoriously difficult challenge. It's 7 exercises, 300 reps performed in a race against the clock. One of the movie's stars, Andrew Pleavin, reportedly finished in 18 minutes, 11 seconds. Can you beat his time? Can you even finish? You've *got* to try . . . for Sparta!

Perform these exercises—in this order—as quickly as possible.

EXERCISE 1: Pull-Ups
Do 25 repetitions.

EXERCISE 2: Barbell Deadlift with 135 pounds
Perform 50 reps.

EXERCISE 3: Push-Ups:
Do 50 reps.

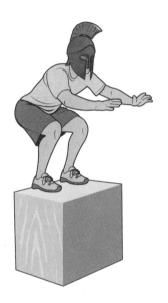

EXERCISE 4: Box Jump onto a 24-inch Box
Total of 50 reps.

EXERCISE 5: Floor Wipers
Do 50 reps. (Lie faceup holding a barbell over your chest. Keeping your legs straight, lift your feet over to the left edge of the bar, then the right.)

EXERCISE 6: Single-Arm Clean and Press with a 36-pound Kettlebell
Perform 50 reps with each arm.

EXERCISE 7: Pull-Ups
Do 25 reps.

PADDLE 260 MILES IN THE WORLD'S TOUGHEST CANOE RACE

If an overnight ultramarathon or a multi-day bike camping trek sounds like an adventure, but you aren't sure you've got the knees for it, use your arms instead: The Texas Water Safari challenges teams of six racers to paddle 260 miles of river in less than 100 hours. Participants must carry all the supplies they'll need, except water and ice, which can be resupplied along the shore.

This is not a leisurely paddle: While there are stretches of open water, the race features meanders that force racers to work for every inch, more than half a dozen dams requiring them to carry their boats, and spiders, alligators, scorpions, and more. In one edition of the race, an alligator gar—a prehistoric-looking sea monster—leapt out of the water and smashed into a woman's chest, breaking two of her ribs. On top of all that, it's hot—the race is held in June, when temperatures often hit triple digits.

Despite all this, 176 boats entered the 2019 edition of the race. But, thanks to all the stuff listed above, plus choppy, 3-foot waves in the race's final 10 miles, 34 of those crafts didn't finish. Of the 142 crews who did complete the trip, 43 of them paddled for more than 72 hours—three solid days.

It's not called the "world's toughest canoe race" for nothing. But if you've got some paddling experience and a screw loose, joining the few who have finished this grueling challenge may be for you. Visit www.texaswatersafari.org.

RUN (OR SKI OR PEDAL) AMERICA'S COLDEST RACE

Only 120 entrants brave the Arrowhead 135 each year, and 80 percent drop out. No wonder: You can choose any mode of transportation you like at the event, but there's one thing you can't choose—you're going to be cold. The race is in northern Minnesota—along the Canadian border in International Falls—and it's in January. So we're talking *really* cold.

That's why not just anyone can join the race: You'll need to apply, and include bona fides showing experience in ultra-endurance events—like another 100-mile running race or a 24-hour bike race—*and* cold weather. The selection process keeps the race safe—so they can keep running it—and allows for solitude on the trail, as participants crunch through the snow of pine-forested hinterlands on this self-supported, keister-freezing endeavor. Think you can finish? Visit www.arrowheadultra.com.

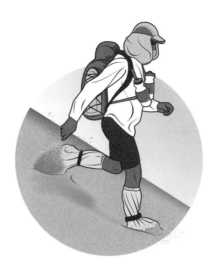

RUN THROUGH THE SAHARA FOR SIX DAYS IN THE "TOUGHEST FOOTRACE ON EARTH"

Running one marathon is tough enough. How about six . . . in six days . . . in the Sahara?
The Marathon des Sables is sheer madness, but 1,000 people are mad enough to try it each year. The 156-mile, six-day journey through the sands of southern Morocco has been called the "toughest footrace on Earth."

"It's 130 degrees. You're carrying a rucksack and you're going to climb 1,000 meters," says Rory Coleman, a coach and speaker who has run the race 15 times. But even though there's a day of 57 miles, Coleman says it's not the running that makes the MdS tough. "It's how you manage yourself over those six days. How do you manage your water? Your food? Your mood?"

Water is provided each night, but only so much. Racers are required to bring their own sleeping materials and food, and carry it with them throughout. Coleman says it's worth doing, though—sure, you'll get bragging rights. But the experience is even more valuable. "I've cried with laughter in the middle of MdS tents, just being with like-minded people, and being in the moment," he says. He's still in contact with people he ran with in his first MdS in 1999. Oh, and he met his wife along the route.

Those experiences aren't cheap: The race costs about $3,500 to enter. But if you're ready for a hot, dry run you'll never forget, the race is run each April. Visit www.marathondessables.com/en.

ACKNOWLEDGMENTS

Thank you, first, to anyone who picked up *The Workout Bucket List* and opened it: Your time and attention are valuable, and the fact that you've spent even a moment of either getting inspired to pursue more adventure through these pages is gratifying.

I've also been privileged to be surrounded by brilliant, interesting people throughout my life, and especially in the course of compiling this list. After more than 300 workouts, I'd like to take a few hundred words to thank some of them.

First, a huge thanks to everyone at Running Press who made *The Workout Bucket List* the gorgeous, illustrated guide you're holding. From the fact checkers to copy editors, from the art department to marketing gurus, thank you. You've made my fever-dream visions a reality.

There are more than 300 illustrations in this book. Peter Sucheski is the brilliant artist who created them. Thank you, Peter, for giving this *List* its signature look.

And thank you to Jordana Hawkins, my patient and kind editor, who believed in this project and shared my enthusiasm for it right from the start. You're a star.

If you tested or tried a workout or challenge from this list, thank you. Your insights helped me hone what I hope became the best *Bucket List* I could make. I'm looking at you, Albert Presto, Joe Gabel, Stephen Majors, Yates Jordan, Emily Norton, Chris Price, Bryan McCann, Matt Stroud, Greg Londino, Vinny Londino, and too many others to list here.

I interviewed hundreds of people to bring this project to life; without their recollections of their experiences, creativity in developing workouts, and most of all, their generosity with their time to tell me about it, this book could not exist. I can't list you all here, but if you were interviewed for this book, thank you.

I'm not sure where I'd be without the guidance, advice, and counsel of my friend, sometimes boss, and—whether he knows it or not—mentor, Steve Madden. Your help in making this book a reality is incalculable. Thank you, Steve.

Another blessing in my life are the many talented editors I've worked with and become friends with during my career—and I'm grateful to those who acted as readers for parts of this book when it was still just a Word doc. Special thanks here to Mike Foss, Nick Schwartz, and Nina Mandell.

Justin Park: Thank you a million times for 14 years of counsel, advice, creativity, and patience in dealing with me . . . and my stressed alter ego. You're an incredible professional partner, a better friend, and a true artist.

Thanks to the Library of Congress, where much of the research for the historical work-outs in this book was done. The Jefferson Reading Room is breathtaking, and it's free to become a reader at the Library. If you visit Washington, DC, go sign up.

To my agent, Rick Richter, thank you for your representation, your good humor, your awesome name, and for always being frank—and letting me be frank, too.

I don't always toot my own horn, but I did a pretty good job picking great parents. Thank you to Albert and Maria Presto for your constant support and encouragement, and for not being too mad when I hit that turkey with Albert's car.

And the most important thanks of all: When I wake up on my best mornings, I ask myself, "How can today be an adventure?" The answer starts and ends with my brilliant wife, Sara Melillo, without whom I could accomplish nothing. I am grateful for your love, support, guidance, straight talk, humor, and indomitable spirit every day.

Index